Aesthetic Rejuvenation Challenges and Solutions

Series in Cosmetic and Laser Therapy
Published in association with the *Journal of Cosmetic and Laser Therapy*
Series editors: *David J Goldberg, Nicholas J Lowe, and Gary P Lask*

1. David J. Goldberg
   Fillers in Cosmetic Dermatology, ISBN 9781841845098

2. Philippe Deprez
   Textbook of Chemical Peels, ISBN 9781841842954

3. C. William Hanke, Gerhard Sattler, Boris Sommer
   Textbook of Liposuction, ISBN 9781841845326

4. Paul J. Carniol, Neil S. Sadick
   Clinical Procedures in Laser Skin Rejuvenation, ISBN 9780415414135

5. David J. Goldberg
   Laser Hair Removal, Second Edition, ISBN 9780415414128

6. Benjamin Ascher, Marina Landau, Bernard Rossi
   Injection Treatments in Cosmetic Surgery, ISBN 9780415386517

7. Avi Shai, Robert Baran, Howard Maibach
   Handbook of Cosmetic Skin Care, Second Edition, ISBN 9780415467186

8. Jenny Kim, Gary Lask
   Comprehensive Aesthetic Rejuvenation: A Regional Approach, ISBN 9780415458948

9. Neil Sadick, Paul Carniol, Deborshi Roy, Luitgard Wiest
   Illustrated Manual of Injectable Fillers, ISBN 9780415476447

10. Paul Carniol, Gary Monheit
    Aesthetic Rejuvenation Challenges and Solutions: A Global Perspective, ISBN 9780415475600

11 Neil Sadick, Diane Berson, Mary Lupo, Zoe Diana Draelos
    Cosmeceutical Science in Clinical Practice, ISBN 9780415471145

12. Anthony Benedetto
    Botulinum Toxins in Clinical Dermatology, Second Edition, ISBN 9780415476362

13. Robert Baran, Howard Maibach
    Textbook of Cosmetic Dermatology, Fourth Edition, ISBN 9781841847009

14. David J. Goldberg, Alexander L. Berlin
    Disorders of Fat and Cellulite, ISBN 9780415477000

15. Ken Beer, Mary Lupo, Vic Narurkar, Wendy Roberts
    Cosmetic Bootcamp Primer, ISBN 9781841846989

Aesthetic Rejuvenation Challenges and Solutions

A World Perspective

Edited by

Paul J Carniol, MD, FACS
President- New Jersey Chapter of American College of Surgeons
Clinical Associate Professor
New Jersey Medical School-UMDNJ
Newark
Cosmetic Laser and Plastic Surgery
Summit, New Jersey, USA

and

Gary D Monheit, MD
Past President- American Society of Dermatology
Clinical Associate Professor
Departments of Dermatology and Ophthalmology
University of Alabama at Birmingham
Total Skin and Beauty Dermatology
Birmingham, Alabama, USA

CRC Press
Taylor & Francis Group
Boca Raton London New York

CRC Press is an imprint of the
Taylor & Francis Group, an **informa** business

First published 2010 by Informa Healthcare

CRC Press
Taylor & Francis Group
6000 Broken Sound Parkway NW, Suite 300
Boca Raton, FL 33487-2742

First issued in paperback 2018

ISBN-13: 978-0-415-47560-0 (hbk)
ISBN-13: 978-1-138-11204-9 (pbk)

Visit the Taylor & Francis Web site at
http://www.taylorandfrancis.com

and the CRC Press Web site at
http://www.crcpress.com

Dedication

This book is dedicated to my wife and best friend, Renie, without whom it would not be possible.
— Paul J Carniol

This book is dedicated to my wife and best friend, Judy, without whom it would not be possible.
— Gary D Monheit

Contents

CONTENTS

List of Contributors

Glynis Ablon
Ablon Skin Institute
Manhattan Beach
and Department of Dermatology
UCLA School of Medicine
Los Angeles, California, USA

Stephen C Adler
Adler Facial Plastic Surgery, P.A.
Stuart and Miami, Florida
and Temple University School of Medicine
Philadelphia, Pennsylvania, USA

Eric T Adler
Adler Facial Plastic Surgery & Wellness Center, P.A.
San Juan, Puerto Rico

Murad Alam
Department of Dermatology, Otolaryngology, and Surgery
Northwestern University
Chicago, Illinois, USA

Sterling S Baker
Ophthalmology
Oklahoma City, Oklahoma, USA

Alfonso Barrera
Department of Plastic Surgery
Baylor College of Medicine
Houston, Texas, USA

Cheryl Burgess
Center for Dermatology and Dermatologic Surgery
Washington, D.C., USA

Paul J Carniol
Cosmetic, Laser and Reconstructive Plastic Surgery
Summit, New Jersey, USA

Mohamed L Elsaie
Department of Dermatology
NRC Cairo, Egypt
and Department of Dermatology and Cutaneous Surgery
University of Miami
Miami, Florida, USA

Daniel Ganc
Cosmetic Laser & Plastic Surgery
Boca Raton, Florida, USA

Vijay Kumar Garg
Department of Dermatology and Venereology
Maulana Azad Medical College and Lok Nayak Hospital
New Delhi, India

Steven A Goldstein
Department of Otolaryngology- Head & Neck Surgery
University of Pennsylvania
Philadelphia, Pennsylvania, USA

Greg Goodman
Dermatology Institute of Victoria
South Yarra, Victoria, Australia

Mary Gorman
Department of Otolaryngology-Head & Neck Surgery
University of Tennessee Health Science Center
Memphis, Tennessee, USA

Issam R Hamadah
Department of Dermatology
King Faisal Specialist Hospital & Research Center
Riyadh, Saudi Arabia

Natalie A Kim
Department of Dermatology
Northwestern University
Chicago, Illinois, USA

Amanda Klinger
Cosmetic, Laser, and Reconstructive Plastic Surgery
Summit, New Jersey, USA

Edward S Kwak
ESK Facial Surgery and Department of Otolaryngology
New York Medical College
New York, New York, USA

Samuel M Lam
Willow Bend Wellness Center
Lam Facial Plastic Surgery Center & Hair Restoration Institute
Plano, Texas, USA

Phillip R Langsdon
Division of Facial Plastic and Reconstructive Surgery
University of Tennessee Health Science Center
Memphis, Tennessee, USA

William Lawson
Mount Sinai School of Medicine
New York, New York, USA

Amit Luthra
Ishira Skin clinic
Phase III,
New Delhi, India

Harish Kumar Malhotra
UMDNJ-New Jersey Medical School
and Department of Psychiatry
Overlook Hospital
Summit, New Jersey, USA

Harry Mittelman
Stanford University Medical Center
and Mittelman Plastic Surgery
Los Altos, California, USA

Gary Monheit
Total Skin and Beauty Dermatology
Birmingham, Alabama, USA

Vic A Narurkar
Bay Area Laser Institute, San Francisco
University of California Davis Medical School
and Department of Dermatology
California Pacific Medical Center
San Francisco, California, USA

Mark Steven Nestor
Center for Cosmetic Enhancement
Center for Clinical and Cosmetic Research
Aventura, Florida
and Department of Dermatology and Cutaneous Surgery
University of Miami
Miami, Florida, USA

Jung I Park
Section of Plastic Surgery
Indiana University School of Medicine
Indianapolis, Indiana, USA

Munish Paul
Skin Laser Centre
Pashchim Vihar
New Delhi, India

Randal Pham
Division of Ophthalmic Plastic & Reconstructive Surgery
Department of Ophthalmology
Stanford University
Palo Alto, California, USA

Chad Prather
Department of Dermatology
Louisiana State University
New Orleans and Dermasurgery Center
Baton Rouge, Louisiana, USA

Christopher La Riche
Center for Clinical and Cosmetic Studies
Aventura, Florida, USA

Eva Ritvo
Center for Clinical and Cosmetic Studies
Aventura, Florida, USA

Rashmi Sarkar
Department of Dermatology and Venereology
Maulana Azad Medical College and Lok Nayak Hospital
New Delhi, India

Sigmund Sattenspiel
UMDNJ-Robert Wood Johnson Medical School
New Brunswick, New Jersey
and Mount Sinai Medical Center
New York, New York, USA

Anita B Sethna
Facial Plastic Surgery
Emory Facial Center
Emory Healthcare
Emory University
Atlanta, Georgia, USA

Mark A Stillman
Center for Clinical and Cosmetic Studies
Aventura, Florida, USA

Konstantin Vasyukevich
NY Facial Surgery
New York, New York, USA

Gregory J Vipond
Lifestyle Lift of the Inland Empire
Ontario, California, USA

Heather Woolery-Lloyd
University of Miami Cosmetic Medicine and Research Institute
and University of Miami Department of Dermatology and
    Cutaneous Surgery
Miami, Florida, USA

Seth A Yellin
Facial Plastic Surgery
Emory Facial Center
Emory Healthcare
Emory University
Atlanta, Georgia, USA

Preface

As physicians, regardless of where you practice, you will have patients with diverse social backgrounds or expectations. This diversity can add significant challenges to aesthetic rejuvenation procedures, since patients' goals can vary significantly depending on their backgrounds, social requirements, and cultural expectations. Furthermore, factors related to ethnicity, medical history, and age can affect how patients will respond to procedures.

In this book, our multiethnic and multinational authors address how to approach patients with due consideration of these differences and how to individually design solutions for them, to optimize the results. There are sections dedicated to procedures for patients with African, Asian, Hispanic, Indian, Middle Eastern, and Pakistani heritage.

Furthermore, there are chapters which address how to solve problems raised by the management of patients who may be among our most challenging for other reasons. This includes chapters on dealing with challenging patients who: have limited time for recovery, require revision procedures, have unrealistis expectations, or, are dissatisfied.

With increasing globalization and no decline in demand for rejuvenation, the need for an understanding of how to tailor personalized aesthetic procedures to a diverse group of patients will only increase. This first edition of *Aesthetic Rejuvenation Challenges and Solutions* will be a valuable addition to the personal reference library of all physicians who perform these procedures.

Paul J Carniol

Acknowledgments

We would like to thank Robert Peden, Commissioning Editor of Informa Healthcare, for all his efforts on behalf of this book. His dedication and expertise are unsurpassed for medical publications.

1   Evaluating the aesthetic patient

Paul J Carniol, Daniel Ganc, and Amanda Klinger

INITIAL CONSULTATION

The initial consultation is very important in the evaluation of an aesthetic patient. During this visit, the physician has the opportunity to meet the patient, listen to the patient's concerns, review the medical history, examine the patient, and arrive at a treatment plan. As part of this process, it is also important for the physician to reach a decision as to the likelihood that the patient will be happy with the probable outcome of the procedures being considered.

Each physician has a personal preference as to how to start this process. The first author has each new patient fill out a medical and psychosocial questionnaire. After this is completed, a member of the office staff reviews it with the patient and asks why the patient came in for consultation. The staff member then presents an assessment of the patient to the first author before his entering the consultation room. In this way the staff member acts as the initial "eyes and ears" for the physician. Therefore, before actually meeting the patient, the physician has information from two sources: the patient's answers to the information sheet and a staff member.

At the start of the consultation the physician should ask the patient what concerns prompted the visit. It is important to elicit the motivations and expectations of the patient.(1) It is also useful to enquire about any prior cosmetic procedures, the patient's assessment of both the results, and the physician who performed the procedure.

It is important to discern the patient's attitudes toward prior treating physicians, as if you decide to treat this patient, you yourself may soon become a prior-treating physician. As patients discuss their concerns, the first author either gives them a mirror or has them stand in front of a mirror so they can point to whatever concerns them.(2)

The first author finds that the use of a mirror can be indispensable. For example, he had a patient who came in for removal of a "bump" on his nose. On examination he found two protuberances on the patient's nose: a larger one over the osseous dorsum and a smaller one over the cartilaginous dorsum.

Before handing the patient a mirror, the first author assumed that the patient wanted both of these removed. However, when the patient looked in a mirror, he pointed to the smaller protrusion over the cartilaginous dorsum. When asked about the larger dorsal hump, at the rhinion, the patient said that he did not want that removed as he was proud of it. This dorsal hump was family trait, which had been present for generations. At surgery, only the cartilaginous hump was removed; the larger hump was left untouched, and the patient was pleased with the results.

Another important issue is how long the patient has had these concerns and considered having treatment. This is helpful in establishing how concerned the patient is about this issue.

Understanding the patient's goals is an important part of the process. As part of the consultation, the physician should discuss with the patient the likelihood of attaining the goal, the variability of potential results, as well as the associated risks.

The patient's medical history should also be reviewed. This should include the past medical history, past surgical history, psychiatric history, social history, medications, and allergies. The social history should include but not be limited to the patient's marital status, employment, work or interpersonal stressors, as well as habits including smoking, alcohol, and substance abuse.

PATIENT MOTIVATION AND GOALS

Understanding the patient's motivations and goals for a procedure is important. If these are inappropriate or not attainable, then it is in the surgeon's best interest to not perform a procedure. Patients seeking aesthetic procedures fall into one of two categories generally based on age. Frequently, younger patients are interested in altering their appearance. These patients may be interested in procedures such as: rhinoplasty, otoplasty, genioplasty, or body contouring procedures. Patients aged 30 and above frequently are looking for procedures to counter age-related changes.

When speaking with the patient, the physician should try to assess the patient's true motivations and issues. For example, the first author had a young patient come in for a revision rhinoplasty consultation several years ago. On speaking with the patient, it became apparent that besides wanting to improve her appearance, she was depressed and hoped that the surgery would make her feel better. As discussed in chapter 25, this patient should be referred for psychiatric treatment before consideration of aesthetic surgery.

In addition to assessing the internal factors motivating the patient, there may also be others encouraging the patient to have a procedure. This could include a significant other, parent, or employer. It is important to identify these patients as they are at significant risk for being unhappy after surgery, since the best surgical result probably will not enhance their personal or work relationships.

PSYCHOLOGICAL ISSUES AND AESTHETIC SURGERY

The psychological issues in relation to aesthetic procedures are discussed in detail in chapter 25. Currently there is controversy over whether patients seeking cosmetic procedures have a greater prevalence of psychopathology.

Some prior studies using standardized measures to assess psychopathology had inconsistent results. Several investigations of cosmetic patients using tests such as the MMPI (Minnesota Multiphasic Personality Inventory), a commonly used and sensitive test for personality disorders, found no significant disorder in patients seeking rhytidectomy or rhinoplasty.(3–6) One older study found increased neurotic and obsessive traits versus a control group of hospital nurses.(7) A more recent study found cosmetic patients to be no more dissatisfied with their general appearance than normal. However, these patients were more dissatisfied than normal with the specific body feature that they sought to correct with surgery. Patients scored normally on tests evaluating patients' preoccupation and satisfaction with their body image.(8)

During the past decade, aesthetic surgery has gained widespread social acceptance. Furthermore, with medical advances, many procedures can be performed in an office or outpatient environment. As such, it is less likely that the average patient seeking a cosmetic procedure has more psychopathology than the general population. Older literature addressing this issue in relation to aesthetic procedures does not take these factors into consideration.

PREOPERATIVE FACIAL ANALYSIS

The evaluation of a patient for a facial aesthetic procedure should begin as soon as the patient starts to speak. Notice the face in repose as well as the changes with facial motion. Next, systematically examine the patient, taking note of characteristics such as facial proportions, asymmetries, skin, soft tissue, bone structure, musculature, and individual facial characteristics. When considering possible rhytidectomy surgery, assessment of the overall osseous framework is important.(9) If there is inadequate osseous support, then the use of alloplastic or other implants should be considered as part of the facial rejuvenation procedure.

FACIAL PROPORTIONS

Concepts of facial beauty can be found in art dating back to antiquity. European scientists and artists, including Leonardo da Vinci and the German artist Albrecht Dürer, used mathematical models for evaluating facial characteristics. Some of these concepts are still used today, such as the concept of facial thirds of the Roman architect Marcus Vitruvius Pollio. More recently, the phi ratio of 1:1.1618 has also been used to describe facial harmony. This has been advocated by Dr. Stephen R. Marquardt. This researcher of human attractiveness has created a two-dimensional "Golden Decagon Mask" using geometrical lines of the face based on this ratio.(10)

Models of facial proportions are useful starting points in facial analysis. However like most guidelines, they have their limitations, including that most were not designed to be applicable across the spectrum of racial groups. Recent anthropomorphic studies have highlighted these differences.(9)

Certain facial characteristics which are considered desirable are gender specific. It has been shown that males prefer females with thin jaws, small chins, large widely spaced eyes, small noses, high cheekbones, and short upper lips. Females have been shown to prefer males with prominent chins, deep-set eyes, heavy brows, and abundant hair.(10)

The determination of an individual's target aesthetic should be tailored by the patient's goals, facial structure and racial makeup, as well as the aesthetic sense of the patient and surgeon. Studies have shown that when humans look at others' faces they see the entire figure, instead of the individual features of the face. This

is important for the aesthetic surgeon. A facial feature should be evaluated in the context of the entire face and individual, not as an isolated part, when performing cosmetic procedures.(11)

Facial proportions can be useful in assessing a patient, but it is important to consider that there can be significant variation between individuals. From a frontal view, the face can be vertically divided into thirds from the hairline to the menton by two horizontal lines. One passes through the browline or glabella and the other through the subnasale.(12, 9) Typically the height of the lower lip down to the menton is twice the distance of the upper lip to the subnasale.(9)

In width, the face can be divided into fifths, each fifth being equal to the horizontal width of the eye as measured from the medial canthus to the lateral canthus. The width of the nose at the ala in the Caucasian individual should approximate the distance between the medial canthi of the eyes.(9)

The shape of the face is another variable that the surgeon should also consider. A width to height ratio of 3:4 is considered ideal, but this is highly variable. The most common shapes of faces are oval, square, triangular, and round. Round and square faces frequently have shorter and wider noses. When evaluating patients' appearance, it is useful to view them in multiple positions, including frontal, oblique, and lateral views.

FACIAL AGING

There are multiple factors that contribute to changes that we traditionally have attributed to facial aging. These changes can involve the skin, subcutaneous layer, musculature, and underlying facial bones. Among the factors contributing to these visible changes are photoaging, cellular biochemical changes, volumetric changes (soft tissue and osseous), tissue changes, and long-term gravitational effects.

The photoaging effects of exposure to the sun's ultraviolet rays are cumulative. The rate of these changes of the skin varies directly with the amount of sun exposure as well as individual skin sensitivity to the sun, which varies by skin type. (Table 1.1) The higher the skin type, the less reactive to sun exposure.

Other classifications have been devised to account for the effects of sun damage and aging. The Fitzpatrick wrinkle scale classifies the extent of wrinkles, (Table 1.2) (13) and the Glogau scale uses a scale that combines photoaging and wrinkling. (Table 1.3)

Table 1.1 Fitzpatrick's Skin Types.

Skin Type	Skin Color	Tanning Response
I	Caucasian; blond or red hair, freckles, fair skin, blue eyes	Always burns, never tans
II	Caucasian; blond or red hair, freckles, fair skin, blue eyes or green eyes	Usually burns, tans with difficulty
III	Darker Caucasian, light Asian	Sometimes burns, tans average
IV	Mediterranean, Asian, Hispanic	Rarely burns, tans with ease
V	Middle Eastern, Latin, light-skinned black, Indian	Very rarely burns, tans very easily
VI	Dark-skinned black	Never burns, always tans

Note: The Fitzpatrick Skin Types separates skin types by reaction to sun exposure.

Table 1.2 Fitzpatrick wrinkle assessment scale.

Class	Wrinkling	Score	Degree of Elastosis
I	Fine wrinkles	1–3	Mild (fine textural changes with subtly accentuated skin lines)
II	Fine to moderate-depth wrinkles, moderate number of lines	4–6	Moderate (distinct popular elastosis [individual papules with yellow translucency under direct lighting] and dyschromia)
III	Fine to deep wrinkles, numerous lines with or without redundant skin folds	7–9	Severe (multipapular and confluent elastosis [thickened yellow and pallid] approaching or consistent with cutis rhomboidalis)

Note: The Fitzpatrick Wrinkle Assessment Scale separates patients by degree of wrinkling and elastosis in facial skin.

When considering facelift surgery, it can be helpful to separate the extent of changes as a guide to selection of the optimal facial rejuvenation procedure. Baker's classification assesses patients' likelihood of obtaining a good result. It includes extent of laxity, skin folds, and platysma banding. (Table 1.4)

Although the effects of age follow a fairly standard pattern, the rate at which these changes occur varies between individuals. Multiple factors can contribute to this variation. These include genetic make-up, body fat content, weight changes, nutrition, and social habits.

GENDER

When considering facial rejuvenation procedures, it is important to consider the anatomical differences between males and females. Even when injecting botox or fillers it is important to take these into account. A more masculine profile has greater projection of the chin and nose, with less rotation of the nasal tip. The brow in males is straighter and lies over the superior orbital rim, whereas the female brow is more curved and lies superior to the rim. A women's face is rounder with more gentle contours, whereas a man's face is more angular.

Hairline differences should be considered in planning incisions in brow and rhytidectomy surgery. The male hairline has some temporal recession, which frequently increases over time. In planning incisions for men, progression of temporal recession should be considered. For women, management of the temporal hairline tuft is important whereas for men, postoperative sideburn and beard pattern should be considered.

RACE AND ETHNICITY

there are multiple components to addressing ethnic variations which are addressed in this book. With increasing greater proportions of non-Caucasians requesting cosmetic surgery (15), these issues should be considered during the planning process. Patients' ethnic backgrounds and cultures can play a role in influencing their perception of beauty and desired surgical goals. An aesthetic result that may be considered desirable in one culture may be less attractive in another. Even individuals within an ethnic group can differ in their goals and expectations.(15) Additionally, with the increasing prevalence of ethnic mixing, patients may have varied genetic factors as well as varying concepts of beauty.

Ethnic individuals tend to be more satisfied with cosmetic surgery if postoperatively there is a high degree of facial harmony as well as a preservation of their ethnic facial characteristics.(16) Frequently, they want to refine certain areas of their appearance without sacrificing their ethnic identity.(15) This must be taken into account by the surgeon when planning surgery.

Differences in the underlying structure of the face, such as will be discussed with rhinoplasty, should be considered when planning surgery. Furthermore, differences in healing and potential for scarring or dyschromia across racial groups should be considered preoperatively. These issues are discussed in detail in the following chapters.

HAIRLINE

Considerations of the shape, density, and location of the hairline are useful in planning incisions for face and brow lifts. For example, patients with a high hairline and large foreheads are better candidates for pretricheal brow lifts. Coronal brow lifts may be preferred in patients with low hairlines. Patients with a receding hairlines or androgenic alopecia are better approached with incisions that avoid the hairline, including direct, mid-forehead, and endoscopic brow lifts. Gender-related issues pertaining to the hairline are previously discussed in this chapter.

FOREHEAD AND PERIORBITAL REGION

The forehead and periorbital region develop rhytids and creases over time. There are multiple factors contributing to these changes, the main factor being the action of their musculature. Patients may express concerns about the appearance of these features. The location and severity of the rhytids and creases should be identified when planning injectable, radiofrequency, or surgical treatment of the musculature.

Table 1.3 Glogau's photoaging classification.

Characteristic	Type I	Type II	Type III	Type IV
Degree of photoaging	Early	Early to moderate	Advanced	Severe
Pigmentation	Mild pigmentary changes	Early senile lentigines	Obvious dyschromia, telangiectasia	Yellow-gray color of skin
Keratosis	None	Palpable but not visible	Visible	Prior skin malignancies
Wrinkles	Minimal or none	Parallel smile lines; wrinkles in motion	Wrinkles present even when not moving	Wrinkled throughout; no normal skin
Patient age	20–39	35–49	50+	60–79
Makeup usage	Minimal or none	Usually wears some foundation	Always wears heavy foundation	Makeup cakes and cracks

Note: Glogau's Photoaging Classification separates patients into four different types based on degree of photoaging and other skin characteristics.

Table 1.4 Daniel Baker's classification system for rhytidectomy patients.

Classification	Age	Characteristics
Type I: the ideal candidate	Early to late 40s	Slight cervical laxity Good cervical skin elasticity Early jowls Submental and submandibular fat +/-Microgenia +/-
Type II: good candidate	Late 40s to late 50s	Moderate cervical skin laxity Moderate jowls Submental and submandibular fat Microgenia +/- No platysma bands with animation
Type III: fair candidate	Late 50s, 60s, early 70s	Moderate cervical skin laxity Significant jowls Submental and submandibular fat Microgenia +/- + platysma bands with animation
Type IV: poor candidate	60s to 70s	Poor cervical skin elasticity Significant jowls Submental and submandibular fat Microgenia +/- + platysma bands with animation Skin folds below cricoid Deep cervical creases

Note: Baker's classification system determines the likelihood of obtaining a good facial rejuvenation result based on a patient's age and certain physical characteristics.(14)

NOSE

Pitanguy stated that the nose "must be in harmony with the rest of the face and the race of the individual."(17) The nose occupies the center of the face geographically, and it aesthetically functions to provide balance to the face.

Dissatisfaction with the nose is one of the more frequent complaints of patients presenting to aesthetic surgeons. Achieving an aesthetically appealing nose while addressing the concerns of the patient is a demanding challenge. Related to this are two issues which the surgeon may have to consider: the surgeon's aesthetic concept and the patient's. In general the surgeon should keep in mind that the patient's goals should take priority over the personal preferences of the surgeon.(15) However, if the surgeon believes that the patient's goals and the surgeon's concept of the ideal aesthetic result are not congruent, then this should be resolved before surgery is performed. If the patient and the surgeon cannot reach goal congruence, then surgery should be deferred.

Concepts of ideal nose may change over time. For example, in the 1950s, patients wanted rhinoplasties that produced more upturned noses with a narrower tip. However by the 1990s, patients wanted a nose with a wider tip and fuller bridge. Overall, the current rhinoplasty patients frequently want a change in their nose that appears more natural and less operated.(15) The surgeon should keep in mind these changes in patient ideals but should strive to produce a surgical result that outlasts the trends.

Ethnicity has a significant effect on surgical intervention because it can make rhinoplasties more challenging. One classification scheme based on anthropomorphic measurements divides nasal structure into three groups: leptorrhine (thin, more projected nose), found more typically in Caucasians; mesorrhine (middle-projected nose), characteristic of East Asians; and platyrrhine

(flat nose), more predominantly in patients of African descent. (18) For patients of African descent, more recently, Ofodile et al. have devised a more descriptive classification of African American noses. He divides them into three categories: African, Afro-Caucasian, and Afro-Indian.(16)

Frequently, non-Caucasian noses have less osseous and cartilaginous support than Caucasian noses. There can be a wider dorsum, a wider pyriform aperture, thicker skin with a larger tip fibrofatty pad, and less tip projection.(17)

A survey of African-American patients found that most patients did not want "Caucasian" noses; they wanted to keep some ethnic characteristics.(17)

The surgeon's analysis of the nose should be performed from multiple angles. The overall shape of the nose can be appreciated from a frontal view. Major septal deviations can create a curvature of the cartilaginous dorsum.

In the Caucasian patient, the ideal inter-alar width is roughly equal to or slightly greater than the distance between the medial canthi. However, an aesthetically appealing nose of a black patient may extend beyond this distance.

Vertically, the nose is traditionally broken down into the upper osseous third, the middle supra-tip third, and the lower third (nasal tip).

The osseous upper third of the nose consists of the nasal bones and frontal processes of the maxilla. It can be evaluated in terms of the nasofrontal region, height and width of the dorsum including possible dorsal hump, if present. The upper lateral cartilages in the middle third of the nose provide the support for the internal nasal valve. Excessive weakness or narrowing of the middle third, either congenital or from prior rhinoplasty, can cause nasal valve narrowing and airway obstruction.

Evaluation of the lower third, or nasal tip, includes an analysis of the tip shape, projection, rotation, and definition. From the frontal view, tip rotation can be initially noted by observing the nares, which should be barely visible. The convexity of the dome and lateral crura should also be noted—ideally they should be convex but not bulbous. The tip-defining points are observed from the frontal view by the light reflex, which should be symmetric. The edge of the nasal columella should just be visible below the level of the nares on a lateral view.

The lateral view is also useful for evaluating other characteristics addressed during rhinoplasty. Beginning superiorly, the first nasal feature noted is the radix, or the root, of the nose. There is no consensus as to the optimal horizontal height for the radix. The ideal level of the radix is generally considered to be between the supratarsal fold and eyelashes of the upper eyelid.(19) Guyuron advocates a target radix location on straight gaze to be at the lower aspect of the upper lid margin.(20) Sheen allows the radix to be placed even lower—to the level of the pupils—when a softer profile is desired.(21)

The ideal height of the radix has been calculated by various methods as well. Goldman described the target radix height as between 15 and 20 mm from the medial canthus. One study based on the profiles of models calculates the target horizontal distance from the anterior border of the cornea to the radix to be 28% of the ideal horizontal nasal length, ranging between 9 and 14 mm.(22) Another paper describes the ideal height of the radix to lie between 4 and 6 mm posterior to the glabella.(20)

The nasofrontal angle, or the angle between the glabella, radix, and nasal dorsum, has been described as ideally being between 110 and 130°.

Further details of nasal analysis and surgical technique are described in chapter 14.

CONCLUSION

To perform aesthetic procedures it is important to first evaluate the patient. The results of this evaluation will vary depending on numerous factors. While planning a procedure, it is important to consider the patient's goals and ethnicity. Another complex issue is dealing with the patient with unrealistic goals. Many of these and other details will be discussed in the following chapters.

REFERENCES

1. Hasan JS. Psychological issues in cosmetic surgery: a functional overview. Ann Plast Surg 2000; 44: 89–96.
2. Rees TD, Latreuta GS. Aesthetic plastic surgery. 2nd ed. Philadelphia: WB Saunders, 1994.
3. Goin MK, Burgoyne RW, Goin JM, Staples FR. A prospective study of 50 female face-lift patients. Plast Reconstr Surg 1980; 65: 436–42.
4. Micheli-Pellegrini V, Manfrida GM. Rhinoplasty and its psychological implications: applied psychological observances in aesthetic surgery. Aesthetic Plast Surg 1979; 3: 299–319.
5. Wright MR, Wright WK. A psychological study of patients undergoing cosmetic surgery. Arch Otolaryngol 1975; 16: 145–51.
6. Goin MK, Rees TD. A prospective study of patients' psychological reactions to rhinoplasty. Ann Plast Surg 1991; 27: 210–5.
7. Hay GG. Psychiatric aspects of cosmetic nasal operations. Br J Psychiatry 1970; 116: 85–97.
8. Sarwer DB, Wadden TA, Pertschuk MJ et al. Body image dissatisfaction and body dysmorphic disorder in 18 cosmetic surgery patients. Plast Reconstr Surg 1998; 16: 1644–9.
9. Krause CJ, Pastorek N, Mangat DS. Aesthetic Facial Surgery. Philadelphia: JB Lippincott, 1991.
10. Adamson P, Zavod M. Changing perceptions of beauty: a surgeon's perspective. Facial Plast Surg 2006; 22: 188–93.
11. Eisenthal Y, Dror G, Ruppin E. Facial attractiveness: beauty and the machine. Neural Computat 2006; 18: 119–42.
12. Beeson WH, McCollough EG. Aesthetic Surgery of the Aging Face. St. Louis: C.V. Mosby, 1986.
13. Weiss RA, Harrinton AC, Pfau RC et al. Periorbital skin resurfacing using high energy erbium: YAG laser: results in 50 patients. Lasers Surg Med 1999; 24: 81–6.
14. Kridel RW, Liu ES. Techniques for creating inconspicuous face-lift scars: avoiding visible incisions and loss of temporal hair. Arch Facial Plast Surg 2003; 5: 325–33.
15. Davis R. Rhinoplasty and concepts of facial beauty. Facial Plast Surg 2006; 22: 198–203.
16. Slupchynskyj O, Gieniusz M. Rhinoplasty for African American patients. Arch Facial Plast Surg 2008; 10: 232–6.
17. Romo T, Abraham M. The ethnic nose. Facial Plast Surg 2003; 19: 269–77.
18. Hinderer KH. Fundamentals of Anatomy and Surgery of the Nose. Birmingham, AL: Aesculapius; 1971.
19. Daniel RK, Farkas LG. Rhinoplasty: image and reality. Clin Plast Surg 1988; 15: 1.
20. Guyuron B. Precision rhinoplasty. Part I: The role of life-size photographs and soft-tissue cephalometric analysis. Plast Reconstr Surg 1988; 81(4): 489–99.
21. Sheen JH. The radix as a reference in rhinoplasty. Perspect Plast Surg 1987; 1: 33.
22. Byrd HS, Hobar PC. Rhinoplasty: a practical guide for surgical planning. Plast Reconstr Surg 1993; 91: 642.

2   Patients with unrealistic expectations
Eva Ritvo, Christopher La Riche, and Mark A Stillman

"Beyond Appearance: Reflections of a Plastic Surgeon," Dr. Robert Goldwyn: Cosmetic surgery is difficult, less because of the technical demands, than the personalities and *expectations of many aesthetic surgery patients.*

Over the years, a clear distinction has been drawn between "medical patients" and "aesthetic patients." Medical patients come into a physician's office or an emergency room with some immediate or ongoing physiological problem, complaint or illness and are in *need* of medical attention and treatment. They often times will perceive their physician as *the* expert and place him/her on a pedestal because of their education and expertise. As such, they are clearly physically vulnerable, and as a result, often bear accompanying feelings of dependency. The sicker the patient, the more dependent they will be. Physicians, are thus, ethically bound to treat the patient and the fee is secondary. Medical patients may change physicians, but cannot avoid treatment.

Conversely, aesthetic patients are seeking self-improvement and are often times attempting to fight the effects of aging.(1) These patients come in with an aesthetic concern, and they are less physically vulnerable; however, as discussed later, they are often times more psychologically vulnerable. They view the physician as *an* expert and are typically more aware of their alternative choices. The doctor-patient relationship is hence less dependent with aesthetic patients. Aesthetic patients do not have an immediate need for medical treatment, and the practitioner is, therefore, not ethically bound to treat the patient. The fee becomes a larger issue in this relationship, and the patient can change physicians and/or avoid treatment all together.

Aesthetic patients commonly expect to enhance their appearance for an appropriate fee with minimal complications, distress, and discomfort. Realistic expectations would include, for instance, fuller lips, fewer lines, decreased pigmentation, enhanced symmetry to facial features, improved or more youthful appearance and, as a result, enhanced self-esteem. Unrealistic or excessive expectations (discussed later in greater detail) would include the assumption of significantly enhanced self-esteem, increased social standing (friends, dates, spouse, etc.), job security, and/or a reversal of the aging process.

According to one author, cosmetic surgery patients comprise largely of white females: 97% between the ages of 19 and 64; nearly half of them will have more than one procedure.(2) Others, including the editors, have found an increased interest in cosmetic surgery among members of all ethnic groups. The nonsurgical aesthetic demographics are similar but with a pronounced skewing toward younger ages due to the popularity of laser hair removal and similar non-age-related treatments.(2) Consistent findings across procedures (i.e., rhinoplasty, rhytidectomy, blepharoplasty, etc.) reveal that, as compared to the general population, aesthetic patients appear to be more dissatisfied with the specific body feature for which they are seeking surgery, as opposed to a more global dissatisfaction with the entire body.(3) Interestingly, aesthetic patients appear to actually have less overall body dissatisfaction than the average American.

Grossbart and Sarwer (1999) defined cosmetic surgery as: "The use of surgical procedures, in absence of disease or physical trauma, to alter the physical appearance of the body in pursuit of psychological benefit." In other words, the pursuit of improved physical appearance is simply a means to a psychological end. Therefore, patient satisfaction will depend on whether the surgery has met their expectations of both the costs as well as the benefits of the procedure.

Sarwer et al. (1998) discussed the interaction between valence (the degree of importance that body image has on ones self-esteem) and value, or range of dissatisfaction with a particular body feature (from "normative discontent" to psychopathological dissatisfaction), as influencing one's decision to pursue aesthetic treatment. (4) They noted that the majority of aesthetic patients place a high degree of importance on their appearance and are dissatisfied with a specific feature. These patients may experience some postsurgical psychosocial benefit, and are likely to have realistic expectations. It is those patients whose valence is extremely high and who express excessive dissatisfaction, such that thoughts about their appearance overly distress and preoccupy them, who may not benefit from cosmetic procedures and may have unrealistic expectations.(5) As explained later, these patients may be better suited for psychological/psychiatric treatment, not aesthetic.

In some studies it has been reported that aesthetic patients have a rather high prevalence of psychiatric disorders. Ishigooka et al. (1998) conducted an investigation of the psychiatric demographics of 415 aesthetic patients.(6) Of the 415 patients, 47.7% were found to have a mental disorder and 56% had poor social adjustment. Male patients were characterized to have a greater number of mental disorders. They noted that 18% were using psychiatric medication at the time of consultation, as compared to noncosmetic patients, whose reported usage is about 5%. This may have changed during the past decade with the advent of new procedures and technology, which have broadened the scope of what can be achieved, are frequently performed in a physician's office, and have a minimal associated recovery.

Of all the psychiatric disorders affecting individuals presenting for aesthetic procedures, the most commonly found, and hence studied, has been Body Dysmorphic Disorder (BDD). The incidence of BDD among this population has been reported to range from 12 to 20%. Bellino et al. (2005) conducted a clinical investigation of dysmorphic concern symptoms and personality disorders in patients seeking cosmetic surgery. They defined BDD as a somatoform disorder in which the patient presents with a significant preoccupation with a defect in appearance. Either the defect is imagined, or, if a slight anomaly is present, the individual's concern is markedly excessive. The Diagnostic and Statistical Manual of Mental Disorders, 4th Edition (DSM-IV) diagnostic criteria specify that the preoccupation must be present for at least 1 hour each day, and cause significant distress or impairment in their social or occupational functioning.

BDD patients repeatedly pursue aesthetic treatment for an imagined defect. BDD has proved responsive to SSRI antidepressant medication and Cognitive-Behavioral Therapy (CBT), but patients often seek plastic surgery.(7) Patients rarely benefit from the procedures; in fact, often times the severity of the BDD is unchanged or worsened after surgery.(7) Tignol et al. (2007) found that the majority of BDD patients receive the cosmetic surgery they seek, often times as a result of their unrelenting search and "craving" for correction. Also, diagnosis of BDD is difficult in a cosmetic surgery setting. Patients with BDD are significantly younger; therefore, young age combined with a preoccupation over a minimal defect may serve as a sign toward possible BDD diagnosis.

BDD is frequently associated with other Axis I disorders such as, major depressive disorder, panic disorder, substance abuse, obsessive-compulsive disorder and social phobia. The majority (53–87%) of BDD patients have a coexisting personality disorder.(8)

According to Meningaud et al. (2002), cosmetic surgery is statistically ineffective as a treatment for depressive disorders.(9) Therefore, the question is posed: "How should providers respond to requests for surgery in reaction to a job loss, an emotional disturbance, or bereavement?" Meningaud et al. (2002) suggest that the practitioner should, generally, advise the patient to wait for the event to settle first, even if it means reconsidering the request later to improve the patient's self-confidence.

In Napoleon's 1993 article: "The presentation of personalities in plastic surgery," he found the following incidence of personality disorders in a cosmetic surgery practice in Southern California over a 1.5-year period (n = 133): Narcissistic: 25%, Histrionic: 9.75%, Borderline: 9%, Obsessive-Compulsive: 4%.(10)

Data were gathered on patients' expectations in this sample, using the Napoleon Preoperative Test (NPT). He found that expectation was significantly related to patient satisfaction. He assessed postoperative patient satisfaction and found that patients who met criteria for borderline personality disorder were the least satisfied, followed by obsessive-compulsive personality disorder and Narcissistic. Idealistic expectations were found to lead to potential postoperative problems. Napoleon found that 0% of the OCD patients had realistic preoperative expectations and therefore were very dissatisfied with surgery. Only 2% of the narcissistic patients and 8% of the borderline patients were found to have realistic expectations. As patients age, he noticed that their expectations become more realistic. (These and other issues are also discussed in more detail in chapter 25.)

AESTHETIC PRACTITIONERS, COSMETIC SURGEONS
The term *cosmetic surgeon* designates a truly heterogeneous body of medical professionals comprising a wide variety of specialties. A lucrative patient market has lured more physicians to enter the field and added to the growing heterogeneity of physicians who perform procedures. Practitioners may include plastic surgeons, facial plastic surgeons, dermatologists, otolaryngologists, oculoplastic surgeons, maxillofacial surgeons, ophthalmologists, and general surgeons–not all of whom have been trained in performing cosmetic procedures, *per se.*

The result has been increased competition, turf wars, and a deeper inquiry into the purpose and definition of aesthetic practice and the rules governing it. Aesthetic practitioners vary greatly in their training, the fellowships they have earned and membership in professional societies. Aesthetic practitioners do, however, all perform some elective cosmetic/surgical procedures on their patients–in the absence of pathology–to aid in the patient's "pursuit of psychosocial benefit"(3)

The term *elective* describes a critical aspect of the cosmetic surgeon's practice; elective implies a choice on behalf of both the patient and the physician to proceed with an optional—nonessential—procedure. The patient has chosen (or is perhaps offered, then chooses) to undergo an intervention, she deems to be to her psychosocial benefit, and has sought out a specialist to perform that intervention. The cosmetic surgeon must make a dual decision: first, s/he must evaluate the patient's unstated, underlying reason for requesting the procedure, and then, considering a number of complex factors comprising a risk/benefit profile, come to his/her own decision to offer, defer, or refuse the procedure.

A chapter on *unrealistic expectations* must necessarily explore the unique measures of success and failure in aesthetic practice. Success in cosmetic surgery is fundamentally different from success in, for example, general surgery or psychiatry. Success in a patient with acute appendicitis means surgical removal of the appendix without complications and with a return to normal functioning. A patient with major depressive disorder expects improved sleep, increased energy, and a full remission of neurovegetative symptoms if the treatment is deemed successful. The measures of success of a patient status postrhinoplasty are *not* a smaller, shorter, or straighter nose—but a *subjective* feeling of increased attractiveness. Aesthetic goals are inherently subjective and it is the subjectivity of success criteria that puts the cosmetic practitioner on unstable ground.

Grossbart and Sawyer (11) report how little awareness we have, as human beings, of our own attractiveness; in fact, they say, through a discussion of Feingold's earlier work, that self-rating of our attractiveness is quantifiable. We are only 6% accurate when rating how attractive we are when we compare it to external (other people's) measures. Attractiveness, then, is a bifurcating path leading to two, distinct experiences: an inner, subjective experience and an outer, objective experience.

However, at first blush it would seem that neither cosmetic surgeons nor their patients are shy about voicing the "inner" and "outer" experiences. The first exchange in the initial consultation is some version of: "What don't you like about yourself?" followed by the patient reporting his/her area(s) of concern, often asking for the surgeon's opinion. But this exchange rarely goes to the heart of the some patients' real motivation: they want the surgery to change something—not on their bodies—but in their life.

The desired life changes are the key to managing *unrealistic expectations.* Does the patient hope that rhytidoplasty will increase self-esteem or infuse her marriage with passion? It is the clinician's job to assess the realistic/unrealistic desires of their patients. According to Grossbart and Sarwer (3) the cosmetic surgeon has three roles: the *corrective surgeon,* reconstructing deformities and trauma, the *social engineer,* maintaining youthful appearances and "moderating stigmatized appearances" and *surgical psychotherapist,* alleviating the "mental anguish" of the patient's "constant realization of the defect". Grossbart and Sawyer conclude by saying "the fundamental link between emotional pain and the desire for cosmetic surgery remains."

That "emotional pain" and "mental anguish" are understandably nothing new. Cosmetic surgeons are aware, some begrudgingly so, of their role as surgical psychotherapists. But if the goal is to identify patients with unrealistic expectations and decrease liability, then our task is not to shy away from the emotional pain but—indeed—to examine it, explore it, parse it into subject and predicate, and bring with us that newly gained awareness—in an act of conscious will—into our decision-making process. A thorough history (see below for specific questions) will serve us greatly in exploring the "fundamental link between emotional pain and desire for cosmetic surgery" and identifying the patient with unrealistic expectations.

DECISION-MAKING PROCESS
(MANAGING LEGAL LIABILITY)

We live in legal times, and each clinical decision is—essentially and implicitly—a legal decision. However, all cosmetic surgeons of disparate backgrounds and attitudes will agree on a single, unifying principle: the desire to reduce liability. Whereas patients with unrealistic expectations *must* be seen in emergency departments for urgent conditions, the nonurgent nature of cosmetic procedures allows practitioners—electively—to refuse them.

In 2007, Cook et al. (12) explored the factors driving cosmetic surgeons' decisions to offer elective surgeries to 366 patients presenting for consultations in the United Kingdom. Low-cost procedures (e.g., minor skin procedures) were the most frequently listed for surgery as were those of extreme abnormality of appearance. However in its findings surrounding patients requesting cosmetic surgery with significant "psychological distress," the British study was equivocal. While psychologically stable patients with a good quality of life were preferentially offered procedures, the patients in "emotional distress" met with inconclusive results regarding the offer of surgery. The UK's caregivers work under quite a different health-care system than US physicians, and although some surgeons balk at treating patients in considerable distress, the issue of surgically treating patients in "emotional pain" is still unanswered. The study came up with no functional rubric or screening device to help in our deliberations. The question of how to successfully manage patient expectations continues to be of concern. One practitioner gave voice to his frustration in an opinion piece: "It's a 'double whammy'…so much of our work is: elective; subject to the vagaries of individual healing properties; influenced by the patient's individual perception of success or failure; and marketed by a specialty that invites plaintiffs' verdicts by its mindless encouragement of untrammeled marketing…".(13) The writer's exasperation is common to many clinicians and shows how many considerations factor into the decision to perform a procedure. He mentions the biological uncertainties ("vagaries of individual healing properties"), the personal perception "of success or failure" and—predictably—underlines the legal implications of every decision made in the field.

Given the present legal climate, cosmetic surgeons find themselves practicing medicine defensively, performing a higher number of low-risk procedures (12) and choosing their patients more shrewdly. And while the climate may be changing, there are three medicolegal principles that haven't changed since we were in medical school. Good physicians will prepare patients and their families for the eventuality of two of the three.

All medical interventions imply *risk.* The risks may be common, infrequent or rare, but a good physician will never downplay the risk to an intervention. First, the consumer model of medicine demands that we provide the patient (and family, where appropriate) with all the necessary pros and cons of a medical decision and let him/her decide. Second, procedures involve possible *complications*—both expected and unexpected. A thorough physician will have reviewed the expected complications with the patient. Managing unexpected complications will depend largely on the rapport a doctor has built with the patient and family. Physicians providing treatment within *established* standard of care should not have to concern themselves further.

Rapport is a recurring *leitmotif* throughout the legal literature on cosmetic surgery. The literature links poor communication and lack of rapport to legal liability in multiple studies. The list is long and not particularly surprising: Coon et al. (14) surveyed the telephone interviews of more than 800 women who reported problems with their breast implants to the FDA, and found that 89% wished their health-care professionals would provide them with more accurate and honest information. Another survey (15) of malpractice defense attorneys attributed 70% of their malpractice suits to miscommunication between physician and patient. Adequate time talking to patients and even answering their phone calls (16) correlate with a lower incidence of suits filed. The age of technology is here, but there's no (legal) substitute for time spent with patients.

With the advent of computer imaging, cosmetic surgeons add another arrow to their quiver of communication tools. Imaging creates for the patient a picture of the end product, and as such, is a step toward creating (and managing) patient expectations. Prudent use of computer imaging warns against "overzealous representation" of a surgeon's skill and should "depict less favorable outcomes" (17) to depict a full range of results. This new technology becomes a legal liability when the surgeon "manages up" expectations without providing a realistic picture of risks and benefits. On the nonsurgical end of the spectrum, another tool exists to help patients understand possible outcomes of Botox/BoNTA procedures. The FLO Questionnaire (17) has been developed to successfully measure patient satisfaction. The tools above, and more like them, should help move patient expectations toward more realistic goals. Take it upon yourself to educate and groom the patient toward taking her own informed, realistic, and "eyes-wide-open" decision about her surgery. Ask her to read articles and brochures about procedural options, look at photos of a range of outcomes, and be able to verbalize all the possibilities inherent in a cosmetic procedure before performing it. If an informed patient is a happy patient, and a happy patient makes a happy doctor, then it would seem that the syllogism holds: an informed patient certainly makes a happy doctor.

The consumer model of medicine received a legal fillip in the 2005. A Florida dentist and oral surgeon lost their claim of slander against a disgruntled former patient's website, dentalfraudinflorida.com.(18) Since 2005 a myriad of sites has opened, providing "medical consumers" an opportunity to critique the quality of their physicians and "rate their doctor". Patient-driven sites such as drscore.com, ratemds.com, healthcarereviews.com, and doctorscorecard.com have joined more sensational sites such as awfulplasticsurgeries.com to give disgruntled (or satisfied) patients a forum–and, by extension, an audience–to voice their opinions of caregivers. Though it is difficult to predict how far-reaching an influence the Internet will have on cosmetic surgical/health-care practices at present, it remains a powerful influence in other consumer/political arenas, and its progress should be monitored.

IDENTIFYING PATIENTS WITH UNREALISTIC EXPECTATIONS

The measurement standards for who is an appropriate candidate for aesthetic surgery seem to have relaxed considerably over time. For instance, in the 1980s, a patient who presented with a history of antidepressant use may have been turned away at an aesthetic practitioner's door. In today's competitive environment, however, knowledge of this would likely be inconsequential.(19)

Assisting patients in establishing realistic psychosocial expectations is critical to their overall satisfaction. Having realistic psychosocial expectations is as vital as having realistic physical expectations. Grossbart and Sarwer (1999) suggest a variety of means to assess patient's psychosocial expectations for surgery. For instance: What are the patient's psychosocial goals? Are they pursuing aesthetic treatment to improve their emotional state? Are they hoping to diminish feelings of appearance-related depression, social anxiety, unlovability? Are they pursuing treatment to save a marriage, or to get a promotion at work? Are they seeking aesthetic surgery to gain employment? To modify perceived stereotyped age, race, or ethnic group characteristics?

At the onset of patient screening, before moving forward with the procedure, it is imperative to obtain a thorough mental health history. Ask the patient about any past or present psychiatric diagnoses.(2) If they have a past history, it may be advisable for them to reestablish contact with their former mental health-care provider. If they are currently in treatment, is their provider aware of the patient's interest in aesthetic surgery? Moreover, it is advisable to consult with the patient's current psychiatrist/psychologist. Screening will also be useful in identifying patients who may be a management problem (i.e., risk of legal action or violence).

During the patient screening process, it is essential to ensure that their postoperative expectations can be met. The American Society of Plastic Surgeons (2008) describes a number of warning signs that suggest that a patient may not be a suitable candidate for cosmetic surgery.
These include:

- expectations of retarding aging itself
- expectations of an appearance enhanced beyond possibility
- unrealistic expectations of lifestyle/career/relationship effects
- unrealistic expectations of the duration of effects
- an unwillingness to learn the risks

- the patient is in crisis due to death of a loved one, divorce, loss of a job, or other major disrupting life event
- an unwillingness to change the behavior that led to the problem (e.g., a liposuction candidate who continues to overeat)
- an obsession with a very minor defect
- mental illness
- the patient is impossible to please (generally this can be inferred from prior behavior, such as ongoing or previous difficult relationships with staff)

The American Society of Plastic Surgeons (2008)

They further assert that unrealistic goals like finding a mate, salvaging a doomed relationship, or achieving a promotion at work call into question the patient's suitability for any type of procedure, as does an expectation of surgical improvement beyond the realm of possibility.(20)

As discussed earlier, patients with BDD, as well as certain personality, mood, and psychotic disorders are generally not suitable candidates for aesthetic procedures and will present with a variety of unrealistic expectations. Therefore, it is vital that the provider screens for these patients so that they are properly identified, diagnosed, and referred for appropriate treatment. In attempting to conduct an accurate screening, Grossbart and Sarwer (1999) offer the several recommendations:

First, ask the patient directly: "What is it about your appearance that you do not like?" What the patient reports should be visible to the physician with little effort. Patients who are very distressed about minor defects that are not readily noticeable may have BDD and may not be good candidates for aesthetic procedures.

Second, assess their degree of dissatisfaction. Ask the patient, "When does it bother you? Are there times when it upsets you more/less? Do you avoid certain activities? Do you try to camouflage?"

Patients with BDD will be markedly distressed and a great deal of time and energy will be spent surrounding the distressing body area.(2) Moreover, they may report that their thoughts are difficult to resist or control and they will spend ample time checking, examining, and hiding the "defect." They may report engaging in avoidance behaviors, like not looking in the mirror. Also, a predominant feature of this type of condition is that they are convinced that they need medical, not psychological, intervention. Two percent of the population and 7% of women presenting for cosmetic surgery will meet this description.(21)

Finally, they discuss the importance of assessing the patient's postoperative expectations. Specifically, how will their life be different after the surgery? What will the procedure do for them? What will they be able to accomplish as a result of procedure? What are the patient's fantasies about their new appearance? Is the procedure being kept a secret from friends, family? Table 2.1 lists additional issues and questions to explore regarding postoperative expectations.(22) If the patient states, "I won't be depressed," or "People will love me," this should raise a red flag for the physician to consider referring to a mental health professional. If the patient provides specific appearance concerns which are easily noticeable, and is internally motivated, there is a greater chance for realistic expectations and a higher degree of postoperative satisfaction.

Table 2.1 Assessing Patients' Post-Operative Expectations.

Is the body part an intrinsic part of the patient's identity?

Does the patient have a realistic outlook on the impact that seeing a different image of themselves in the mirror will have on their identity? Are they attempting to change *who they are* by changing their appearance?

Does the patient expect the procedure to automatically make them confident around others, when they have otherwise been recluse?

While aesthetic rejuvenation may have a positive effect on the patient's self-esteem, it is not realistic to expect that long standing, possibly maladaptive, patterns of social behavior will automatically correct themselves without the aid of either cognitive and/or behavioral modification strategies.

Are they expecting plastic surgery to change the way others react to them, or the way others treat them?

It is realistic to expect that the people in the patient's lives will notice a change in their physical appearance and may react positively. It is not realistic, however, to believe that their new appearance will offer them the respect they may have been lacking from friends, workmates, colleagues, etc. Nor is it realistic to expect others to treat them differently based solely on their appearance.

Are they using aesthetic rejuvenation as a diversion to keep from having to face a painful part of their life?

If the patient is undergoing a major aesthetic procedure because she/he fears her/his spouse has been (or will be) disloyal, it is unrealistic for them to expect the treatment to save their marriage.

Are they looking to plastic surgery as a way to erase the pain of past teasing and torment in their childhood?

Teasing about appearance in childhood and adolescence has been found to be significant predictor for motivation to undergo aesthetic treatment.(23) It is, however, unrealistic to believe that cosmetic alteration will erase the trauma of early childhood experiences.

If it appears, based on the issues described thus far, that the patient is presenting with unrealistic expectations, it may be necessary to consult with a mental health professional. A consulting or on-staff psychologist/psychiatrist can assist in recommending if a patient is a suitable candidate for aesthetic treatment, or if they may benefit from mental health intervention, either before, after or in place of undergoing the aesthetic procedure. As discussed, there are various risk management and legal implications involved in treating patients with unrealistic expectations; therefore, it behooves the aesthetic practitioner, the patient, and the medical and public community to properly identify such individuals before they commit to a life-changing decision. In properly selected candidates, results are much more likely to be positive. Findings have demonstrated that, among appropriately chosen patients, mental health and quality of life improve following aesthetic surgery on a number of dimensions, including physical health, physical appearance, social life, and inner life.(24)

REFERENCES

1. Luftman D, Ritvo E. The beauty prescription: the complete formula for looking and feeling beautiful. United States, McGraw-Hill: 2008.
2. Barson J. Cosmetic surgery demographics by patient age. MedicalspaMD.com 2/11/2006, http://www.medicalspamd.com/the-blog/2006/11/2/cosmetic-surgery-demographics-by-patient-age.html
3. Grossbart TA, Sarwer DB. Cosmetic surgery: surgical tools—psychosocial goals. Semin Cutan Med Surg 1999; 18(2): 101–11.
4. Sarwer, DB. The psychology of cosmetic surgery: a review and reconceptualization. Clinl Psychol Rev 1998; 18(1): 1–22.
5. Glogau, RG. Cosmetic dermatology: no apologies, a few regrets. Arch Dermatol 1998; 134: 1204–6.
6. Ishigooka J, Iwao M, Suzuki M et al. Demographic features of patients seeking cosmetic surgery. Psychiatry and Medical Neurosciences 1998; 52(3): 283–7.
7. Tignol, J, Biraben-Gotzamanis L, Martin-Guehl et al. Body dysmorphic disorder and cosmetic surgery: evolution of 24 subjects with a minimal defect in appearance 5 years after their request for cosmetic surgery. European Psychiatry 2007; 22: 520–4.
8. Bellino S, Zizza M, Paradiso E et al. Dysmorphic concern symptoms and personality disorders: a clinical investigation in patients seeking cosmetic surgery. Psychiatry Res 2006; 144: 73–8.
9. Meningaud J, Benadiba L, Servant J et al. Depression, anxiety and quality of life: outcome 9 months after facial cosmetic surgery. J Craniomaxillofac Surg 2003; 31: 46–50.
10. Napoleon A. The presentation of personalities in plastic surgery. Ann Plast Surg 1993; 31: 193–208.
11. Grossbart T, Sawyer D. Psychosocial issues and their relevance to the cosmetic surgery patient. Semin Cutan Med Surg 2003; 22(2): 136–47.
12. Cook S, Rossner R, James M, Kaney S, Salmon P. Factors influencing surgeons' decisions in elective cosmetic surgery consultations. Med Decis Making 2007; 27: 311–29.
13. Gorney, M. Gluttony at the bar: suing for fun and profit. J Plast Reconstr Surg Nurs 2000; 105(1): 451–2.
14. Coon SK, Burris R, Coleman EA, Lemon SJ. An analysis of telephone interview data collected in 1992 from 820 women who reported problems with their breast implants to the food and Drug Administration. Plast Reconstr Surg 2002; 109; 2043–51.
15. Avery JK. Lawyers tell what turns some patients litigious. Med Malpract 1986; 5: 35.
16. Charles SC, Gibbons RD, Frisch PR et al. Predicting risk for medical malpractice claims using quality-of-care characteristics. West J Med 1992; 157(4): 433–9.
17. Cliff SH. Patient satisfaction measures: clinical data. Cosmet Dermatol 2007; 20(7): 27–31.
18. Lynch D. Former patient's online complaints draw slander suit. Law.com 1/26/2005, http://www.law.com/jsp/article.jsp?id=1106573725914.
19. Lewis W. The cosmetic commodity. PlasticSurgeryPractice.com 9/12/2008, http://www.plasticsurgerypractice.com/issues/articles/2007-10_05.asp
20. The American Society of Plastic Surgeons. Physician's guide to cosmetic surgery: overview of cosmetic surgery. PlasticSurgery.com 8/15/2008. http://www.plasticsurgery.org/medical_professionals/publications/Physicians-Guide-to-Cosmetic-Surgery-Overview.cfm#
21. Sarwer, DB, Wadden TA, Pertschuk MJ et al. Body image dissatisfaction and body dysmorphic disorder in 100 cosmetic surgery patients. Plast Reconstr Surg 1998; 101: 1644–9.
22. Kita N. Unmet and unrealistic expectations. About.com 12/20/2007 http://plasticsurgery.about.com/od/psychologyethics/a/expectations.htm
23. Soest T, Kvalem IL, Skolleborg KC et al. Psychosocial factors predicting the motivation to undergo cosmetic surgery. Plast Reconstr Surg 2006; 117(1): 51–62.
24. Chahraoui K, Danino A, Frachebois C, Clerc AS, Malka G. Aesthetic surgery and quality of life before and four months postoperatively. Annals of Plastic Surgery and Aesthetic 2006; 3: 207–10.

3   Deciding whom to perform a procedure on, which procedure, and how to say "no"

Phillip R Langsdon and Mary Gorman

There is little doubt that every surgeon should have a high level of surgical talent, experience, and ability. Technical surgical expertise is a necessity. However, success requires more of a surgeon than skill in hand-eye coordination. Appropriate patient selection and surgical planning are essential to the success of a cosmetic surgical practice.

The surgeon must be able to determine if the potential patient is a good psychological and physical candidate. S/he must be able to properly select the best procedure for the condition in question. It will also serve well if s/he is able to separate the realistic from unrealistic patients. Unrealistic outcome expectations do not foster postoperative satisfaction, no matter how outstanding a result might be accomplished. The surgeon bears the burden of selecting both the patient and the appropriate procedure, providing patient education, and declining surgery when indicated.

DECIDING WHOM TO PERFORM A PROCEDURE ON

One of the first questions a surgeon asks him/herself is "does the patient have a cosmetic condition that can or should be altered". Assuming that a patient presents with a physically improvable cosmetic condition, there are many conditions that simply cannot be altered to the extent or manner that the patient imagines attainable. It is necessary to determine if the patient comprehends the surgeon's assessment and expected outcome; and that the patient accepts and understands the realities of the venture.

A second, but no less important concern of every potential surgical candidate should be that the patient is psychologically fit to undergo the contemplated procedure. There are multiple psychotic, neurotic, and normal variants of the human mental state. Additionally, some of these states change over time and with personal circumstance.

Psychotic individuals can be unrealistic and dangerous. Normal conditions of the face, ears, nose, etc. can be viewed as grossly flawed. The opposite can also be true. But, one thing is for sure; a surgeon can never accurately guess how an outcome will be viewed by an unstable individual. Nor can we assume that their response to a surgical outcome will be reasonable.

Psychotic patients are sometimes relatively easy to identify, but neurotic individuals can be more of a challenge than the outright psychotic patient. Neurotic people are occasionally better at hiding the eccentricities of their psychological condition until after a surgical procedure has been performed. Even if the neurotic individual is identified before surgery and the surgeon feels it is safe to operate, the degree and direction of the patient's view of his/her outcome cannot be predicted with any level of certainty. Their response, when negative, has the potential to be troubling or outright dangerous.

One of the cautionary signs that presents repeatedly is the patient who is overly obsessed with a minor detail. The imagined defect, the inflated problem, the out of proportion impact upon his/her social, family, or business life is a sign that this particular patient might never attain satisfaction with even the most flawless surgical result. Surgery on such an individual should either be avoided entirely or undertaken only with the expectation of constant repeated reassurances and explanations during the postoperative course. Even after great effort, they may never achieve satisfaction.

Normal individuals with no apparent psychotic or neurotic conditions should also be approached with caution. Some individuals simply cannot be satisfied, whereas others seek surgery for the wrong reasons. An inventory of the patient's motivation, expectations, and ego strength helps determine if the patient might obtain a satisfactory result.(1) Surgery will not win friends, lovers, jobs, or general approval that one might seek. If surgery is sought for any reason other than the patient's own dissatisfaction with a real flaw, one that is reasonably improvable, then surgery should be reconsidered. Family members should also be included in the patient evaluation process. It may be prudent to have the spouse, adult child, or close friend to sit in on preoperative sessions. It only takes one negative remark about the outcome from a spouse to turn a flawless surgical success into a failure in the eyes of an individual with weak ego strength. And, many times, those most influential on the patient may not have had the opportunity to sit in on the consultation and learn about the normal expectations. Educating the patient's support network on realistic outcomes and the normal variations of the postoperative course avoids misunderstandings and promotes realistic expectations. This relatively simple step promotes, but does not guarantees, postoperative patient satisfaction.

Some "normal" individuals can border on neurotic and find fault with even the best result realistically obtainable. The most difficult normal patients are those who will simply find fault with everything in their lives; surgery is not excluded.

However, with good communication and patient follow-up, reassurance of the healing process and outcome....description of what is normal and expected (before, during, and after the initial healing process) will usually help the normal individual understand when to be satisfied.

Information from the electronic and print media, as well as the views of friends or family members, taints a patient's expectations. This outside information is often flawed and interferes with normal patient expectations. One of the most difficult tasks a physician faces is to educate the patient on what is realistically obtainable, as well as the process necessary to obtain that result. Some patients listen, some don't; then some listen but decide on their own what they want regardless of what the surgeon tries to explain. Every cosmetic surgeon struggles with the challenge. Repetition of realistic expectations and accurate documentation remain the most effective tools for promoting postoperative patient satisfaction.

Potential patients should also be willing to follow instructions. Failure to do so may ruin an otherwise excellent surgical outcome. If a patient exhibits the early warning signs of an inability to cooperate or conform to office protocols, it might be wise to reconsider agreeing to operate.

The ideal situation is a psychologically normal patient, in good health, with an improvable flaw, motivated by his/her own wish to improve the condition in question, who complies with office protocols, policies, and programs. Not all factors can be directly addressed by the physician and a combination of intuition and experience are necessary to develop the appropriate sensitivities to warning signs in the patient's initial consultation and history.

WHICH PROCEDURE TO PERFORM

Deciding which procedure to perform requires close attention to the patient's area of concern. While a myriad of potential improvements may be obvious to the trained clinician, patient satisfaction is most effectively achieved by specifically addressing the concerns expressed by the patient and then providing patient and caregiver education on how that specific concern can be addressed and what the realistic expectations for outcomes are in that particular patient's situation. If patient desires appear unrealistic, then surgery should be reconsidered.

The three main manifestations of the aging face include the development of 1) excess sagging tissues, 2) thinning skin with wrinkle development, pigment abnormalities, and keratosis, and 3) facial deflation. Each manifestation may require a different treatment type. The treatment or combination of treatments recommended depends on the degree of aging manifestation present in the three main categories. For example, facelift, blepharoplasty, cervicoplasty, and forehead lifting may improve sagging tissues, but they cannot remove wrinkles or re-inflate the face.

If rhytids are present they may require facial skin exfoliation and hydration. Exfoliation may be accomplished with daily use of exfoliation agents such as glycolic acid or retinoic acid. Resistant rhytids may necessitate the addition of superficial, moderate depth, or deep peeling or light-based treatments, depending on the degree of treatment required. Rhytids that are the result of dynamic facial muscular movement may benefit from chemodenervation.

Areas of facial deflation, such as the orbital cheek groove, oblique cheek depression, nasolabial and mentolabial regions may benefit from facial fillers.

Surgical procedures designed to alter the architectural structure of the face such as rhinoplasty, otoplasty, or mentoplasty are selected based upon the condition in question, the options available, and the other criteria described above.

Repeated patient education helps the patient understand that one procedure will not address all three manifestations of facial aging.

While some patients state specifically what part of the aging process or what part of an anatomical structure bothers them most acutely, other patients may have a more nebulous sense of dissatisfaction, such as the statement, "I just look too old" or "I just don't like how my nose looks." All patients require clear, repeated descriptions of the expected results of a cosmetic surgical procedure to avoid postoperative disappointment. Clear elucidation of what can and can't be expected is provided to the patient in the initial consultation, the preoperative visit, then reinforced again by the physician the day of the procedure, preferably with a companion present who can remind the patient of the conversation when the details are forgotten. Written materials describing the given procedures, intended results and limitations, and the postoperative course and care involved may help if distributed to the patient preoperatively and important points highlighted by the physician or nurse with the patient's caregiver present.

WHEN TO SAY NO

If in the surgeon's judgment, the patient's desired result cannot be reasonably attained or is surgically unobtainable or unrealistic, the option of surgery might be reconsidered. Aesthetic perfection is an unrealistic expectation. Patients who expect perfection should not be accepted as surgical candidates. In the case of the psychologically unstable patients, any sort of operative intervention is best delayed or avoided outright if prolonged psychological stability cannot be achieved. The postoperative recovery period may pose serious challenges to the psyche of the "stable" patient and such stress exerted on patients without the mental resiliency to rebound may be catastrophic to the patient and the physician. Patients with a previous history of attempted suicide or serious depression treated with shock therapy or who refuse to see a counselor for preoperative clearance or depressed patients who secretly hope to die from the procedure should be refused surgery.(2)

Any active medical conditions are best stabilized before elective cosmetic surgery. Certain medical conditions may contraindicate surgery.

Telling a patient "no" can be done by stating that the physician does not believe he/she can achieve that results desired by the patient or by explaining the issues of concern. One should cautiously assess the best method, manner, and location when declining surgery.

REFERENCE

1. Beeson WH, McCollough EG. Aesthetic Surgery of the Aging Face Ch 2 Patient Selection (William H Beeson), Mosby Company, St. Louis MO, 1986: 10–12.
2. Anderson & Ries, Rhinoplasty: Emphasizing the External Approach, Ch 4, p 17-28, Patient Selection: Phychologic and Physical Considerations, Thieme Inc., New York, 1986.

4 Minimal recovery procedures
Mark S Nestor and Glynis R Ablon

INTRODUCTION

It is human nature to want more and more for less and less. This is certainly true when it comes to aesthetic procedures. Patients are hoping for the greatest degree of improvement with minimal recovery, risks, and of course minimal cost. From the patient's standpoint, it would be ideal to apply a cream every night and in doing so erase both the intrinsic and extrinsic signs of aging. Minimal recovery procedures, the so-called "no downtime procedures," offer patients significant aesthetic options with minimal or no recovery time and for the most part, minimal risks. Results though are conservative and require repeat procedures and/or maintenance treatments. Patients must understand both the upsides—instant gratification with little down time and the downside which is conservative results. Minimal recovery procedures including the use of botulinum toxin, fillers, laser, light, and radiofrequency and peels are among the most popular and widely utilized aesthetic procedures. New minimally invasive procedures are also being developed to enhance contours of the body by dissolving body fat. In addition to the aesthetic benefit, clinical benefits in conditions such as rosacea, acne, and melasma, as well as actinic damage may also be gleaned from procedures that may be originally developed for the aesthetic patient. The popularity of these procedures has opened up the potential of aesthetic enhancement to a wide range of individuals, both expanding the appropriate age range of the patients benefiting from aesthetic procedure as well as including all socioeconomic classes of individual. With the advent of minimal recovery procedures, aesthetic enhancement is no longer necessarily reserved for older, affluent individuals.

The older paradigm for cosmetic surgery was aggressive, surgical and resurfacing procedures for significant facial and photoaging skin with major cosmetic results, 4 to 6 week down times and risk factors. This was during our era where cosmetic patients were only of an affluent class, scheduled a major "make-over" and planned for a prolonged recovery. Patients kept their procedures secretive but reemerged at a later date looking not only younger but "different".

Now patients do prefer a much more conservative approach with natural results. The demand of "no down time" with little to no risk factors are a result of a more active working population with time and monetary restraints. Rather than "turning back the clock" our patients would rather "look my best for my age".

For minimally invasive procedures to be successful, physicians must evaluate the needs, desires, and expectations of the aesthetic patient. The degree of aging including intrinsic aging and photoaging must be assessed and put in the context of the anticipated goals for the patient. When it comes to minimally invasive procedures, it is especially important that goals are realistic and the patients are not expecting degrees or types of improvement that can only be accomplished by surgical or other invasive procedures. Although significant risks of minimally invasive procedures are for the most part fairly rare, patients still need to understand both recovery time and risks for the type of procedure that they may choose. Patients still wish to turn back the clock and to remove years of both intrinsic and extrinsic aging to look and feel better. Physicians have many choices at their disposal. Peels, laser and light treatments including intense pulse light, infrared lasers, fractionated laser resurfacing, visible light lasers including 532 nm, 585 nm, Q-switch Ruby and Q-switch Yag lasers and radiofrequency can offer aesthetic benefits to a wide variety of patients.

A variety of hair removal laser systems can remove unwanted hair gently and effectively. The use of botulinum toxin type A (Botox or Dysport) can relax dynamic folds and rhytides, and the use of variety of dermal fillers can smooth static lines and folds, and replace lost volume. Many physicians use combination therapy which includes multiple devices and procedures. An example is the use of fillers and toxins used simultaneously to dramatically improve the patients' aesthetic appearance. Finally, combination therapy with pharmaceuticals, including tretinoin and hydroquinone, and an array of cosmeceutical products, including proteins, peptides, and growth factors can also enhance the final result. This chapter will highlight the most frequently utilized minimal recovery procedures and discuss their role in clinical practice.

PROCEDURES

Chemical Peels

A variety of peeling agents have been available for aesthetic enhancement dating back to Cleopatra and her sour milk (lactic acid) cleansing ritual. Chemical peels effectively target photodamaged skin, pigmentary disorders, superficial growths and superficial scarring as well as acne. Superficial, medium depth, and deep peeling agents have been available for decades.(1) Deeper peeling agents or combinations of medium depth agents can yield significant results, but cannot truly be considered minimal recovery procedures. Efficacy of peels is divided as follows:

Peel	Agent	Depth of Penetration	Recovery Time
Light	10–20% TCA Salicylic Acid Glycolic Acid Jesner's Peel	Partial or Complete Epidermal destruction	24–72 hours
Medium Depth	Jesner's + 35% TCA Glycolic 70% + 35% TCA	Epidermal destruction + inflammation of upper dermis	5–7 days
Deep	Phenol Peels	Destruction of epidermis to reticular dermis	10–14 days

The use of repetitive superficial peels has become one of the most popular cosmetic procedures to improve skin color, texture, fine lines, pores, and active acne. It is a useful complement for other laser and injectable procedures. These procedures are repetitive with results cumulative over time.

Trichloracetic acid (TCA) is effective with varying concentrations leading to different depths of penetration, but it remains very user dependent leading to a broad range of results and complications. Milder chemical peeling agents such as glycolic acid or beta hydroxy acids are usually the agents of choice for "lunchtime" peels. These agents provide reproducible but usually minimal improvement in dispigmentation and very fine lines in sun damaged skin. Superficial peels are frequently simple procedure performed monthly or bimonthly to keep the skin looking fresh and thus more youthful. Combining peeling agents with prescription and nonprescription creams can also lead to enhanced results.(2) The medium depth peel—Jessner's + 35% TCA or the "Monheit procedure"—is a very reliable reproducible procedure that will accomplish significant skin texture change, remove sun damaged growth, and give skin a brighter more uniform color in one procedure rather than multiple repetitive light peels. It is ideal for patients who have had treatment with cosmoceuticals and repetitive light peels and now request greater results with a more aggressive technique.

Ablative Lasers

Lasers have been used for the aesthetic patient since the late 1980s and early 1990s. It was the advent of the pulse and scan CO_2 laser in the early 1990s that brought the use of the laser to the forefront of aesthetic medicine.(3, 4) CO_2 lasers could reproducibly and dramatically improve fine and deep lines and wrinkles albeit with significant downtime and risks of scarring, hyper, and hypopigmentation. Physicians looked to modify the CO_2 laser by a variety of methods to decrease both downtime and risks to the patient. Scanning devices, (Feather Touch, Sharplan) and single-pass CO_2 techniques allowed for more superficial resurfacing with less down time and risk, along with less dramatic results.(3, 4)The advent of the Erbium laser was initially thought to be the answer for decreased downtime and risk but it became clear that there was a one-to-one relationship between overall effectiveness and downtime and risks. Short-pulse Erbium lasers also had the disadvantage of not allowing for hemostasis which further limited its effectiveness. The advent of the long-pulsed Erbium laser allowed for hemostasis and improved outcomes but with inherently greater downtime and risk. A series of superficial Erbium laser treatments (Microlaserpeels) (4) did improve outcome with minimal recovery for each treatment although the patient had to undergo a series of "weekends with a red peeling face". Over the past few years, CO_2 and Erbium laser have made a type of reappearance as platforms for fractionated laser procedures, again with the hope of having significant effects with minimal downtime and risks.(5, 6)

Fractionated Lasers

Fractionated lasers have been developed for both ablative and nonablative treatment and have proven to be effective for conditions such as melasma, acne scarring, as well as aesthetic enhancement.(7) Microscopic thermal zones are created with fractionated lasers, instead of full skin thermal damage. The difference between the ablative and nonablative fractional machines is directly related to the type of energy (wavelength) and amount of heat delivered by these new devices. Similar to nonfractionated devices, ablative fractionated lasers cause tissue vaporization, causing a greater degree of heating, leading to thermal molecular changes and subsequent tissue tightening. Thus, the more heat the more dramatic the results, but likewise the more recovery needed. Nonablative devices such as the 1550 nm Fraxel Restore (Reliant Technologies) or Lux 1540 (Palomar) improve actinic damage, rhytids and superficial acne scaring with minimal recovery through a series of treatments.

Ablative fractionated lasers come in many different wavelengths and thus vary on the degree of recovery time. The longer wavelengths such as 12600 nm CO_2 devices (DOT therapy Fraxel Repair or Pixel) and 2904 nm Erbium devices (ProFractional or Lux2940) can leave patients with 2–7 days of spreckling or crusting.(7, 8)

The results of fractional ablative laser can approach those previously seen with CO_2 lasers with less down time and theoretically less risk of pigmentary problems or scarring. The destroyed microthermal zones within the dermis will give results of tissue tightening and ablation of fine rhytids.

Intense Pulsed Light

The advent of intense pulse light in the mid 1990s offered new way of improving vascular and pigmented conditions such as diffuse telangiectases and lentigines, as well as having some minimal effect on the fine lines, wrinkles and tightening with minimal or no downtime.(9, 10) Photorejuvenation or FotoFacials had and have become a very popular option for aesthetic enhancement. Intense pulse light (IPL) offers a variety of wavelengths of light in one pulse, which, by theory of selective photothermolysis, allows treatment of pigmented lesions, vascular lesions, and allows for collagen remodeling simultaneously. So called "Photorejuvenation Treatments" or "PhotoFacial", performed with Intense Pulsed light, are usually performed as a series allowing for maximal improvement with minimal downtime. Photorejuvenation is also very effective for clinical conditions with aesthetic component such as acne vulgaris, rosacea, and melasma.(9, 11, 12) Better overall results are observed when wavelengths (cut-off filters), pulse durations, and energy levels are adjusted and customized to each patient's clinical needs.

Photodynamic Therapy

The use of lasers and light in combination with topical photosensitizer such as 5-aminolevulinic acid (Photodynamic Therapy, PDT) has not only boosted the aesthetic benefit of procedures such as IPL photorejuvenation, but also have had significant clinical affects on reduction in precancerous actinic keratoses and even skin cancers.(13) The photosensitizer is applied to clean skin for different incubation periods, generally 30 minutes to 1 hour, followed by dynamic activators such as IPL or LED technology (red or blue light). Patients experience 48 hours of photosensitivity and have a minimal amount of redness and peeling. A series of treatments are used for the best results.(14) PDT has also been shown to be effective in a variety of conditions from acne to keratosis pilaris.(15, 16)

Light Emitting Diodes

LED (Light Emitting Diode) light at variety of wavelengths can yield minimal improvement in the patients with photodamage, acne vulgaris, and rosacea who are searching for aesthetic enhancement with virtually no downtime or risk.(17) LED technology found in devices with varying wavelengths (Omnilux and Gentlewaves) affect the skin using photobiomodulation (18) (cells absorb light from emitting diode wavelength and cause a biochemical reaction). Unlike lasers, the effects are seen without heating of tissue through noncoherent, monochromatic light, with spontaneous emission. Omnilux offers 415 nm, 633 nm, 830 nm with 20 minute duration (Phototherapeutics). Gentlewaves (Light BioScience) is 585 nm with short pulse 35-second treatment duration. While hand-held units of LED technology for home use have become available, and have some effect on acne, facial erythema, rosacea, and mild photodamage, due to the small head size, they currently won't replace the office-based unit. LED results are very minimal and probably best for patients with very little photodamage—Glogau I or II—with little need or demand for change.

Vascular and Pigment Specific Lasers

The use of wavelength specific lasers including vascular lasers with wavelengths of 532, 585, and 1064 allow for treatment of vascular anomalies, diffuse erythema, facial telangiectases, and leg venules generally with minimal downtime and risk. These superficial vascular lesions are targeted by specific laser wavelengths: the longer the wavelength, the deeper/larger vessel absorption occurs. Very superficial vessels respond to potassium titanyl phosphate (KTP), or pulse dye lasers, whereas larger leg veins may respond to Nd-Yag 1064 nm.(19, 20)

Pigment Specific lasers, such as Q-switched Ruby or Q-switch Yag, absorb in the superficial pigment spectrum. While these lasers have been shown to improve photodamage, they do appear to work best when hitting their specific target. Those targets are lentiginous, ephelides, lentigos and thin seborrheic keratoses. Using a Q-switch Yag laser at 52 or 1064 nm most lesions can be removed or improved in one treatment session. The shorter the wavelength, again, the more superficial lentigines are targeted. (21, 22) Deeper pigment abnormalities, such as Nevus of Ota, respond better to the Ruby laser or alexandrite.(23, 24)

Endovenous Procedures

The nonablative use of lasers to treat cutaneous leg veins has lead to the development of endovenous leg vein therapy, using 810 nm, 940 nm, and 980 nm, and 1320 nm lasers. This procedure has revolutionized the difficult realm of varicose vein treatment. Without destroying incompetent larger perforating veins, the success with sclerotherapy remains poor. With endovenous lasers, we can now provide patients with outpatient, virtually painless procedures with excellent, long-lasting results.(25) While vein ligation and stripping may lead to common recurrence of varicosities, failing to treat the origin of the vein reflux, infection, and neurosensory loss, endovenous laser ablation distributes thermal energy causing tissue damage and collapse of venous walls with success rates reported at 90–100%.(26) The veins are resorbed over a period of 3 to 4 months. Complications tend to be minimal including eccymoses, phlebitis, and edema. Rare side effects include cellulitis and deep venous thrombosis (DVT). Frequently a combination of endovenous vein treatment followed by superficial vascular treatment for telangiectasias and matting can give patients extremely satisfying results.

Infrared Lasers

Nonablative, infrared lasers including wavelengths such as 1319, 1320, and 1550 can be utilized to improve fine lines as well as scars such as acne scars.(27) These wavelengths allow penetration into the dermal tissue while bypassing any epidermal absorption. Patients have no recovery, and higher fluences have led to greater improvement in skin tightening. Epidermal cooling and topical anesthetics alone provide sufficient comfort throughout the procedure. Heating of the dermal collagen and elastin leads to shrinkage of these fibers, which gives these lasers their facial-lifting abilities.(28) Significant improvement can also be seen using infared lasers for the treatment of fresh acne and injury scars, including recent stretch marks.

Laser Hair Removal

Laser hair removal has become one of the most popular procedures in aesthetic medicine and certainly can allow for permanent removal of unwanted hair.(29) Idiopathic hirsutism is common in some ethnic groups, and true hirsute women can also be seen with hormone abnormalities. The majority of individuals however undertake laser hair removal strictly for cosmetic reasons. A detailed patient history and sun avoidance education is important to assure safety and benefit. It is necessary to choose a laser specifically based on each individual patient's skin type to enhance clinical benefit and minimize risk. While multiple laser purchases may be cost prohibitive, choosing one based on your general skin type population is best, making sure to refer out patients that have higher risks with the wavelength chosen. Alexandrite lasers 755 nm and Nd:Yag 1064 nm work well on darker skin types, with moderate improvement on lighter skin. The risks of laser hair removal complications still remain, especially for the patient who has had significant recent sun exposure as well as Fitzpatrick skin types IV, V, and VI.

Radiofrequency

One of the so-called holy grails of minimally invasive procedures is the ability to tighten lax skin without the use of invasive procedures. The use of unipolar radiofrequency has certainly shown some benefit in this area; however it is clear that the procedure does not take the place of surgical rhytidectomy. Unipolar radiofrequency, such as the Thermage (Thermage Corp.) procedure, can be utilized both on and off the face to cause significant three-dimensional skin tightening by affecting not only the collagen fibers in the dermis but also the fibers in the so-called fibroseptae that links deeper structures such as fascia to the skin.(30) In this way, skin can benefit from toning and tightening not just by two dimensionally decreasing the lax surface area but also by actually pulling the skin closer to the deeper structures. Radiofrequency allows the thermal energy to pass directly into the dermal tissue layer, and with superficial cooling spares most epidermal risk. Shallow treatment tips have even allowed tissue tightening of upper eyelid skin, an area typically restricted to resurfacing lasers or surgery.(31) New techniques using multiple passes at lower energies yield promising, and significantly less painful, results.(32) The larger tips with an intermittent radiofrequency delivery have improved safety and efficacy for treatment of the face. Now areas of cellulite, skin redundancy and flaccidity can be tightened and smoothed on arms, abdomen, buttocks, and thighs. Bipolar radiofrequency, which generates lower energies than unipolar radiofrequency, when used in conjunction with IPL, the so-called Elos procedure also has been shown to have an effect on skin tightening. Even with the low incidence of complications, improper use, energies and handling of radiofrequency devices can lead to skin damage and scars.(33)

Botulinum Toxin Type A

The use of botulinum toxin, initially developed for the treatment of spastic muscles has evolved into the most widely used minimally invasive aesthetic procedures available.(34) In the mid- to late 1990s, it was noted that the use of botulinum toxin can significantly reduce the appearance of glabella lines and wrinkles, and overtime, the procedure has evolved to become the number one treatment option for the upper face including the glabella, forehead, periorbital region. Treatment of dynamic wrinkles—those dependent on muscle movement—will flatten and smooth with appropriate doses of Botulinum toxin-A placed into proper injection points. In addition it is noted that treatment of the glabella and lateral brow will in fact raise the eyebrows 2 to 3 mm creating a "chemical brow lift". Treatment of periorbital wrinkles or crows feet also open the eyes creating a more youthful appearance. These treatments have given us a greater understanding of the dynamism between "elevator and depressor" muscles, useful in lifting sagging structures. This concept has led to the use of Botulinum toxin-A to treat the depressor angularis oris to lift the corner of the mouth and platysmal injections to smooth a sagging jawline. Thus botulinum toxin has been utilized in treatment of dynamic rhytides in the lower face and neck. It appears that regular dosing with botulinum toxin can lead to muscle relaxation, or retraining of muscle movement leading to prolonged results. Over the years the use of botulinum toxin has been modified, working toward a relaxation of muscles as opposed to a frozen appearance. We also know now that this toxin can even improve migraines. Additionally, the botulinum toxin aesthetically is used in hyperhidrosis or in the patients who just "do not want to sweat". Properly administered, botulinum toxin is incredibly safe and effective. There is virtually no downtime and the effects last somewhere between 3 and 5 months. The aesthetic benefits of botulinum toxin seem to much greater than the aesthetic benefit of a smooth glabella, forehead, or periorbital region and in fact it appears that the inability to frown or scowl causes the acquaintances viewing the treated subject to view them as less angry, sad, and overall happier.(35) Interpersonal relationships may indeed benefit in ways that transcend the aesthetic benefit.(36) The use of Botulinum toxin-A (Botox®) has become the most commonly used cosmetic procedure as documented by surveys of American Society of Plastic and Reconstructive Surgery (ASPRS) and the American Society of Dermatologic Surgery (ASDS). Most recently a second Botulinum toxin-A (Dysport®) has been FDA approved for the use of glabellar lines. It has been used over the past decade in Europe for cosmetic usage and found to be equally effective as Botox®. It is suggested by experienced users to have an earlier onset (1 to 3 days) and so may be more suitable for patients requiring a procedure with minimal recovery time before an imminent social deadline. It may also have a greater "field of effort" or "diffusion". Often botulinum toxin is used in conjunction with a variety of light laser or laser procedures and/or the use of dermal fillers.(37)

Dermal Fillers

Second only to botulinum toxin, the use of dermal fillers has revolutionized the treatment of the aesthetic patient as well as aesthetic marketplace.(38, 39) In the United States, collagen was approved in the 1980s and Zyplast and Zyderm were used to treat deeper lines and folds as well as fine lines and wrinkles. Bovine collagen had significant limitations, most notably the patients with allergic reactions, therefore the need for skin testing, as well as duration of only approximately 3 to 6 months. Human collagen was developed in the late 1990s and early part of this millennium and while reactions were not an issue persistence was still limited to 3 to 5 months. New forms of collagen such as Glymatrix porcine collagen offer improved persistence, no or minimal allergic reactions, and absolute minimal recovery. The lack of inflammation, swelling, and purpura makes it an ideal soft tissue filler for nasolabial folds.

The first hyaluronic acid filler was approved in the United States in 2004. The present hyaluronic acid fillers have significantly increased clinical efficacy based on better crosslinking that decreases the breakdown of hyaluronic acid in the skin. This has increased longevity and ability of the filler to lift and volume fill. Hyaluronic acid fillers have become the most widely used fillers for the treatments of both lines and folds as well as replacement of lost facial volume. Aesthetically, hyaluronic acid fillers are used to fill deeper folds and wrinkles such as the nasolabial fold and mesolabial fold, deeper notches including the pre-jowl sulcus, replace volume in tear troughs, replace and enhance volume for lips, and finally to replace volume associate with the aging face in the mid face, cheeks, and other areas. We are even now able to perform nonsurgical nasal reconstruction with fillers to lift the sagging nasal tip and treat depressions and bumps.(40) Recent studies have also shown that when hyaluronic acid fillers are inject in areas such as the nasolabial folds and then optimized by re-injection in 4 to 6 months, persistence may last 18 to 24 months, probably caused by decreased breakdown of the filler as well as the stimulation of integral collagen.(41) Thicker variations of hyaluronic acid can be used to replace deep volume loss, while lower concentrations of hyaluronic acid can by used for more superficial filling, especially around the eyes and lips.(42) With the array of new hyaluronic acid products on the market (Restylane®, Juvederm®, Prevelle Silk®, Perlane®) the variables of each product such as particle concentration, crosslinking, degree of hardness or G' and fluid saturation can be used for different locations and clinical needs. For example softer, less crosslinked hyaluronic acid gives a more natural appearance for lips whereas a stiffer more robust hyaluronic acid with a high G' is better for vertical lift in deep nasolabial folds. In addition to hyaluronic acid, calcium hydroxyapatite (Radiesse) is a useful synthetic volume filler for 1 year duration. PLA or polylactic acid (Sculptra®) produces volumetric filling through collagen synthesis in the dermis and subcutaneous tissue. The fibroplasia induced by PLA is a natural thickening of the skin and soft tissue regenerating aging facial atrophy as well as correcting skin texture. This treatment though requires multiple injection sessions with final results gradually appearing after 4 to 6 months.

The permanent injectable fillers—Artefil which is polymethyl methacrylate beads in collagen—have recently appeared on the market. They are reserved for the expert injector as the results are permanent leaving little margin for error. Injectable silicone is also available for off-label usage for tissue augmentation. The microdroplet technique has been used successfully but nodules and silicone granulomas have been reported a year or so after injections.(39, 43–45)

Soft tissue fillers are a major tool in the portfolio of the cosmetic surgeon and is used in combination with Botulinum toxin-A, lasers, peels and cosmoceuticals

Minimally Invasive Fat Removal

A trim, toned body is the new fashion statement for the millennium and as is with all the aesthetic procedures, patients are looking to reshape their bodies with a minimal amount of recovery. The gold standard for body shaping is liposuction. Tumescent liposuction has been shown to be very safe and effective and can, at least to some, be thought of as a minimal recovery procedure. Patients, however, are looking for new procedures with improvement similar to liposuction but with less invasive characteristics and minimal recovery time. Laser lipolysis has become very popular over the past 3 to 4 years whereby a laser fiber is used within a canula to melt away fat.(46) A very small incision, usually 1 to 2 mm is made and the small catheter with the laser fiber is inserted into the fatty layer. The laser lipolysis is used both with and without concomitant liposuction. The benefits of laser lipolysis are theoretically a lessening of bleeding and bruising, and significant tissue tightening. Small areas can certainly be treated with minimal recovery time. Many wavelengths have been approved for laser lipolysis including 1064, 1320, and 980. Recently, devices are used with combinations of these wavelengths to maximize fat dissolution and dermal tightening. Two or three other types of device may be utilized in the future to dissolve unwanted fat. Radiofrequency has been known for some time to cause, mostly as a side effect, dissolution of fat. New unipolar radiofrequency devices and tips can penetrate deep into the fat layer and theoretically have the potential of melting away fat in a completely noninvasive method. High-energy focused ultrasound is being studied extensively to significantly decrease fat and recontour abdominal and other areas. One of the most advanced devices is called the Liposonix device which uses high energy focused ultrasound placed on the skin to heat and destroy fat approximately 1 cm below the dermis. Other studies in Europe show a reduction in abdominal girth of anywhere between 2 and 8 cm with a single treatment.(47) Treatment optimization studies are being performed to maximize treatment efficacy.

Cryolipolysis, using a device called Zeltiq (48), takes advantage of the fact that fat hardens and the fat cells undergo apoptosis at a higher temperature than other tissue. Using a special suction device the fatty tissue is noninvasively cooled and over the next 90 days the dead fat cells are taken away by macrophages. The procedure is basically painless and noninvasive. At this point it is being used primarily for areas such as love-handles and pockets of fat on the back. Over time these minimally invasive procedures may be used in combination to totally remodel and remold unwanted fat, especially in individuals who are toned but genetically have fat pockets. The terms Mesotherapy and phosphatidylcholine

have been used interchangeably to describe a method of injecting compounds subcutaneously for localized fat reduction, yet the two terms are quite different. Mesotherapy is a therapy recognized in Europe for the treatment of joint pains. It is frequently a concoction of drugs including vitamins, antiinflammatories, methylxanthines, and frequently phosphatidylcholine/deoxycholate (PC/DC) combination. The first US-based study demonstrated the success and safety of pure PC/DC mixture for infraorbital fat pads.(49) Direct injection of DC into lipomas supported lipolysis and laboratory studies have shown that deoxycholate, the bile salt used as a stabilizer in these compounds, is likely the active ingredient causing fat dissolution.(50) While large-scale studies and FDA approval are still lacking, the apparent moderate success, noninvasive nature, and low product cost keep these injectables in the hands of anxious and often unqualified injectors. Even though side effects appear to be minimal in published data, dosing regimen, and frequency of injections remain undetermined. We continue to anticipate large double-blinded clinical trials to support and establish clinical efficacy and subsequent FDA approval.

COSMECEUTICALS AND PHARMACEUTICALS

The use of cosmeceuticals and prescription topical creams allow physicians to maximize the benefits of minimal recovery procedures. One of the first pharmaceutical products shown to have significant benefit for the aesthetic patient was tretinoin.(51) The use of retinoids has been known for the past 15 to 20 years to enhance the appearance of the patients and decrease the signs of aging. Retinoids such as tazarotene, adapalene, and tretinoin are often used alone or in combination with hydroquinone, glycolic acid, and another peeling agents of afford significant benefits to the patient. The use of hydroquinone has also been touted for its clinical effect on hyperpigmentation, which is often significant concern in the aesthetic patient. Combination product such as Tri-Luma allows for significant overall improvement in hyperpigmentation especially in condition such as melasma and may be utilized with laser and light treatments to improve the overall affect on the skin.

Topical antioxidants such as Revale (Coffeeberry), L-ascorbic acid, Prevage (Idebenone), and alpha-lipoic acid fight free radicals prevent inflammation, and improve skin texture and tone. Human growth factors such as TNS from Skin Medica, Neocutis, as well as plant growth factors have demonstrated wound healing and stimulation of collagen. Peptides and proteins such as Strivectin interrupt neuromuscular junction and relax facial muscles Pentapeptides decrease collagen breakdown, while hexapeptides (DMAE) contract muscle, improve skin tone, alter cellular communication at the neuromuscular junction. Enzymes such as Dimercine recognize DNA damage and repair it, to prevent skin cancer and improve photodamaged skin.(52) It is important that patients understand that topical agents in the right concentration, pH, and delivery base can be effective. Expectations must be explained clearly as topical products are not the same as lasers or injections. When patients are made aware of the true potential of topical agents, and how they can enhance cosmetic procedural dermatology, satisfaction improves dramatically.

CONCLUSIONS: MINIMAL RECOVERY PROCEDURES AND COMBINATION THERAPY

Ultimately the maximum benefit aesthetically can be reached by combining a number of minimally invasive procedures.(53) The use of nonablative lasers and lights to improve many aspects of photoaging including telangiectases and lentigines along with fractionated lasers for scarring and fine lines can maximize the clinical appearance of the skin. Newer lasers work on other body parts including varicosities and fat deposits with more successful results, and little recovery. The use of dermal fillers and botulinum toxin can decrease both dynamic rhytides as well as replace lost volume and fill lines and folds, while radiofrequency and other tightening procedures can enhance tightening and toning of the skin. Finally, the addition of topical products, both prescription creams and cosmeceuticals, can help maintain the overall aesthetic improvement. In combination, minimal recovery procedures can effectively reverse many signs of intrinsic and extrinsic aging and offer dramatic benefits to the aesthetic patient with minimal downtime, side effects, and risks. In the future it is clear that both new and enhanced, existing procedures will continue to minimize risks and maximize aesthetic benefits.

REFERENCES

1. Clark E, Scerri L. Superficial and medium-depth chemical peels. Clin Dermatol 2008; 26(2): 209–18.
2. Garg VK, Sarkar R, Agarwal R. Comparative evaluation of beneficiary effects of priming agents (2% hydroquinone and 0.025% retinoic acid) in the treatment of melasma with glycolic acid peels. Dermatol Surg 2008; 34(8): 1032–9.
3. Ramsdell WM. Carbon dioxide laser resurfacing. Arch Facial Plast Surg 2009; 11(1): 62–3.
4. Nestor MS. Ablative laser resurfacing, in Photoaging. editors: Rigel DS, Weiss R, Lim HW, Dover JS, Marcel Dekker Press 2004.
5. Berlin AL, Hussain M, Phelps R, Goldberg DJ. Treatment of photoaging with a very superficial Er:Yag laser in combination with a broadband light source. J Drugs Dermatol 2007; 6(11): 1114–8.
6. Chapas AM, Brightman L, Sukal S et al. Successful treatment of acneiform scarring with CO_2 ablative fractional resurfacing. Lasers Surg Med 2008; 40(6): 381–6.
7. Alexiades-Armenakas MR, Dover JS, Arndt KA. The spectrum of laser skin resurfacing: nonablative, fractional, and ablative laser resurfacing. J Am Acad Dermatol 2008; 58(5): 719–37.
8. Tanzi EL, Wanitphakdeedecha R, Alster TS. Fraxel laser indications and long-term follow-up. Aesthet Surg J 2008; 28(6): 675–8.
9. Nestor MS, Goldberg DJ, Goldman MP, Weis RA, Rigel DA. Photorejuvination: non-ablative skin rejuvination using intese pulsed light. Skin and Aging March 1999.
10. Taub AF, Battle EF Jr, Nikolaidis G. Multicenter clinical perspectives on a broadband infrared light device for skin tightening. J Drugs Dermatol 2006; 5(8): 771–8.
11. Chan HH, Kono T. The use of lasers and intense pulsed light sources for the treatment of pigmentary lesions. Skin Therapy Lett 2004; 9(8): 5–7.
12. Sami NA, Attia AT, Badawi AM. Phototherapy in the treatment of acne vulgaris. J Drugs Dermatol 2008; 7(7): 627–32.
13. Alexiades-Armenakas M. Aminolevulinic acid photodynamic therapy for actinic keratoses/actinic cheilitis/acne: vascular lasers. Dermatol Clin 2007; 25(1): 25–33.
14. Gold MH. Continuing medical education article-skin treatment: photodynamic therapy: indications and treatment. Aesthet Surg J 2008; 28(5): 545–52.
15. Nestor MS, Gold MH, Kauvar AN et al. The use of photodynamic therapy in dermatology: results of a concensus conference. J Drugs Dermatol 2006; 5(2): 140–54.
16. Nestor MS. The use of photodynamic therapy for the treatment of acne vulgaris. Dermatol Clin 2007; 25(1): 47–57.
17. Baez F, Reilly LR. The use of light-emitting diode therapy in the treatment of photoaged skin. J Cosmet Dermatol 2007; 6(3): 189–94.
18. DeLand MM, Weiss RA, McDaniel DH, Geronemus RG. Treatment of radiation-induced dermatitis with light-emitting diode (LED) photomodulation. Lasers Surg Med 2007; 39(2): 164–8.
19. Nestor MS. Role of millisecond domain lasers and intense pulsed light in the treatment of vascular anomalies and ectasis, in Controversies and Conversations in Cutaneous Laser Surgery, Editors: Arndt KA, Dover JS, AMA press, 2002.
20. Galeckas KJ, Ross EV, Uebelhoer NS. A pulsed dye laser with a 10-mm beam diameter and a pigmented lesion window for purpura-free photorejuvenation. Dermatol Surg 2008; 34(3): 308–13.
21. Galeckas KJ, Collins M, Ross EV, Uebelhoer NS. Split-face treatment of facial dyschromia: pulsed dye laser with a compression handpiece versus intense pulsed light. Dermatol Surg 2008; 34(5): 672–80.
22. Ortonne JP, Pandya AG, Lui H, Hexsel D. Treatment of solar lentigines. J Am Acad Dermatol 2006; 54(5 Suppl 2): S262–71.
23. Sadighha A, Saatee S, Muhaghegh-Zahed G. Efficacy and adverse effects of Q-switched ruby laser on solar lentigines: a prospective study of 91 patients with Fitzpatrick skin type II, III, and IV. Dermatol Surg 2008; 34(11): 1465–8.
24. Trafeli JP, Kwan JM, Meehan KJ et al. Use of a long-pulse alexandrite laser in the treatment of superficial pigmented lesions. Dermatol Surg 2007; 33(12): 1477–82.
25. Johnson CM, McLafferty RB. Endovenous laser ablation of varicose veins: review of current technologies and clinical outcome. Vascular 2007; 15(5): 250–4.
26. Brasic N, Lopresti D, McSwain H. Endovenous laser ablation and sclerotherapy for treatment of varicose veins. Sem in Cut Med and Surg 2008; 27(4): 264–75.
27. Taub AF. Fractionated delivery systems for difficult to treat clinical applications: acne scarring, melasma, atrophic scarring, striae distensae, and deep rhytides. J Drugs Dermatol 2007; 6(11): 1120–8.
28. Alexiades-Armenakas M. Nonablative skin tightening with a variable depth heating 1310-nm wavelength laser in combination with surface cooling. J Drugs Dermatol 2007; 6(11): 1096–103.
29. Gold MH. Lasers and light sources for the removal of unwanted hair. Clin Dermatol 2007; 25(5): 443–53.
30. Dover JS, Zelickson B. 14-Physician Multispecialty Consensus Panel. Results of a survey of 5,700 patient monopolar radiofrequency facial skin tightening treatments: assessment of a low-energy multiple-pass technique leading to a clinical end point algorithm. Dermatol Surg 2007; 33(8): 900–7.
31. Biesman BS, Pope K. Monopolar radiofrequency treatment of the eyelids: a safety evaluation. Dermatol Surg 2007; 33(7): 794–801.
32. Sukal SA, Geronemus RG. Thermage: the nonablative radiofrequency for rejuvenation. Clin Dermatol 2008; 26(6): 602–7.
33. Paasch U, Bodendorf MO, Grunewald S, Simon JC. Skin rejuvenation by radiofrequency therapy: methods, effects and risks. J Dtsch Dermatol Ges 2009; 7(3): 196–203.
34. Dayan SH, Maas CS. Botulinum toxins for facial wrinkles: beyond glabellar lines. Facial Plast Surg Clin North Am 2007; 15(1): 41–9.
35. Fagien S, Carruthers JD. A comprehensive review of patient-reported satisfaction with botulinum toxin type a for aesthetic procedures. Plast Reconstr Surg 2008; 122(6): 1915–25.
36. Dayan SH, Lieberman ED, Thakkar NN, Larimer KA, Anstead A. Botulinum toxin a can positively impact first impression. Dermatol Surg 2008; 34(Suppl 1): S40–7.
37. Carruthers JD, Glogau RG, Blitzer A. Facial Aesthetics Consensus Group Faculty Advances in facial rejuvenation: botulinum toxin type a, hyaluronic acid dermal fillers, and combination therapies—consensus recommendations. Plast Reconstr Surg 2008; 121(5 Suppl): 5S–30S.
38. Hirsch RJ, Cohen JL. Soft tissue augmentation. Cutis 2006; 78(3): 165–72.
39. Fitzgerald R, Vleggaar D, Burgess C. Facial dermal fillers. Aesthet Surg J 2008; 28(6): 699–701.
40. Siclovan HR, Jomah JA. Injectable calcium hydroxylapatite for correction of nasal bridge deformities. Aesthetic Plast Surg 2008; 9.
41. Narins RS, Dayan SH, Brandt FS, Baldwin EK. Persistence and improvement of nasolabial fold correction with non-animal stabilized hyaluronic acid 100,000 gel particles/mL filler on two retreatment schedules: results up to 18 months on two retreatment schedules. Dermatol Surg 2008; 34(Suppl 1): S2–8.

42. Andre P. New trends in face rejuvenation by hyaluronic acid injections. J Cosmet Dermatol 2008; 7(4): 251–8.

43. Piacquadio D, Smith S, Anderson R. A comparison of commercially available polymethylmethacrylate-based soft tissue fillers. Dermatol Surg 2008; 34(Suppl 1): S48–52.

44. Narins RS, Beer K. Liquid injectable silicone: a review of its history, immunology, technical considerations, complications, and potential. Plast Reconstr Surg 2006; 118(3 Suppl): 77S–84S.

45. Buck DW 2nd, Alam M, Kim JY. Injectable fillers for facial rejuvenation: a review. J Plast Reconstr Aesthet Surg 2009; 62(1): 11–8.

46. Kim KH, Geronemus RG. Laser lipolysis using a novel 1,064 nm Nd:YAG Laser. Dermatol Surg 2006; 32(2): 241–8.

47. Murray E. The use and mechanism of action of high-intensity focused ultrasound for adipose tissue removal and non-invasive body sculpting. (Abstract) ASPS Meeting Chicago, Illinois, September 2006.

48. Manstein, Laubach H, Watanabe K et al. Selective cryolysis: a novel method of non-invasive fat removal. Lasers Surg Med 2008; 40: 595–604.

49. Ablon G. Rotunda, AM E. Treatment of lower eyelid fat pads using phosphatidylcholine: clinical trial and review. Derm Surg 2004; 30: 422–7.

50. Rotunda AM, Suzuki H, Moy RL, Kolodney MS. Detergent effects of sodium deoxycholate are a major feature of an injectable phosphatidylcholine formulation used for localized fat dissolution. Dermatol Surg 2004; 30: 1001–8.

51. Singh M, Griffiths CE. The use of retinoids in the treatment of photoaging. Dermatol Ther 2006; 19(5): 297–305.

52. Draelos ZD. The cosmeceutical realm. Clin Dermatol 2008; 26(6): 627–32.

53. Nestor MS. Combination therapy in clinical and cosmetic dermatology: the marriage of device and drug. J Drugs Dermatol 2004; 3(5 Suppl): S4–11.

5 Patients who only want natural, nonoperated-appearing results
Harry Mittelman and Gregory J Vipond

INTRODUCTION

The desire of cosmetic surgery patients to maintain a natural, nonoperated appearance is extremely common. With increasing awareness of cosmetic surgery and rejuvenation procedures comes a heightened knowledge of their complications and telltale signs. Many patients are adamant about avoiding these stigmata and will stress this sentiment at the initial consultation. It is frequently stated that they desire a natural, "refreshed" look and consequently may want a less dramatic result. Some of the happiest postoperative patients share comments from friends and family on how they look like they have returned from a relaxing vacation, or have started a new diet or exercise regimen. Very few patients want their acquaintances asking who their surgeon was.

Geographic location of the patient may also influence expectations and preferences. It is not uncommon for people from various regions within the United States to actually want a taut or "pulled" appearance after a rhytidoplasty. Although this may sound unusual to the facial plastic surgeon, one possible explanation is that such an appearance may be a status symbol or reflection of social standing. In California, there exists such a dichotomy. Within the bay area of northern California, a natural appearance is emphasized, whereas in southern California, around the Los Angeles and Palm Springs areas, a more surgical appearance is the vogue.

Previous experience with cosmetic surgery and procedures also influence patient expectations. A patient with previous complications or stigmata or who has a friend or family member with such sequelae may have a great deal of fear and misconception.

The wishes of the patient must be elicited at the initial consultation. Many patients will volunteer their desire for a natural look, otherwise this can be elucidated by the surgeon. The patient comments should be documented verbatim in the medical chart as it is not uncommon for these requests to be forgotten postoperatively. Showing patients the notes from their consultation refreshes their memory and helps to improve their satisfaction with the result. If a patient still insists on a more dramatic change, then secondary procedures may be performed after the acute recovery period.

The route to obtaining natural postoperative appearances involves several key principles: the preoperative evaluation, a conservative approach to structures of the face, volume preservation, and avoidance of telltale surgical signs. Each of these will be discussed in detail.

PREOPERATIVE EVALUATION

The preoperative evaluation is essential for developing a professional relationship between the patient, the surgeon, and the surgical practice, clarifying patient expectations and goals, analyzing the patient pathology, and determining an individualized treatment plan which addresses both this pathology and achieves the patient's goals. Depending on the style of practice, commonly, a trained consultant will see the patient before the surgeon's evaluation. This consultant should be professional in appearance and manner, friendly and able to assuage any reservations. The medical history should be reviewed, including any previous cosmetic or rejuvenation procedures, the reason for the consultation discussed, a brief background of the surgeon, and basic treatment descriptions given before the surgeon meets the patient. Commonly, the patient will feel more relaxed with the consultant and a more honest description of his or her expectations can be obtained. Preoperative photos may be taken at this time and should include anteroposterior, right and left oblique, and right and left lateral views. This preconsultation should last approximately 10 to 15 minutes and should make the patient feel completely at-ease with the practice. It should set the tone and lay the groundwork for the subsequent surgeon consultation. The surgeon needs to review the preconsultation before meeting the patient to deliver an optimal first physician-patient interaction.

After quickly establishing rapport with the patient, it is useful to then address the patient's concerns and expectations, thereby validating them. If the patient is amenable to a global assessment, it is valuable to do this in a systematic, consistent manner. The senior author uses a standard evaluation form for every patient consultation (Figure 5.1). A numerical scale allows for quantification of the patient's findings while also allowing comparison between patients and is essential in operative planning and technique selection. The individualized nature of the patient evaluation cannot be over-emphasized. By objectively assessing the patient's individual pathology, treatment can be customized which helps ensure a more natural postoperative appearance.

A complete discussion of the preoperative patient evaluation may be found in chapter 1. However, several important aspects will be discussed here. Starting in a superior to inferior fashion, the first key area occurs at the brow-periorbital zone. With advancing age, the brow descends, especially in its temporal aspect. This is due to a combination of forehead dermatochalasis, fascial laxity, and hypertrophy of the brow depressor muscles. The accepted ideal brow configuration (1) varies with patient gender. In both men and women, the medial edge of the brow begins at the intersection of a vertical line drawn from the lateral edge of the nasal ala with the medial canthus. It is described as club-shaped. In women, it arches over the supraorbital rim with its peak at the lateral limbus or lateral canthus. The lateral edge of the brow is at the same vertical height as the medial edge and ends at the intersection of a line drawn through the lateral aspect of the nasal ala intersecting with the lateral canthus. The thickness of the eyebrow may vary by person, but generally tapers from the thick medial edge to a thin lateral edge. In men, the length of the eyebrow is similar, but the shape varies. The position is relatively flat and lies along the supraorbital rim. The thickness also remains relatively constant without any discernable taper. However, it is

Hairline   Low   Medium   High   Male Pattern Baldness 1 2 3 4 5
Forehead Lines   1 2 3 4 5   Nasoglabellar Lines   1 2 3 4 5
Crow's Feet   1 2 3 4 5   Nasion Lines   1 2 3 4 5
Lower Lid Rhytids   1 2 3 4 5   Diagonal Malar Lines   1 2 3 4 5
Eyebrow Ptosis   R 1 2 3 4 5   L1 2 3 4 5
Upper Lids
  Excess Skin   R 1 2 3 4 5   L1 2 3 4 5
  Fat Protrusion Medial   R 1 2 3 4 5   L1 2 3 4 5
                 Central   R 1 2 3 4 5   L1 2 3 4 5
                 Lateral   R 1 2 3 4 5   L1 2 3 4 5
  Excess Muscle   R 1 2 3 4 5   L1 2 3 4 5
  Lateral Bony Excess   R 1 2 3 4 5   L1 2 3 4 5
  Peripheral Visual Loss   R 1 2 3 4 5   L1 2 3 4 5
Lower Lids
  Excess Skin   R 1 2 3 4 5   L 1 2 3 4 5
  Fat Protrusion R Medial   1 2 3 4 5   L 1 2 3 4 5
                 R Central   1 2 3 4 5   L 1 2 3 4 5
                 R Lateral   1 2 3 4 5   L 1 2 3 4 5
  Excess Muscle   R 1 2 3 4 5   L 1 2 3 4 5
  Laxity   R 1 2 3 4 5   L 1 2 3 4 5
  Scleral Show   R _____ mm   L_____ mm
  Lateral Rounding   R 1 2 3 4 5   L 1 2 3 4 5
  Nasojugal Groove   1 2 3 4 5
  Malar Bags   1 2 3 4 5
Malar Area
  Hypoplastic   1 2 3 4 5   Sub-Malar Cheek Hollow 1 2 3 4 5
Facial Cheek Area
  Cheek Skin Laxity   1 2 3 4 5
  Nasolabial   Groove   1 2 3 4 5   Crease 1 2 3 4 5   Fold 1 2 3 4 5
Chin-Mandible Line
  Hypoplastic   1 2 3 4 5   Protruding   1 2 3 4 5
  Pre-Jowl Sulcus   1 2 3 4 5
  J-M Elastosis   1 2 3 4 5
  Jowl Fullness   1 2 3 4 5
  C-M   Groove   1 2 3 4 5   Crease 1 2 3 4 5 Fold 1 2 3 4 5
  Depressed COM   R 1 2 3 4 5   L 1 2 3 4 5
Neck Submental
  Skin Elastosis   1 2 3 4 5   Fat 1 2 3 4 5
  Platysmal Banding   C 1 2 3 4 5   R 1 2 3 4 5   L 1 2 3 4 5
  Central Vertical Pleating 1 2 3 4 5
Neck Lower Lateral
  J-M Fullness   1 2 3 4 5   Horizontal Line Depth   1 2 3 4 5
Rhytids
  Perioral   1 2 3 4 5   Upper Lip 1 2 3 4 5 Periorbital 1 2 3 4 5
  Lateral Facial Lines   1 2 3 4 5   Vermilion Loss   1 2 3 4 5
Skin
  Cobblestone   1 2 3 4 5
  Scars _____   Lesions _____   Skin Tone _____
Ears
  Protrusion   1 2 3 4 5

Figure 5.1 Patient analysis form.

important to realize that this configuration needs to be individualized. To maintain a natural appearance, the patient must not be given a shape or position that he or she never had. Reviewing patient photos from 10 to 15 years earlier helps clarify the goal for brow rejuvenation.

Pathology of the periorbital region should also be evaluated on an individual basis and broken down into components. Hooding and decreased upper lid show may be the result of dermatochalasis, orbicularis oculi hypertrophy, orbital fat pseudoherniation, or lacrimal gland ptosis. Lid ptosis must also be evaluated. Surgery should only involve correction of the relevant pathology to restore a natural, youthful appearance.

Similar analysis is necessary for the lower lid: dermatochalasis, orbicularis oculi hypertrophy, orbital fat pseudoherniation. Just as the upper lid must be evaluated for signs of ptosis, the lower lid must be similarly evaluated for malposition. To maintain a natural appearance, the patient needs to have correction of his or her individual pathology. Creation of an ideal lower eyelid position, while conforming to aesthetic standards, may create a dramatically different appearance in that patient. Again, review of photographs from 10 to 15 years earlier may help make obvious the ideal eyelid position for that patient.

The malar and submalar regions also require careful evaluation. With advancing age comes descent and atrophy of the suborbicularis oculi and malar fat pads. There are various techniques to restore volume to these areas, including fillers, implants, and surgical resuspension. To ensure a natural postoperative result, it is imperative to avoid overcorrection giving the patient a different, as opposed to rejuvenated, appearance.

The nose is an area where alterations in anatomy can translate to changed appearance. Because of its central location, it is a key focal point during social interactions. A distinction may be made between primarily aesthetic rhinoplasty and aging rhinoplasty. With regard to the former, a noticeable change is generally the goal, whereas for the latter, the goal is restoration of the patient's youthful nasal appearance. It should be emphasized to any prospective patient that rhinoplasty is more of a beautification than rejuvenation procedure.

Although every surgeon has his or her own approach to the patient evaluation, it is important to adopt a systematic approach to ensure a complete analysis of the patient pathology. Review of photographs from 10 to 15 years earlier may help guide the approach to a natural appearing postoperative appearance. An individualized approach, rather than relying on empirical measurements, will help ensure surgical results that fit the patient and avoid a dramatic, unnatural change.

CONSERVATIVE APPROACH

Another essential aspect of ensuring a natural postoperative result is being conservative in several important areas. The periorbital zone, liposculpture, and skin re-draping are areas where an aggressive technique can lead to unnatural results.

As mentioned in the proceeding section, the periorbital zone, including the brow and upper and lower lid complexes, must be carefully analyzed on an individual basis. Empirically treating a patient based on ideal measurements and position may lead the surgeon down a path to an operated appearance with an unhappy

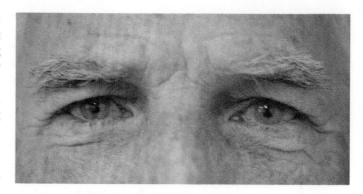

Figure 5.2 Preoperative photo of patient with brow ptosis.

patient. If there is evidence of brow ptosis, then the brow needs to be restored to a more youthful position. The ideal position needs to be assessed with the patient, referring where possible, to patient photographs 10 to 15 years prior. Figure 5.2 shows a preoperative photograph of a male patient who was determined to have brow ptosis. Although a brow lift was discussed, the patient opted not to have this procedure because he believed that it would adversely change his appearance.

There are many different approaches to the aging brow each with their own merits and shortcomings. One approach, favored by the senior author, is the use of Botulinum Toxin (Botox®) to perform a chemical browlift. By weakening the depressor muscles of the eye, the preorbital orbicularis oculi, the procerus, depressor supercilii, and corrugator supercilii, the elevating effect of the frontalis muscle is relatively strengthened and a dependable temporal browlift is achieved which lasts 2 to 3 months in duration.(2) In the senior author's experience, the amount of browlift attained with Botox® is equivalent to that achieved surgically, via a coronal, midforehead, or endoscopic browlift, 1 year postoperatively. The ability to nonsurgically elevate the brow allows a quick, low-risk treatment with a temporary effect. With careful injection technique, elevation can be fairly localized, something which is more difficult surgically. Touch-up injections can be easily performed as needed. Botox® can also be used adjunctively after surgical brow elevation for asymmetry. Whatever the approach used, the surgeon must bear in mind that conservative rather than dramatic elevation is preferable, and that the intended brow position is patient-specific.

Similarly, treatment of the aging lid complex should be customized. As mentioned previously, there are several components to the aging lid and correction not only should be specific but also conservative. Over-resection of skin in the upper lid can lead to ectropion, lid retraction, and a skeletonized orbit with a high degree of lid show. Recently, research by Knoll et al. found that public perception of fatigue was most affected by the length of pretarsal lid height and that simulation of the skin resection of an upper blepharoplasty resulted in a perceived increase in patient fatigue.(3) Thus, conservative skin resection without a high supratarsal crease will preserve a natural, youthful appearance. In the event that both the surgeon and patient feel that an inadequate amount of skin was removed, a revision under local anesthesia is easily performed. With regard to male blepharoplasty, it is even more important to be conservative with skin excision as too much resection can lead to excess lid show which may be a feminizing as

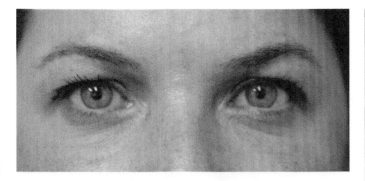

Figure 5.3 Preoperative photo of patient with orbicularis hypertrophy.

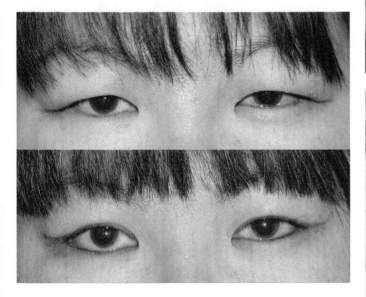

Figure 5.4 Pre and postoperative photo of patient with orbicularis hypertrophy and no supratarsal crease.

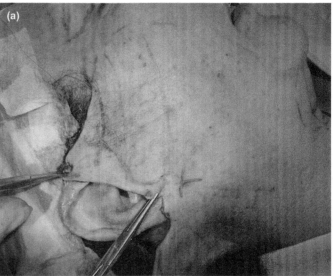

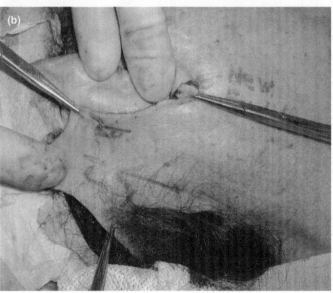

Figure 5.5 (A) Pre-auricular skin redraping. (B) Post-auricular skin redraping.

well as an aging feature. In the lower lid, excess skin resection can lead to scleral show, lateral rounding, and ectropion. Conservative treatment of pseudoherniated orbital fat is also extremely important and will be discussed in detail later. When addressing the orbicularis oculi, it is essential to avoid unnecessary resection. Resection is necessary if the patient presents with muscle hypertrophy (Figure 5.3), or if there is a need to create or accentuate the supratarsal crease (Figure 5.4). Unnecessary resection of the orbicularis oculi may lead to postoperative dyskinesia as well as lid skeletonization.

A conservative approach is vital in the redraping of the skin following a rhytidoplasty. Excess skin tension can lead to poor wound healing, scar hypertrophy, and widening postoperatively. While a fair degree of tension may be placed on the superficial musculoaponeurotic system, or SMAS, limited tension should be placed on the skin (Figure 5.5). The manner of closure has been modified by the senior author during his career as the result of careful scrutiny of his postoperative patients. It is felt that the ear lobule is the key area of the incision where tension must absolutely be minimal. Consequently, the incision is closed preauricularly to the level of the anti-tragus, and then closed postauricularly. The lobule is closed last, allowing any tension to be distributed elsewhere. The minimum possible tension on the lobule will help

reduce any postoperative changes to its appearance as the result of wound healing and scar contracture.

Although many patients may approach rejuvenation surgery with the desire to do as much as possible to completely correct any pathology, it is important to emphasize a conservative approach to maintain a natural postoperative appearance. Proper discussion of treatment goals and the benefits of such an approach will help the patient to better understand the surgical expectations and will ensure a pleasant postoperative experience.

VOLUME PRESERVATION

There has been a change in thinking in cosmetic surgery with a shift away from volume reduction and toward volume preservation. Currently, it is recognized that a youthful face is one with that is full without features of skeletonization. Conversely, a face that has lost volume has a harder appearance with easily seen borders between the different anatomic zones. The number of adipocytes within a body is determined at the time of puberty. Subsequently,

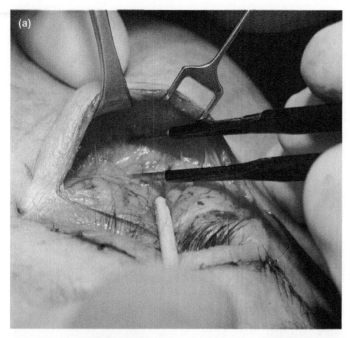

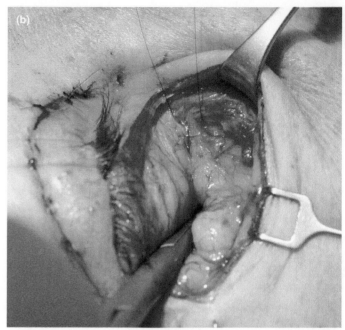

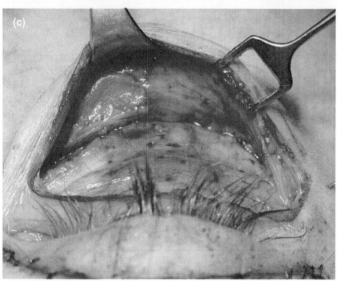

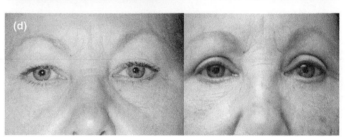

Figure 5.6 Sub-Orbicularis Oculi Fat Pad (SOOF) Repositioning: A) Exposure of the inferior orbital rim, SOOF, and lower lid fat pads. B) Redraping of the lower lid fat pads over the inferior orbital rim with 6-0 Prolene sutures. C) Completed lower lid fat pad redraping. D) Pre and postoperative photo of a patient after upper and lower lid blepharoplasty with SOOF repositioning.

any postpubertal gain or loss of body mass is reflected by a concurrent increase or decrease in adipocyte size, not number. Any treatment which results in the reduction of adipose tissue permanently reduces the number of adipocytes. Most surgeons will agree that it is vital to preserve or restore volume to the face in order to create a natural, rejuvenated result.

The concept of volume preservation initially should start with preserving whatever volume a patient has. Once volume has been removed or lost from a face, it cannot regenerate and additional treatment is necessary. Submental and jowl-mandibular liposculpture and pseudoherniation of orbital fat are all areas where judicious reduction is needed.

To some extent, the face reflects the overall fat composition of the body, and patients with a higher body mass index, or BMI, commonly accumulate fat in the submentum, along the jowl-mandibular border, and in the neck. One of the most common

reasons for a patient to seek rejuvenation procedures is to improve a perceived loss of cervicomental definition. Surgical correction, via submentoplasty, is the most direct and effective approach to submental adiposity. During both the evaluation and surgery, it is important to distinguish subcutaneous (supraplastysmal) fat from subplatysmal fat. Removal of subcutaneous fat is easily performed under direct visualization with either liposuction cannulas or via direct excision. The surgeon should avoid skeletonization of the platysma and midline neck structures such as the strap muscles, laryngeal cartilages, and hyoid bone. Even if not completely removed, it is conceivable that some of the adipocytes may be devitalized during submentoplasty and subsequently will undergo apoptosis leading to a further reduction in fat volume. If too much subcutaneous fat is removed, postoperative contraction may cause unsightly visualization of muscle edges. Subplatysmal fat may also lead to loss of an acute cervicomental angle and should be addressed if present. The method favored by the senior author is to make very small buttonhole incisions in the platysma or its decussation. Similar to transection of the septum orbitale, excess fat will prolapse through these violations. A liposuction cannula then easily removes the fat while leaving the platysma and its decussation intact. Conservative removal of subplatysmal fat will help reduce the risk of a postoperative cobra deformity, or submental skeletonization. The surgeon should recognize and reassure the patient that some submental firmness and contour irregularity is to be expected during the early postoperative period. However, with time and light finger massage, where necessary, this should resolve after a few months.

In patients with heavy necks, fat accumulation along and inferior to the mandibular border leads to loss of demarcation between the jawline and neck. Consequently, it is necessary to remove some of this volume. Again, the surgeon should only remove enough volume to improve the mandibular contour as excess liposuction will lead to skeletonization. The senior author frequently uses microliposuction cannulas so to be conservative with fat removal as well as achieve a soft feathering, or transition, from the areas of liposuction to untreated areas. The microliposuction cannula may also be used to achieve a gradual transition from the submentum to the lateral neck which helps to avoid postoperative stigmata. One risk that is encountered with jowl-mandibular liposuction before rhytidoplasty is that the areas that have undergone liposuction may subsequently be elevated above the mandible, leading to volume deficiency along the inferior jawline. The surgeon may avoid this risk by delaying liposuction along the mandibular border until the SMAS and platysma have been resuspended. The key principle in facial liposculpture is that it is better to be conservative and leave too much volume than to be excessive and cause postoperative volume deficiency. If required, further removal can be easily performed under local anesthetic after the acute postoperative period.

During the resuspension of the SMAS/Platysma complex, the surgeon is faced with the choice of plication or imbrications techniques. Consistent with the emphasis on volume preservation, the senior author performs a multivector SMAS/Platysma plication on the vast majority of his patients. In patients with excessive facial fullness, an imbrication may be performed. It is felt that plication minimizes the volume loss that may occur with resuspension of the SMAS/Platysma and helps reduce the effect of volume loss that occurs with further aging.

Volume preservation in the midface is essential. With aging, there is descent of the malar fat pad, sub-orbicularis oculi fat (SOOF) pad, and buccal fat pads. Although this may contribute to fullness in the lower third of the face, the surgeon must not remove volume. Instead, resuspension of the ptotic tissue should be performed. Loss of midface volume contributes to a hollowed-out, gaunt appearance which then requires additional treatment. The use of alloplastic implants to add volume to the malar and midface regions should be performed conservatively to preserve a natural appearance. If the implant is undersized, it may be easier to persuade the patient to either keep the implant or have it replaced with a larger size. However, if the implant is too large, not only is there an increased risk of neuropraxia and hypesthesia, but the patient is also more likely to refuse any implant rather than accept a smaller size.

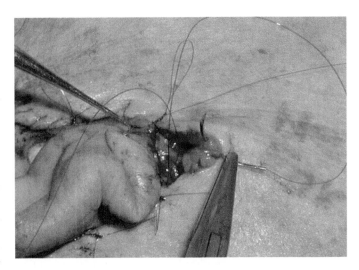

Figure 5.7 Lobule support suture.

In the orbit, resection of pseudoherniated fat during blepharoplasty should similarly be conservative and performed only if pathologic. Loss of volume contributes to orbital hollowing and is difficult to correct. Intraoperatively, the surgeon should minimize any violation of the septum orbitale and should only resect that adipose tissue which prolapses with slight orbital pressure. As mentioned in the previous section, resection of the orbicularis oculi should only be performed if there is preoperative evidence of muscle hypertrophy. Unnecessary resection may contribute to postoperative skeletonization.

With respect to the lower lid complex, fat pseudoherniation may be used to camouflage a prominent nasojugal groove, thereby preserving orbital volume and using the patient's own excess to treat an area of deficiency. Figure 5.6 outlines this procedure. The prolapsed orbital fat is draped over the inferior orbital rim and sutured to the SOOF and orbital rim periosteum. In patients with extensive orbital fat pseudoherniation, it may be necessary to resect some of the fat in addition to repositioning it. This technique offers a potentially permanent method of correction as the transposed fat should remain vital. However, with continued aging, the nasojugal groove prominence may return requiring further treatment.

In patients with insufficient volume, it is necessary to use injectables. There are a great number of fillers, artificial and endogenous, temporary and permanent. Discussion of injectables is beyond the scope of this chapter. Suffice it to say, they are an essential component of the facial plastic surgeon's armamentarium, but conservative technique is necessary to maintain a natural appearance. Areas which are essential to recognize and treat include the nasojugal groove, the melolabial groove, and commissure-mandibular groove. Again, it is much preferable to perform a "touch-up" a few weeks later than to over-inject and need to either remove/dissolve it or suffer an unhappy patient.

And so, volume preservation and conservative restoration is a relatively new concept in facial rejuvenation. However, it is crucial is preserving a natural, nonoperated appearance and keeping happy patients. Future research and techniques which may revolutionize the field include the possibility of autologous adipocyte stem cell transfer from regions outside of the face to potentially restore fullness.(4) Although it may be unlikely that this technique would ever supplant surgery, it may be a very important adjunct.

AVOIDANCE OF TELLTALE SURGICAL SIGNS

While all of the previous sections have focused on techniques to help ensure a natural, nonoperated appearance, there are some postoperative stigmata which serve as an advertisement that facial plastic surgery has been performed. With increasing public awareness of cosmetic surgery, due to numerous television programs, there is a resulting increased awareness of complications and suboptimal results that can accompany such procedures. Fortunately, many of these can be minimized or avoided.

The primary complication to be avoided during a submentoplasty is the cobra deformity. This was discussed previously and may be seen as the result of excessive subcutaneous and, more importantly, subplatysmal fat removal which leads to a volume deficiency in the central neck. Conservative liposuction with use of the platysmal buttonhole technique for deeper fat will help reduce this distortion. Another helpful concept is to minimize trauma to the platysmal muscle, by limiting both unnecessary resection and excessive cautery. Mechanical and thermal damage will lead to amplified wound healing with the potential for increased fibrosis and scar contracture. Avoidance of damage to the superficial layer of the platysma reduces the potential for postoperative adhesion between the muscle and skin.

There are several deformities that should be avoided in the face/neck lift, or rhytidoplasty. One of the most important is the pixie or satyr ear deformity which is an attached lobule without a dependent portion. The preoperative evaluation is essential in determining if the patient has an attached lobule, which is fairly common. If present, it must be pointed out and can be revised intraoperatively through a relatively straightforward V-Y advancement. As mentioned previously, it is essential to minimize any tension on the lobule during reapproximation. Consequently, the lobule closure is left to the very end of the rhytidoplasty closure so that skin tension will be optimal. Another technique which helps is the use of a long-term absorbable or permanent, suture from the dermis beneath the skin flap to the virtually immobile mastoid fascia (Figure 5.7). This provides long-term support along the lobule closure. The pixie ear deformity may not be seen during the early postoperative period and is more commonly seen months to years after surgery as continued descent of facial tissue and scar migration pull the lobule anteroinferiorly. Fortunately, it can be improved through a relatively simple V-Y advancement under local anesthesia.

The peri-tragal incision must also be closed with minimal tension. The senior author uses an apical-tragal incision to camouflage the resultant preauricular scar. During wound closure, half-buried polypropylene sutures are left in place above and below the tragus for 11 to 12 days postoperatively. This prolonged support helps to reduce postoperative anterior migration of the tragus.

The temporal hair tuft is another area which can be adversely changed after rhytidoplasty. Many surgeons opt to carry the temporal skin incision vertically into the temporal hair. When redraping the skin flap after resuspension of the SMAS complex, the temporal hairline is shifted posterosuperiorly. This elevation reduces the normal curvilinear aspect of the temporal hairline and causes it to assume a squared-off appearance. The senior author has modified his incision to avoid any alteration to the temporal hairline (Figure 5.8). The skin incision is brought from

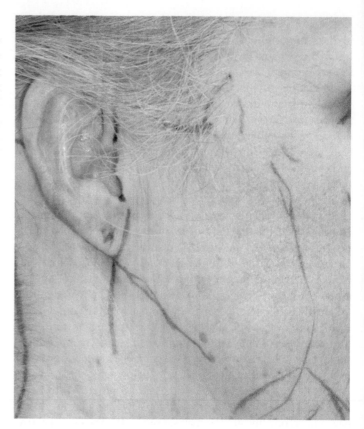

Figure 5.8 Incision marking along sideburn.

its apex at the helical root, anteriorly into the inferior aspect of the sideburn. This allows for skin redraping superior and anterior to the helical root with minimal distortion of the hairline. If needed, the horizontal side burn incision may be extended superiorly around the anterior edge of the sideburn which helps to reduce skin bunching during redraping. However, it is very important to meticulously close the vertical portion of the incision to avoid an unsightly scar.

As mentioned throughout this chapter, it is essential to be conservative when removing volume. Just as excessive liposuction during submentoplasty can lead to abnormal postoperative hollowing, similarly excessive jowl-mandibular liposuction can lead to abnormal skeletonization of the mandible. This was discussed in more detail previously, but is worth repeating. Especially in patients with significant jowl-mandibular elastosis, it may be prudent to delay liposuction in this region until after the SMAS/Platysma has been resuspended. This will avoid elevation of a defatted cervical skin into a supramandibular position. Hollowing above the mandible creates an unnatural appearance and certainly suggests cosmetic surgery as the culprit.

Perhaps the most concerning complication that may result from a rhytidoplasty is alteration of the position of the oral commissure. Many patients express their desire to avoid a "fish hook" or "wind tunnel" appearance after surgery. Often this desire is based upon their knowledge of a celebrity with just such an appearance. To avoid distortion of the corner of the mouth, it is extremely important for the surgeon to be attentive when resuspending the SMAS. If there is any unnatural superior or lateral skin pull after placing a suture, then that suture should be replaced more proximally away

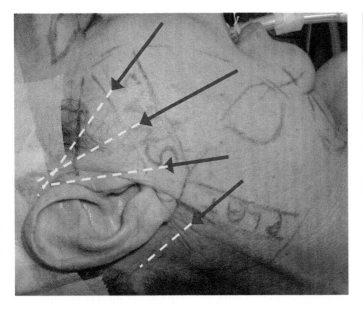

Figure 5.9 Multi-vector SMAS.

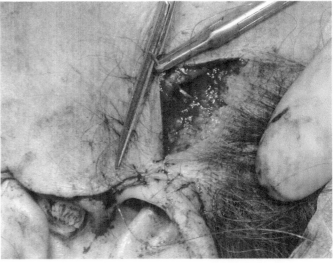

Figure 5.10 Sideburn suspension suture.

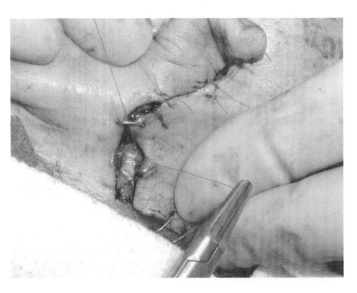

Figure 5.11 Post-auricular suspension suture.

from the modiolus. The risk of this complication is reduced with less extensive rhytidoplasty procedures where the extent of skin undermining is smaller. However, with extensive face/neck lifts, the area of skin undermining may approach the modiolus and the danger of distortion is greater.

Hamra describes the "lateral sweep" as being one of the most common sequelae after a traditional rhytidoplasty.(5) He attributes this complication to the lateral pull of the SMAS/skin complex without a superior vector. He recommends a composite rhytidectomy with a superior-medial repositioning of the orbicularis oculi to avoid this lateral sweep. In contrast, the senior author feels that the increased risk to neurovascular structures, the increased operative time, and increased postoperative edema and ecchymosis does not translate into a noticeably better postoperative appearance. Instead, a multivector resuspension of the SMAS-Platysma complex is performed. The multivector suspension takes into account that different regions of the face require different vectors of pull (Figure 5.9). This is a very individualized approach, but several generalizations may be made. The submentum and upper neck regions are best improved with a primarily vertical vector of pull at the mandibular angle. The midface and cheek are best elevated with a primarily posterior and secondarily superior vector whereas the commissure-mandibular fold is optimally corrected with equal superior and posterior vectors of pull. By adjusting the vectors of SMAS/Platysma resuspension, a natural appearance is preserved and a lateral windswept appearance is avoided.

A final, but essential, point in preserving a natural look during rhytidoplasty involves the surgical incision and wound closure. In performing the incision, it is necessary to anticipate future scar migration. Due to continual aging, the scars will tend to migrate anteriorly and inferiorly, and may also increase in width. Future alopecia must also be anticipated, particularly in the areas of the sideburn and postauricular hairline. If the patient has wispy or thinning hair along the inferior sideburn or along the anterior aspect of the postauricular hairline, then the incision should be made inside these areas where the hair density is greater. This will help avoid the scars become more noticeable as hair loss progresses postoperatively. Similarly the postauricular incision needs to be performed lateral to the postauricular sulcus as the scar will migrate medially.

To provide long-term support and to decrease wound tension and scar widening, the senior author uses three key long-term absorbable or permanent sutures. The first suture is placed along the inferior aspect of the sideburn incision and suspends the dermis on the skin flap to the less mobile temporalis fascia (Figure 5.10). The second suture, described previously, is placed at the apex of the ear lobule and suspends the dermis on the skin flap to the mastoid fascia (Figure 5.7). The final suture is placed at the apex of the postauricular incision and suspends the skin flap dermis to the fixed mastoid fascia superiorly (Figure 5.11). To reduce the incidence of suture reactivity, monofilament suture is used both for these buried sutures and for all skin sutures.

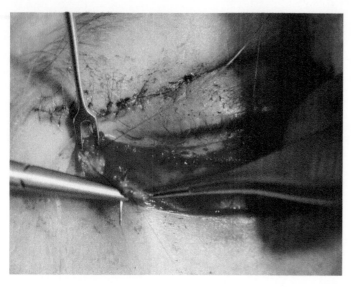

Figure 5.12 Cheek Suspension Suture.

Although much research has been performed on wound healing, there are several factors that are under the surgeon's control. Careful antiseptic technique and perioperative antibiosis can minimize postoperative infection which can contribute to a prolonged inflammatory phase of healing. Foreign bodies in the incision, such as hair, suture ends, and talc must also be avoided to minimize postoperative inflammation. Finally, incisional skin tension must be minimized so to allow optimal delivery of blood and oxygen. Careful postoperative wound care and the use of steroid injections, where necessary, also help achieve optimal healing.

In the brow, it is important to avoid a "surprised" postoperative appearance. This is done through careful preoperative evaluation, thorough discussion with the patient, and preferential elevation of the lateral brow. The use of Botox® for minor brow ptosis may also help to preserve a natural look. In the senior author's experience, a midforehead approach allows more selective elevation of the brow than either an endoscopic or coronal/trichophytic approach.

In the periorbital region, it is necessary to avoid orbital hollowing through a conservative and volume-preserving approach. It is furthermore important to avoid lower lid malposition. Although briefly discussed earlier, careful preoperative evaluation with an operative plan to address any lateral rounding, sclera show, or ectropion must be employed. Skin excision should be conservative and any dissection or cautery on the pretarsal orbicularis should be avoided. If there is any preoperative malposition or laxity, or if there is significant disruption of the orbicularis oculi, then a cheek suspension suture from the inferior edge of the exposed orbicularis to the periosteum of the lateral orbital rim will help prevent future malposition (Figure 5.12).

CONCLUSION

Although it is unrealistic for a patient to expect no noticeable postoperative changes, with a thorough preoperative evaluation and discussion, a conservative approach, attention to volume preservation, and careful surgical technique, most of the stigmata of surgery can be avoided and a natural, nonoperated appearance maintained. However, there will always be factors beyond the surgeon's control, such as genetics and poor patient compliance, which can lead to a complication. In this event, the surgeon must closely follow the patient, give reassurance, and provide any necessary treatment. Fortunately, these events are an exception and excellent healing and results tend to be more the rule.

REFERENCES
1. Ellenbogen R. Transcoronal eyebrow lift with concomitant upper blepharoplasty. Plast Reconstr Surg 1983; 71 (4): 490–9.
2. Ahn MS, Catten M, Maas CS. Temporal browl lift using botulinum toxin A. Plast Reconstr Surg 2000; 105: 1129–35.
3. Knoll BT, Attkiss KJ, Persing JA. The influence of forehead, brow, and periorbital aesthetics on perceived expression in the youthful face. Plast Reconstr Surg 2008; 121: 1793–802.
4. Moseley TA, Zhu M, Hedrick MH. Adipose-derived stem and progenitor cells as fillers in plastic and reconstructive surgery. Plast Reconstr Surg 2006; 118(3 Suppl): 121S–8S.
5. Hamra ST. Frequent face lift sequeale: hollow eyes and the lateral sweep: cause and repair. Plast Reconstr Surg 1998; 102(5): 1658–66.

6 Cosmetic concerns and therapeutic considerations in ethnic skin
Cheryl Burgess

OVERVIEW

It is paramount that cosmetic surgeons and dermatologists acquire the necessary knowledge and instruction so that thorough and comprehensive aesthetic services can deliver the greatest efficacy with the lowest risk of adverse events when using state-of-the-art products and procedures in ethnic skin. To achieve this goal for your patients and your practice requires a rigorous and constant effort. This is especially true in light of daily advances in the cosmetic industry and growing diversity of skin types in ethnic consumers who seek our services. Because of important differences that exist between white skin and ethnic skin, clinicians must be aware of the effects of the aging process that are specific to ethnic skin, and the resulting differences in aesthetic treatments that are used for patients with ethnic skin. To meet this challenge, the following chapter provides a brief overview of skin types in the United States and a quick review of the documented differences between white skin and ethnic skin. The remainder of the chapter is dedicated to providing detailed information about the most common problems in ethnic skin, the aesthetic treatments that are appropriate within this patient population, and the steps to limit any risks for adverse events within this patient population.

Throughout the burgeoning research on ethnic skin, it has been difficult to provide consistent terminology in the medical literature that conveys appropriate categorization and accurate description of skin types. To address this challenge, throughout the chapter, the following conventions have been developed: The term "white skin" is used to refer to skin that has a Fitzpatrick Classification of I, II, and III. The term "Caucasian" is avoided because this term refers to a larger group of skin types, beyond people with white skin. The term "ethnic skin" will be used to refer to skin that has a Fitzpatrick Classification of IV, V, and VI, which applies to skin types in people of Black, Latino, Asian, and Middle Eastern ethnic groups. The term 'Blacks' is used in place of 'African-Americans' because the latter term refers to only a subgroup of a much larger category of people with pigmented skin. These conventions have been selected to provide more consistency, accuracy, and clarity in the following discussion. The terminology conventions are not intended for broad use in the medical literature to substitute for careful, detailed description of classification of skin types.

Learning Objectives

- Recognize diversity among skin types
- Recognize differences between white skin and ethnic skin
- Understand the underlying mechanisms of the aging face
- Recognize tissue response in ethnic skin
- Recognize potential adverse effects in ethnic skin
- Addressing cosmetic concerns in ethnic skin
- Assess therapeutic considerations in ethnic skin

DIVERSITY OF SKIN TYPES

In the United States, individuals with pigmented skin come from a large collection of racial and ethnic groups. The diversity of racial and ethnic groups yields a broad spectrum of pigmented skin types that defy easy categorization. Throughout the years, the fields of dermatology and cosmetics have struggled to characterize pigmented skin types adequately. After its development in the 1970s, the Fitzpatrick Skin Phototype classification became a surrogate classification system for this purpose.

The Fitzpatrick Skin Phototype classification system was originally developed to categorize the skin's response to UV radiation. Over time, dermatologists became accustomed to using the system to classify both UV sensitivity and skin color. However, the system has limited utility for accurately communicating patient information for either research or clinical purposes, and is of almost no value for helping clinicians treat ethnic skin effectively and safely. Patients with ethnic skin would benefit more from a classification system based on the propensity of the skin to scar and/or become hyperpigmented—a unique characteristic of pigmented skin.(1) Several classification systems have been developed or proposed to meet these obvious needs. However, none has risen to an industry standard.(2)

Roberts Skin Type Classification System
The recently introduced Roberts Skin Type Classification System (Table 6.1) may provide the most comprehensive information to meet the needs of clinicians.(2) This system uses a four-part serial profile to characterize the skin's likely response to insult, injury, and inflammation through a quantitative and qualitative assessment that includes a review of ancestral and clinical history, visual examination, test site reactions, and physical examination of the patient's skin. Skin is categorized using a numeric descriptor that provides information on the phototype, hyperpigmentation, photoaging, and scarring characteristics. The Roberts classification system can provide a means to help facilitate study designs and communicate data in the medical literature.(2)

A classification system of the Roberts type is sorely needed to characterize the ever-increasing diversity of skin types among a growing population of ethnic groups in the United States. In 1990, the U.S. Census Bureau listed 6 races with 23 racial subtypes. Only 10 years later, the same 6 race categories now included 67 subtypes.(3)

DEMOGRAPHIC TRENDS AND MARKET GROWTH OF ETHNIC COSMETICS
By the year 2050, Black, Hispanic Asian, and other minorities are expected to make up almost half of the total US population: 25% Hispanic; 14% Black; 8% Asian; 1% other (Taylor/Burgess/

Table 6.1 The Roberts Classification System.

Name (units)	Fitzpatrick Scale (FZ)	Roberts Hyperpigmentation Scale (H)	Glogau Scale (G)	Roberts Scarring Scale (S)
Scale	(measures skin phototypes)	(propensity for pigmentation)	(describes photoaging)	(describes scar morphology)
Categories	FZ_1 White skin. Always burns, never cans	H_0 Hypopigmentation	G_1 No wrinkles, early photoaging	S_0 Atrophy
	FZ_2 White skin. Always burns, minimal tan	H_1 Minimal and transient (< 1 year) hyperpigmentation	G_2 Wrinkles and motion, early to moderate photoaging	S_1 None
	FZ_3 White skin. Burns minimally, tans moderately and gradually	H_2 Minimal and permanent (> 1 year) hyperpigmentation	G_3 Wrinkles at rest, advanced photoaging	S_2 Macule
	FZ_4 Light brown skin. Burns minimally, tans well	H_3 Moderate and transient (< 1 year) hyperpigmentation	G_4 Only wrinkles, severe photoaging	S_3 Plaque within scarred boundaries
	FZ_5 Brown skin. Rarely burns, tans deeply	H_4 Severe and transient (> 1 year) hyperpigmentation		S_4 Keloid
	FZ_6 Dark brown/black skin	H_5 Severe and transient (< 1 year) hyperpigmentation		S_5 Keloid nodule
		H_6 Severe and permanent (> 1 year) hyperpigmentation		

Source: Roberts.(24)

Callender not published, 4). Growing diversity of skin types and shifting trends in US demographics are part of the reason for increased growth in ethnic cosmetics. This is also due to the expansion of product lines to include cosmetic colors and shades that address the whole spectrum of skin colors. In addition, ethnic consumers are increasingly using cosmetic products, specifically designed to address the unique skin care needs of women and men of color. Moreover, the cosmetic industry is using novel mechanisms for marketing directly to ethnic consumers. As a result, the growth of ethnic cosmetic markets has been predicted to reach record $1.8 billion revenue.(5)

Growth in cosmetic procedures

According to recent surveys, 11.7 million cosmetic procedures were performed in 2007 at a cost of $13.2 billion, an overall increase of 8% in surgical procedures. Surgical procedures increased by 114%, and nonsurgical procedures increased by 754%. This represents an increase of 457% in the total number of cosmetic procedures since 1997. Surveys of the American Board of Medical Specialists found that, in 2007, the top five nonsurgical cosmetic procedures were Botox injections (2.8 million), hyaluronic acid (1.5 million), laser hair removal (1.4 million) microdermabrasion (830,000), and skin resurfacing (648,000).(6)

As the number of cosmetic procedures continues to increase, dermatologists and cosmetic surgeons can expect greater numbers of procedures to be performed in specialized ethnic populations. Cosmetic procedures have already enjoyed significant growth from ethnic consumers. Of the total 11.7 million cosmetic procedures performed in 2007, 2.48 million (22%) procedures were performed in ethnic groups. Hispanics accounted for 9%; African-Americans accounted for 6%; Asians, 5%; and other non-Caucasians, 2%. This represents an increase of more than 65% in ethnic groups since 2004.(6)

Products expected to grow in the ethnic markets include fade creams and gels, cleansers, toners, astringents, soaps, emollients, moisturizers, and antiwrinkle products. In the ethnic market, products that target skin discoloration are experiencing the best consumer response. For Black consumers, uneven skin tone, sensitive skin, and acne-prone skin are the most problematic areas. Products targeting the Black market have been most successful when sold at the mass-market and drugstore level, as demonstrated by the success of certain ethnic products sold in Walgreens and Wal-Mart stores. Ethnic skin care lines are handled more often through distributors, compared to general market products. This is because successful marketing of ethnic products requires careful use of finely tuned distribution channels. Cofounder Dr. Cheryl Burgess and representatives of US Black Opal note the success of distributors with operations in the United Kingdom, including destinations in the Caribbean, Botswana, Brazil, and Zaire. Certain ingredients are extremely popular among Blacks, including the use of alpha hydroxy acid (AHA) and cocoa butter; AHA reduces the ashy appearance of skin in some Blacks by speeding up the natural process of sloughing off dead skin cells, and by the emollient properties of cocoa butter. Another indicator of the success of products targeting ethnic populations is the acquisition of cosmetic companies in non-Western countries: For example, L'Oreal's purchase of Yue Sai Kan cosmetics and Carson, Inc.(7)

DIFFERENCES BETWEEN BLACK AND WHITE SKIN

In the skin of Blacks, the stratum corneum layer counts are significantly higher and more compact, with thicker collagen bundles present in the dermis.(8) The most evident difference between ethnic skin and white skin is epidermal melanin content. Although no differences exist in the number of melanocytes, variations do exist in the number and size (9) and packaging and distribution (10) of melanosomes. In the skin of Blacks, melanosomes are larger and more dispersed. Moreover, the epidermal melanin unit in ethnic skin contains more melanin overall and may undergo slower degradation.(9) These differences in melanin and melanosomes provide superior UV protection in ethnic skin. In fact, the minimal erythema dose in Black skin is 30-fold greater than that of white skin (Kaidbey

1979)(10). In addition, Black skin has increased apocrine and sebaceous glands that are associated with increased follicular responses (8), and transdermal water loss is increased in the skin of Blacks .

Because of these differences in skin structure and function, ethnic people suffer less photodamage than whites (10) do. In fact, one study of adults living in Tucson, Arizona, found that the epidermis of Black participants was largely spared the gross photodamage observed in white participants. Most of the white women, aged 45 to 50 years, had wrinkles in the crow's feet and on the corners of the mouth, whereas none of the Black women of comparable age had obvious crow's feet wrinkles or perioral rhytids. The skin of Blacks also felt firmer, and the histology of the dermal elastic fibers in Black skin was similar to the appearance of these fibers in sun-protected white skin .(11)

MOST COMMON COSMETIC CONCERNS OF ETHNIC SKIN

Although differences in the structure of ethnic skin can be beneficial, the photoprotection afforded by differences in melanosome and melanin characteristics also causes frequent hyperpigmentation in ethnic skin, and may be responsible for divergent responses observed in burn injuries.(12) Individuals with darker skin experience frequent postinflammatory hyperpigmentation.(12)

Indeed, one survey found that uneven skin tone was a chief complaint in more than one-third of black women, while another survey found that pigment disorders were the third most commonly treated dermatoses. In a survey of 100 women of color, complaints about dark spots reached 86%, while 49% of women complained of sensitive or very sensitive skin.(9) Causes of hyperpigmentation include melasma, postinflammatory hyperpigmentation, and dyschromia of photoaging .(13) Although the underlying mechanisms of postinflammatory hyperpigmentation have not been well clarified, the intensity and duration of the disease is linked to darker skin hues and to dermatoses with disruption of the basal layer.(11)

Keloidal scarring is thought to occur 3–18 times more often in black persons compared with white persons, because of differences in the composition of fibroblasts. Research suggests that fibroblasts are larger and binucleated or multinucleated in black persons. It is thought that the interaction of cytokines with the large, numerous fibroblasts in black skin may be responsible for overproduction of collagen, and underdegradation of extracellular matrix components.(2)

Oftentimes, black patients will indicate that they want to be treated for a scar. However, in many cases, the purported scars are in fact, affects of postinflammatory hyperpigmentation. It is important to discuss the significant differences between true scarring and postinflammatory hyperpigmentation, such as differences in the specific therapies and relative difficulty between treating true scarring and postinflammatory hyperpigmentation.

Dermatosis papulosis nigra (DPN) presents as small (1–3 mm in diameter), discrete, rounded, brownish-black skin growths on the face, and develop most often, on a person's cheeks, neck, upper chest, and back. Lesions begin to appear in the mid-20s as flesh colored to Black is papules and/or plaques on the face, neck, and

upper torso. The condition is chronic, with new lesions continually developing as the person ages. The exact reason for the growth of these lesions remains unknown. However, researchers are confident that the appearance of DPNs has a hereditary tendency, which leads to DPNs observed on the skin of family members and relatives. Dermatosis papulosa nigra occurs more often in females, and overall, affects one in three Blacks. Although most dermatologists believe that these growths are unique to Black skin, some dermatologists think these same growths occur on the skin of Asians.

Striae distensae (rubra), commonly referred to as red stretch marks, is common in pregnant women, obese or overweight people, adolescents undergoing growth spurts, and body builders. Stretch marks can also occur from prolonged use of topical corticosteroids.

TREATING COMMON SKIN DISORDERS OF ETHNIC SKIN

Dyschromia

Pigmentary disorders are especially prevalent and distressing for Blacks, Latinos, Asians, and Middle Easterners. Postinflammatory hyperpigmentation is caused by various inflammatory skin disorders, such as eczema, allergic contact or irritant contact dermatitis, acne, or other causes. In fact, ethnic patients are commonly more distressed by the resulting dark areas than the initial culprit - the acute acne lesion. Dermal incontinence of pigment also occurs in melasma and hereditary dyschromias. Unprotected sun exposure is also a significant source of additional skin discoloration because it prolongs melanin production in active melanocytes in various inflammatory conditions. Sun protection is typically required during procedures to blend skin discoloration. Chemical (organic) sun protection includes avobenzone, mexoryl, oxybenzone, octinoxate. Physical (inorganic) sun protection includes micronized titanium dioxide, zinc oxide, mineral makeup, clothing, hats, and umbrellas.

Hyperpigmentation can be evaluated to provide a general idea of the prognosis and length of treatment. The evaluation can consist of both qualitative diagnosis and quantitative analysis (Table 6.2). A positive Wood's lamp examination reveals superficial (epidermal) incontinence of pigment, whereas a negative Wood's lamp examination reveals a deep (dermal) incontinence of pigment. Although not commonly used, quantitative analysis can be performed with a colorimeter.

Although disorders of hyperpigmentation may be difficult to treat, several therapeutic agents have been used over the years and others are in development (Table 6.3). Epidermal incontinence of pigment can be seen in postinflammatory hyperpigmentation. Product ingredients of lightening agents containing hydroquinone 4–6%, mequinol, kojic acid, azelaic acid, licorice (glabridin), citric acid, retinol, soy, arbutin, n-acetyl glucosamine, nicotinamide, and mulberry are used once to twice daily (Table 6.4).

Topical agents are generally classified as phenolic or nonphenolic compounds. The goal of these therapeutic agents is to inhibit key regulatory steps of hyperactive melanocytes by regulating: (1) melanin synthesis via transcription inhibition of tyrosinase or TRP-1, (2) the uptake and distribution of melanosomes in keratinocytes, and (3) known and degradation and cell

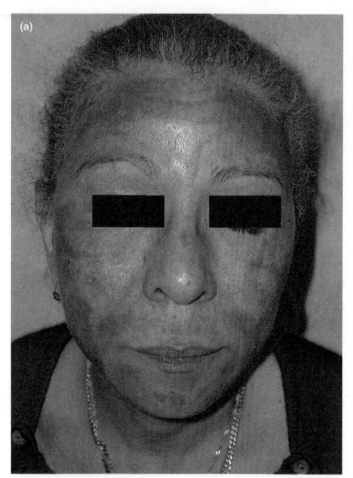

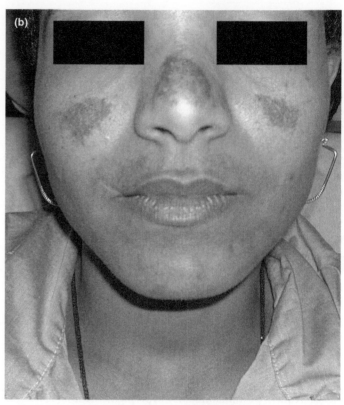

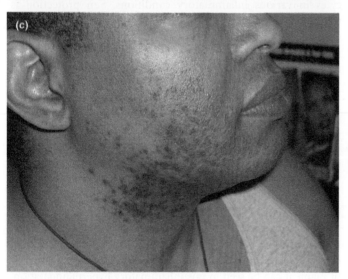

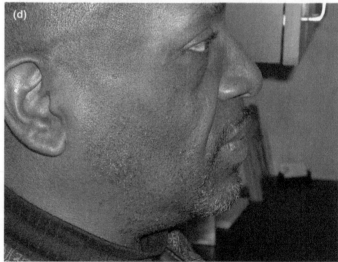

Figure 6.1 Facial dyschromia.

turnover. Hydroquinone has been the standard for many years, but has occasionally been mired in controversy about safety.(16) Lightening agents are also used for pretreatment of areas that will undergo cosmetic procedures. The agents are typically applied in advance as a cautionary measure to minimize any hyperpigmentation that may result from procedures.

Scarring
Keloids are benign, sometimes painful and/or pruritic, proliferative growths of dermal collagen that typically occur in ethnic skin as a result of excessive tissue response to trauma. These growths typically occur between 3 and 18 fold more often than in white skin. Patients with a Fitzgerald phototype of IV-VI are at greater risk for keloid formation and keloid recurrence after treatment. A higher incidence occurs in younger females due to your piercing. People aged 65 years or older seldom experience keloids; however the incidence is increasing as more individuals experience coronary artery bypass surgery and mid-chest operations. Treatment success is variable and the first rule of keloid therapy is prevention. Success rates are low and the rate of recurrence is high, for

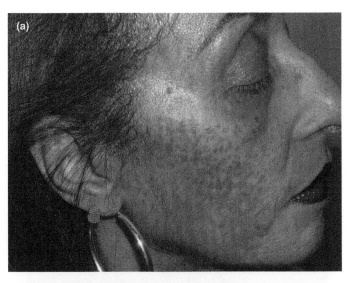

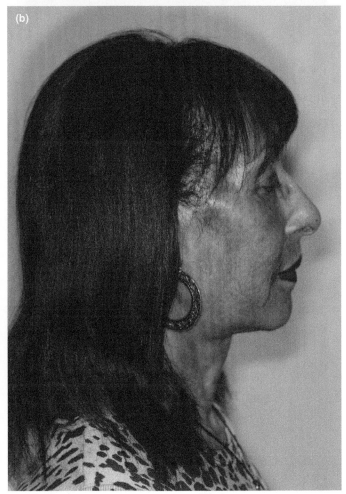

Figure 6.2 (a) Before and (b) after the use of 6% hydroquinone and Jessner's peels (lactic acid 14%, salicylic acid 14%).

Table 6.2 Hyperpigmentation evaluation.

Qualitative Diagnosis:
- + Wood's lamp examination
  – Superficial (epidermal) incontinence of pigment
- – Wood's lamp examination
  – Deep (dermal) incontinence of pigment

Quantitative Analysis: (not commonly used)
- Colorimeter
  – Delta L, a and b
    - L (98.4) white-black
    - a (0.2) red-green
    - b (1.2) yellow-blue

Source: Klaus Wolff.(34)
Shriver MD.(35)

Table 6.3 Most Common Cosmetic Concerns in Ethnic skin

- Dyschromia (postinflammatory hyperpigmentation/hypopigmentation; melasma; vitiligo
- Scarring (acne scars, hypertrophic scars, keloid scars (surgical versus nonsurgical) also discoloration
- Dermatosis papulosa nigra/seborrheic keratosis/acrochordons
- Accentuated facial lines of expression (especially glabellar frown lines)
- Lipoatrophy (deep nasolabial folds, skin laxity and cheek festooning)
- Striae distensae

Table 6.4 Treatment of epidermal dyschromia (postinflammatory hyperpigmentation).

Therapeutic Choices:	Lightening Ingredients:
• Lightening preparations	• Hydroquinone
• Sun protection	• Mequinol
• Chemical peeling agents	• Azelaic acid
– Jessner's Peel (lactic acid 14%, salicylic acid 14%, resorcinol)	• Kojic acid Licorice (glabridin)
– Salicylic acid peel (20–30%)	• Citric acid
– Glycolic acid peel (30–70%)	• Retinol
– Trichloroacetic acid peel (15–30%)	• Soy
• Microdermabrasion	• N-acetyl glucosamine
• Laser (necessary for the treatment of deep dermal pigment)	• Nicotinamide
– Q-Switched Nd:Yag 1064nm	• Mulberry
– Fractionated erbium	• Arbutin
	• Potential topical steroids (Class I, II)

Source: Taylor SC.(29)

example, 50–80% after excision therapy. Patients should be aware of familial keloid history, especially in Blacks. Therapy is more complex for large, nonpedunculated earlobe keloids or keloids with wide bases.

For many years, the standard of care for treating keloids was injection with triamcinolone acetonide (10–40 mg/mL). Patients should be told in advance that injected areas may become hypopigmented for 6–12 months. Pain can be minimized by using topical anesthetic preparations before injection. With the exception of treating midsternal keloids, the current gold standard of treatment is primary excision followed by adjuvant therapy. Excision can be followed up with corticosteroid injection, radiation therapy, and pressure gradient garments. Other primary therapies include lasers and silicone gel-sheeting.

Although nonessential cosmetic surgery should not be performed, nonsurgical procedures have shown no evidence of injection site trauma that causes keloid formation. Performed with appropriate caution, it is typically safe to use botulinum toxin and dermal fillers without causing scarring. However, there is significant risk of hyperactive collagen stimulation or fibroplasia

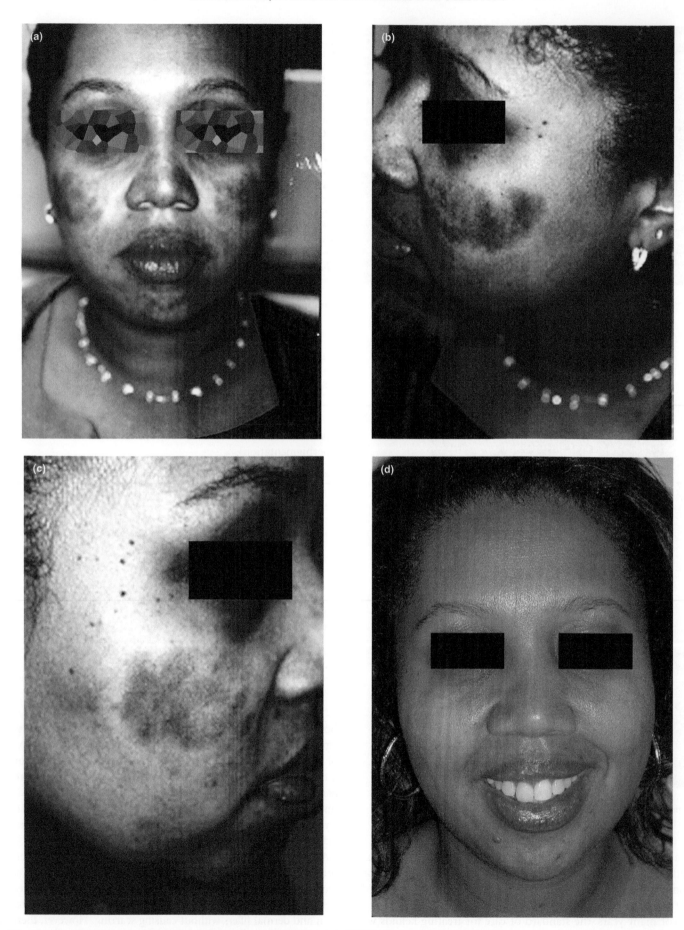

Figure 6.3 Superficial Skin Resurfacing: dermal pigment treatment with Q-switched Nd:Yag 1064 nm. Hydroquinone 6%.

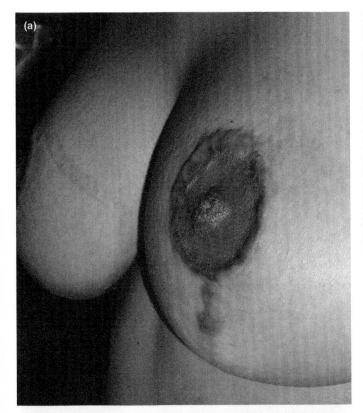

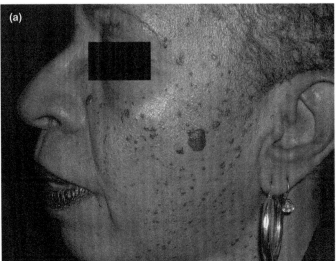

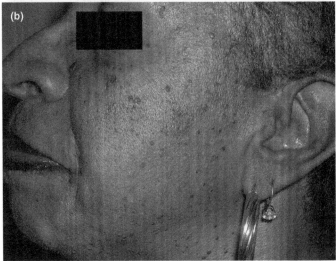

Figure 6.5 Dermatosis papulosa nigra and seborrheic keratosis: Treatment with 2 second spray liquid nitrogen & electrodesiccation (ConMed® Hyfrecator 2000 Monopolar low mode @4.8 watts -1 session).

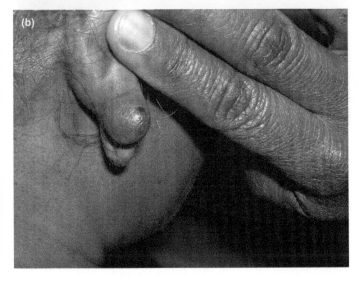

Figure 6.4 (a) Hypertrophic scarring after breast reduction and (b) keloid scarring after ear piercing.

when using stimulator fillers in ethnic skin. To minimize risks, thoroughly access scar history of ethic patients and allow longer followup (6–8 weeks vs. 4–6 weeks). Hyperactive collagen stimulation is potentially more common in patients with a Fitzgerald phototype of IV-VI.

Dermatosis papulosa nigra/seborrheic keratoses/acrochordons

Some persons choose to treat DPNs for cosmetic reasons or as a medical necessity. For example, medical reasons for removing these lesions might include chronic irritations about the neck, caused by chains or collars rubbing on the lesions, or interference with the line of vision, caused by lesions that occur on the eyelids. More commonly, however, these lesions are removed for cosmetic reasons, as the DPNs are histologically and biologically benign. Effective cosmetic therapy is available to treat dermatosis papulosa nigra/seborrheic keratoses/acrochordons. Treatment of these 'skin tags' can effectively reduce the appearance of age by 10 years. Low-voltage electrodesiccation is an effective treatment for more common smaller, flat macules. Electrodesiccation causes very little pain, since the procedure is normally done under local anesthesia using a topical anesthetic cream. In about a week's time, the individual lesions begin to drop off the skin, leaving a normal skin appearance. Advise the patient to not pick at the treated areas. Pedunculated lesions respond well to scissor excision of papules; use local anesthesia to alleviate pain. If a person has hundreds of DPNs, several treatment sessions may be required to completely remove all of the lesions. Although cryosurgery is commonly used to destroy DPNs/seborrheic keratoses, the method has a high incidence of causing hyperpigmentation and hypopigmentation, and therefore, should be considered the last treatment option. Cryosurgery requires significant caution; risks should be minimized; use only short bursts of nitrogen as the risk for discoloration increases with the length of freezing . Trichloroacetic acid (50%) can be used for large seborrheic keratotic plaques.

Accentuated facial lines of expression

The formation of crease lines and rhytids is a natural component of the aging process that can lead to deep furrows and frown/ scowl lines. Such furrows and frown/scowl lines are referred to as dynamic rhytids, because they arise when we laugh, frown, or smile. Dynamic rhytids are caused by the repeated forces generated by hyperkinetic muscles include the frontalis (responsible for forehead furrows), corrugator supercilii (involved in frown/scowl lines), orbicularis oculi (crow's feet), procerus and depressor supercilii (also involved in frown/scowl lines), and nasalis (bunny lines).(18) Although botulinum toxin A has FDA approval for treatment of the glabellar region of the face, it is often used off-label for relaxation of the upper and lower hyperkinetic muscles. Most patients are treated successfully with a minimum of 20 U of botulinum toxin type A in the glabellar region. However, in ethnic skin, there are fewer requests for treatment of crow's feet and perioral rhytids, which rarely develops as seen in white patients.

The demand for botulinum toxin injections and other cosmetic procedures has continued to increase, fueled in part by growth in new sectors of the market. According to the ASAPS, botulinum toxin was the number one procedure performed in 2007 with 2.78 million injections, nearly 25% of all cosmetic procedures. The number of procedures dropped among women (-15.1%) from 2006 to 2007, but increased in men (+9.7%), according to the American Academy of Cosmetic Surgery.(6)

Striae distensae/Red striae

Affected areas can be treated with topical retinoids, fractionated erbium laser, and pulsed dye laser. Tretinoin provides sufficient irritation to stimulate collagen. Topical treatments are less effective and are used less often than other more successful therapies, such as the pulsed dye laser. The fractionated erbium laser is the latest therapeutic development, but has variable results. Very few patients respond to retinoids, but it should not be ruled out, since some patients have had favorable responses.

FIGHTING THE EFFECTS OF AGING IN ETHNIC SKIN

Morphology of Aging

It is becoming widely accepted that volume loss in the skin and soft tissue contributes greatly to the resulting appearance of the aging face. In addition, experts are recognizing that the loss of craniofacial support from aging or disease further contributes to the effects of aging because of diminished surface area for the outer soft tissue to envelope. In fact, the individual and combined effects of fat atrophy, bone loss, changes in musculature, and changes in the skin itself are all factors that bring about the folding and sagging that is observed in the aging face. Changes in

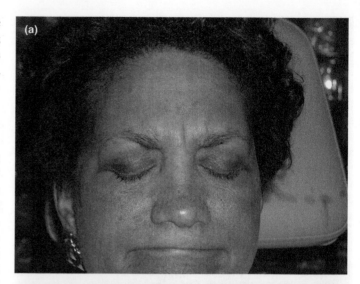

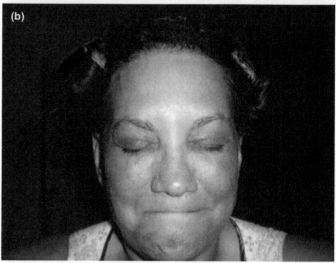

Figure 6.6 (a) Before and (b) after treatment with 20 units of botulinum toxin type A to the glabellar region.

any of these components bring about individual and synergistic effects that result in the aging appearance of the face .(19)

The atrophy/hypertrophy model for aging represents a shift from focusing on wrinkles and gravitational sagging to a more comprehensive approach that treats the aging face from "the inside out." An optimal treatment plan for the rejuvenation of the aging face requires a comprehensive approach. For that reason, it is vital that physicians understand the natural progression of changes in the aging face, the microstructural changes, and especially the macrostructural changes.(19)

In the young face, superficial and deep fat is distributed evenly, creating a homogenous topographical appearance with smooth primary arcs and convexities. With age, the distribution of fat becomes altered by fat atrophy and hypertrophy, producing hills and valleys with demarcations between the cosmetic units. Fat atrophy becomes clinically apparent in the temple and cheek and is followed by fat loss around the chin and mandibular areas. Features become concave, characterized by flat lips, sunken temple and cheek, scalloped mandible, and increased shadowing from hills and valleys. With aging, the most significant change in appearance is the sagging of excess skin, which develops as primary arcs become straight lines. Skin tends to drape inferiorly and diagonally from the temporal area toward the perioral region, creating a central focus on the perioral and mandibular regions. Fat atrophy is the result of decreased fat cell size, diminished fat cell function, impaired fat cell differentiation, and redistribution of fat cells. Fat hypertrophy occurs submentally, in the jowl, lateral nasolabial fold, lateral labiomental crease, and lateral malar areas. The accumulation of fat pulls the excessive skin downward under the force of gravity.(20) With aging, the gradual change from convex cosmetic units to concave regions brings about diminished reflection of light leading to a less radiant appearance. This may sometimes be reported by ethnic patients.

Fat atrophy and hypertrophy are further compounded by bone loss due to aging. Changes in craniofacial skeleton volume occur as a natural process of aging, but may be accelerated due to biological or environmental factors. Morphologic modifications in the appearance of the head, face, and neck become more evident around 50 years of age in both genders. However, bone loss is greater in women, potentially from the effects of menopause. The aging of the craniofacial skeleton is thought to occur from changes in the relative dynamics of own expansion and bone resorption. Significant volume changes are noted in the maxilla and mandible. Maxillary bone remodeling results in diminished support for overlying soft tissue, which leads to sagging skin.(19)

Soft Tissue Fillers in Blacks

In black skin, differences in composition lead to less frequency of certain conditions experienced with white skin, such as perioral rhytids or wrinkling. However, Blacks experience various other issues related to skin sagging and sinking, uneven complexion, loss of volume in skin laxity, and epidermal growths. Based on the particular ethnic skin type, some soft tissue fillers will achieve better results than others will. Histologically, there is less thinning of collagen bundles and elastic tissue in this skin type. As a result, fillers that stimulate collagen production or skin tightening appear to be more effective in ethnic skin.

Because keloid scarring can occur in ethnic patients as a result of invasive procedures such as full or partial facelifts, many patients and practitioners may be uncertain of what to expect from noninvasive procedures, such as soft tissue augmentation. However, careful explanation can increase comfort levels in patients and cautionary measures will alleviate the occurrence of hyperpigmentation in ethnic patients and lead to positive results for restoring a youthful facial appearance.

Soft tissue fillers are excellent for emphasizing cheeks and minimizing cheek festooning, filling accentuated tear troughs, and for treating the pre-jowl sulcus and temples. Volumizing is accomplished in the infraorbital, upper cheek, and lateral cheek regions using crosslinked or larger particle hyaluronic acid, calcium hydroxylapatite, or PLLA. Longevity of the effect varies with the type of substance. Temporary or less-permanent fillers provide immediate or delayed effects that last 9–18 months. For example, PLLA, which requires three sessions with 4–6 week periods between treatments, produces a soft tissue augmentation that lasts between 18 months and 3 years. Around the eyes, laxity of the upper/lower eyelid skin may develop; therefore,

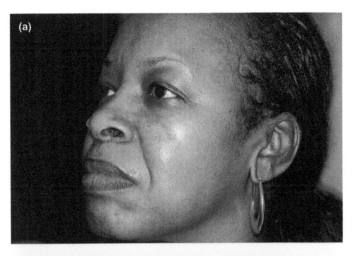

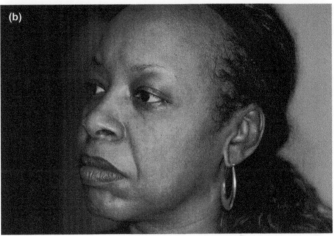

Figure 6.7 Age-related lipoatrophy: cheek festooning corrected with HA in the cheeks.

volume enhancement of the subbrow region can be achieved by injecting the dermal filler just below the eyebrow hair for an instant brow lift.

Safe Effective Use of PLLA

Studies have reported the development of granulomas and nodules after soft tissue augmentation using PLLA. However, reports of adverse events can usually be traced back to poor technique involving injection preparation, incorrect location of injections, and use of a hasty treatment plan. It is crucial for dermatologists and plastic surgeons to recognize and acknowledge the distinct differences between PLLA and other soft tissue fillers. The characteristics that distinguish PLLA from traditional fillers are: (1) the mechanism of action, (2) the treatment plan, (3) the preparation of the injection material, and (4) the injection technique.(21) Poly-L-lactic acid causes a gradual volume restoration that may take 3–6 months to develop. In addition, the rate of dermal thickening increases from the first to last injection. Since immediate correction is not the primary goal, as is the case in most traditional fillers, the use of PLLA requires a markedly different approach and treatment plan. Physicians should treat, wait, assess, and then decide how to proceed. Both patients and physicians need to observe great patience

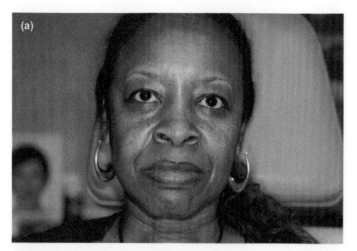

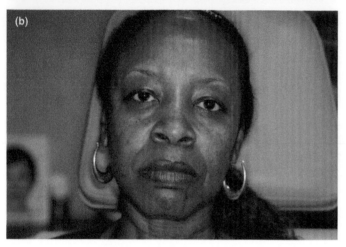

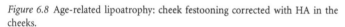

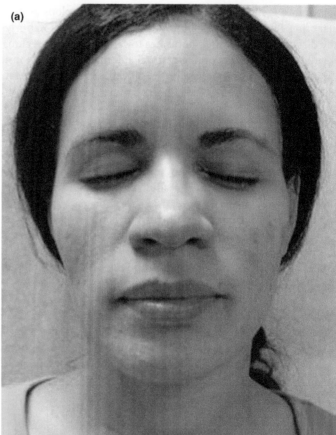

Figure 6.8 Age-related lipoatrophy: cheek festooning corrected with HA in the cheeks.

throughout the span of the treatment sessions. Unlike other cosmetic injectables, PLLA requires reconstitution before use. Although manufacturers recommend diluting in 3–5 mL of sterile water, 5–7 mL of sterile water is the customary reconstitution volume in the United States. In fact, some studies have reported that adverse effects, such as granulomas and nodules, have resulted because PLLA is difficult to dissolve completely (Figure 6.8a–d). However, Dreschnack notes that failure to allow sufficient time for reconstitution is probably the most common clinical error made by clinicians. Dermik laboratories recommend a 2-hour period of stabilization and dissolution of the microparticles after reconstitution. What is most critical for successful outcomes is that physicians receive sufficient training before attempting to inject PLLA. This training should include distinctions in injection technique. For example, as opposed to treating a specific line, the strategy of PLLA treatment is to return volume to a facial area. In addition, PLLA is injected into the dermal-subcutaneous plane, unlike collagen or hyaluronic acids. Finally, it is important that PLLA injection be accompanied by massage of the treatment area and continued by the patient posttreatment.

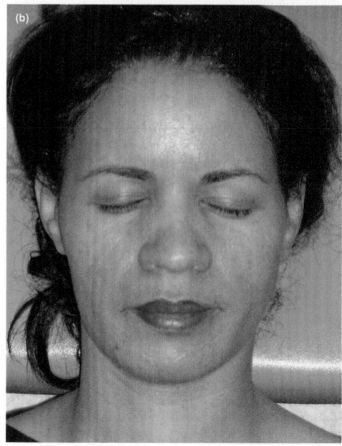

Figure 6.9 Facial enhancement with PLLA 2 sessions (6 mos.).

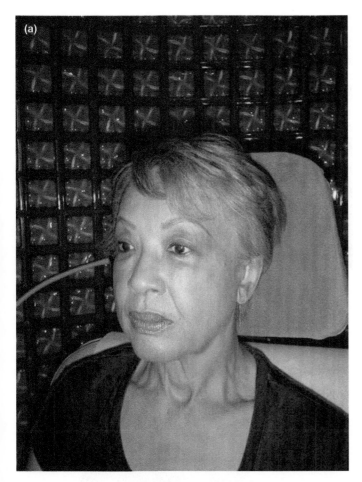

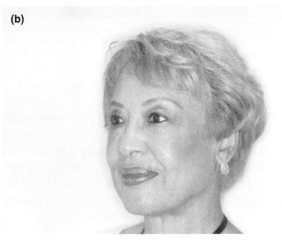

Figure 6.10 Facial enhancement with PLLA 2 sessions (6 mos.).

Poly-L-lactic acid has been used effectively in both the younger and older patient. However, in the older or aging patient the thickness of the dermis plane is diminished, leading to a greater likelihood for bruising that results from increased fragility of blood vessels. In these patients, it is recommended that clinicians allow 8 weeks between treatment sessions, as opposed to the regular 4–6 week waiting period. For clinicians, the learning curve is longer in these patients, due to the concerns associated with treating patients with a thin dermis plane. Experts recommend that physicians acquire sufficient knowledge and training before attempting procedures, and performing less-ambitious corrections before injecting around the orbits or into the perioral region.

Lip rejuvenation

In the 1990s, the desire among white women for full, voluptuous lips began to stimulate the market for collagen injections used to enhance the appearance of lips. Over the years, the desire for full lips has gained widespread popularity and fueled the demand for lip augmentation. By contrast, full lips have historically been viewed as an unattractive feature by most Black women. However, changes in self-perception are motivating more Black women to emphasize the beauty of their lips. As a result, many of these women are now choosing procedures to rebuild an aging lip.(22, 23)

Whereas the typical goal of lip augmentation in white women is to increase the lip size beyond the original volume, Black women generally seek augmentation to only restore the size of the lip to the original volume and appearance. Although the intrinsic aging process causes similar affects to the lips of Black and white patients, some subtle differences are important to note. Whereas in white women, lip aging usually occurs relatively early in life, these effects typically occur later in Black women. In white women, supravermilion rhytides develop above and below the vermilion borders, because of thinning of the dermis, volume loss, loss of vermillion border, and the overactivity of the periorbicularis oris musculature.

The lips of white women appear thin, long, flat, and wrinkled, with down-turned corners of the mouth that appear sad or angry looking. However, for Black women, rhytides occur predominantly in the body of the lip below the vermilion border, in response to loss of volume of the upper lip. In addition, the lower lip usually maintains the same appearance; however, it sometimes becomes flat and more visible. Unlike white women, collagen enhancement of the vermillion border is rarely performed and therefore, the primary treatment consists of rolling the lip up using injections of hyaluronic acid. If there is overactivity of the periorbicularis oris musculature, botulinum toxin A is the preferred method to relax muscles perioral rhytids.(24)

Restoring Elastin in the Aging Face

Although several therapies have been developed to improve the loss of collagen that occurs in aging skin, until recently, no agent has been available to treat the loss of elastin function, which is a significant feature of chronologic aging and photoaging. Two recent studies have demonstrated favorable results by using a cream containing a zinc complex that penetrates the skin and stimulates elastin development through a myriad of molecular pathways. In both studies, the zinc complex cream was applied for 4 weeks. In the first study, improvement was evaluated by snap-test time, which determines the time needed for the skin to snap back to baseline after being pulled a specific distance. Response was also determined by measurement with a DermaLab® suction cup and blinded assessment by

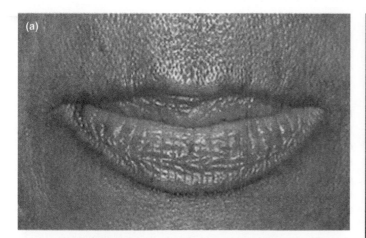

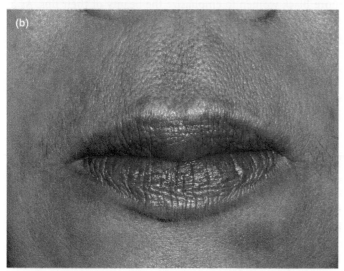

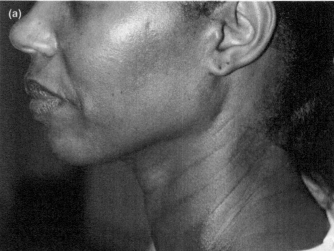

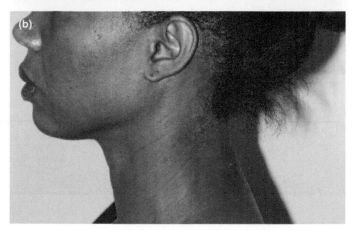

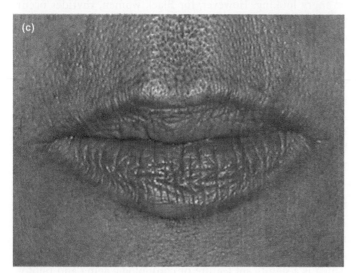

Figure 6.12 Before and after one session of monopolar radiofrequency skin tightening of the lower face, submental and neck regions.

Figure 6.11 Upper age-related lip atrophy. Several days following HA to the upper lip. One month after HA enhancement of the upper lip.

a dermatologist. After 4 weeks of treatment, there was a 40% improvement in snap time, significant improvement in vacuum as measured by the DermaLab® suction cup, and improvement in skin roughness, fine and coarse lines, laxity, puffiness, dark circles, and crepey and sunken appearance. In the second study,

there was a 29% decrease in the number and depth of fine lines and wrinkles around the eyes, following once-daily application for 4 weeks. Results of the study also found a 37% decrease in course wrinkles, 42% decrease in under-eye laxity, 30% decrease in under-eye puffiness, and a 21% decrease in under-eye dark circles.(25) Restoration of elastin is likely to be especially effective in ethnic skin, due to the lower magnitude of elastin loss observed in the aging face of ethnic people.

Skin Tightening

Skin tightening can be accomplished through a number of heat-producing technologies, including radiofrequency (RF), long wavelength laser, and broad-spectrum light sources. These technologies use heat-producing energy, which causes a cascade of molecular and mechanical effects that tighten skin without injury or removal of overlying epidermis. The result is direct and immediate contraction of collagen fibers, as well as a delayed wound-healing response with dermal remodeling and ultimately neocollagenesis.(26) While some FDA approved-devices use only one type of energy, other devices combine energy types, e.g., bipolar RF energy combined with diode laser energy, or RF energy combined with both diode laser and intense pulse light energy.(27)

Early drawbacks to skin-tightening procedures were considerable pain and variable results between patients. However, the treatment parameters reduce the amount of pain so that most of these therapies can be perform under topical anesthesia. Clinicians must also inform patients that 3–6 months are required for the intended effects to fully develop, and that skin laxity without a great deal of muscular attachment yields the most promising clinical outcome from these kinds of procedures .

The various FDA-approved skin-tightening devices have demonstrated different results when used on different parts of the body, with reference to skin laxity, texture, firmness, and effects on volume reduction. For example, the multiple pass, low fluence treatment algorithm for lower face laxity has demonstrated favorable results with RF skin tightening.(28) In addition, the cost of procedure, associated adverse effects, and required treatment length and sessions are a consideration for both clinician and patient.(26, 27, 29)

Skin-tightening technology can be combined with other aesthetic modalities such as soft tissue augmentation; the skin-tightening process can be applied either simultaneously or after receiving the other modality. The combination of modalities was recently tested in a study by England et al. using an animal model. The study found that monopolar RF heating had no observed adverse effects on the filler collagen responses or persistence of the various filler substances, which included crosslinked human collagen (Cosmoplast™), hyaluronic acid (Restylane®), calcium hydroxylapatite (Radiesse™), polylactic acid (Sculptra™), and liquid injectable silicone (Silikon™). Further clinical studies are needed to study the effects on aesthetic outcome.(30)

SUMMARY

In recent years, people with pigmented skin have become an increasingly important market force for the cosmetic industry. Product lines have been expanded to accommodate a broader spectrum of skin colors, and marketing strategies have been specialized to target specific ethnic populations. In addition, it is predicted that people with pigmented skin will eventually comprise a majority of the domestic and international population during the 21st century. Not surprisingly, people with pigmented skin are increasingly seeking out products and procedures to fight the effects of aging, including increases in surgical and nonsurgical cosmetic procedures. In some cases, ethnic patients may be skeptical about the safety of certain cosmetic procedures. Because keloid scarring can occur in ethnic patients as a result of invasive procedures such as full or partial facelifts, many patients and practitioners are uncertain of what to expect from noninvasive procedures, such as soft tissue augmentation. Fortunately, techniques that are specific to ethnic populations can alleviate the occurrence of hyperpigmentation in pigmented skin and lead to positive results for restoring a youthful facial appearance. Clinicians must also be aware of the different manifestations of fat atrophy and hypertrophy that are experienced by patients with pigmented skin. As with patients of all skin colors, a comprehensive approach to assessment and treatment of the face is absolutely necessary. Various injectable reconstructors and fillers exist that can

be used alone or in combination. These fillers differ in composition, mechanism of action, longevity, and price. It is critical that clinicians receive specialized training for specific soft tissue fillers before attempting to treat patients. With proper training and technique, clinicians can provide successful outcomes with little risk of adverse events to patients with pigmented skin.

REFERENCES

1. Taylor SC. Ethnic skin: biology, structure, function, and implications for dermatologic disease. J Am Acad Dermatol 2002; 46(2 Suppl): S41–62.
2. Roberts WE. The Roberts Skin Type Classification System. J Drugs Dermatol 2008; 7(5): 452–6.
3. U.S. Census Bureau 1990, 2000. Available at www.census.gov. Accessed March 01, 2008.
4. Taylor SC, Burgess C, Callender V. The safety and efficacy of Restylane and Perlane in patients with skin of color: results from a perspective, randomized, evaluator-blinded comparative trial (not published yet).
5. Tenerelli. Ethnic skin-care: special products for a special sector. Global Cosmetic Industry 2000; 32–7.
6. Cosmetic Surgery National Data Bank 2007 Statistics. American Society for Aesthetic Plastic Surgery [Internet]. Available at: http://www.surgery.org/download/2007stats.pdf. Accessed July 25, 2008.
7. How does collaboration with supply-chain partners play a role in new product success? Cass Business School [Internet]. Available at: www.cass.citv.ac.uk <http://www.cass.citv.ac.uk>. Accessed September 21, 2004.
8. Christian Oresajo, PhD Scientific Director, Ethnic Skin Research Institute, L'Oreal, Chicago, IL; Howard University College of Medicine, Washington, DC. Second International Symposium sub number 19–21, 2003. Chicago, IL.
9. Baumann L, Rodriguez D, Taylor SC, Wu J. Natural considerations for ethnic skin. Cutis 2006; 78(6 Suppl): 2–19.
10. Kaidbey KH, Agin PP, Sayre RM, Kligman AM. Photoprotection by melanin–a comparison of black and white skin. J Am Acad Dermatol 1979; 1(3): 249–60.
11. Stephens T. Ethnic sensitive skin: a review. Allured Cosmetics and Toiletries 1994; 109: 75–80.
12. Draelos Z. All skin is not the same. Cosmet Dermatol 2006; 19: 99–101.
13. Pigment Matters: Focus on pigmentary disorders. Pigmentary Disorders Academy, by MedSense Ltd, on behalf of Galderma International [Internet]. Available at: <http://www.pigmentarydisordersacademy.org/pigmatters_summer.pdf>. Accessed June 29, 2007.
14. Klaus Wolff, Lowell A. Goldsmith, Stephen I. Katz et al. Fitzpatrick's Dermatology in General Medicine, 7th edition. New York City: McGraw-Hill Publishing, 2008.
15. Shriver MD, Parra EJ. Comparison of narrow-band reflectance spectroscopy and tristimulus colorimetry for measurements of skin and hair color in persons of different biological ancestry. Am J Phys Anthropol 2000; 112(1): 17–27.
16. Badreshia-Bansal S, Draelos ZD. Insight into skin lightening cosmeceuticals for women of color. J Drugs Dermatol 2007; 6(1): 32–9.
17. Taylor SC, Burgess CM, Callender VD et al. Postinflammatory hyperpigmentation: evolving combination treatment strategies. Cutis 2006; 78(2 Suppl): 6–19.
18. Carruthers A, Kiene K, Carruthers J. Botulinum A exotoxin use in clinical dermatology. J Am Acad Dermatol 1996; 34: 788–97.
19. Vleggaar D, Fitzgerald R. Dermatological implications of skeletal aging: a focus on supraperiosteal volumization for perioral rejuvenation. J Drugs Dermatol 2008; 7(3): 209–20.
20. Donofrio LM. Fat distribution: a morphologic study of the aging face. Dermatol Surg. 2000; 26(12): 1107–12.
21. Burgess CM, Lowe NJ. NewFill for skin augmentation: a new filler or failure? Dermatol Surg 2006; 32(12): 1530–2.
22. Burgess CM. Soft tissue augmentation in skin of color: market growth, available fillers, and successful techniques. J Drugs Dermatol 2007; 6(1): 51–5.

23. Garries R. Restoring the fullness: lip rejuvenation in the African American female. Available at: <http://www.plasticsurgeryproductsonline.com/article.php?s=PSP/2006/05&p=7>. Accessed August 24, 2006.

24. Burgess CM. Cosmetic Dermatology. Heidelberg: Springer; 2005.

25. Baumann L. Improving elasticity: the science of aging skin. Cosmet Dermatol 2007; 20(3): 168–72.

26. Technology Report: Tissue Tightening. American Society for Dermatologic Surgery [Internet]. February 2007. Available at: http://www.asds.net/Media/PositionStatements/technology-tissuetightening.html. Accessed June 21, 2007.

27. Mayoral FA. Skin tightening with a combined unipolar and bipolar radiofrequency device. J Drugs Dermatol 2007; 6(2): 212–5.

28. Bogle MA, Ubelhoer N, Weiss RA, Mayoral F, Kaminer MS. Evaluation of the multiple pass, low fluence algorithm for radiofrequency tightening of the lower face. Lasers Surg Med 2007; 39(3): 210–7.

29. England L, Tan M, Shumaker P. Effects of monopolar radiofrequency treatment over soft-tissue fillers in an animal model. Lasers Surg Med 2005; 37: 356–65.

30. Sadick NS, Makino Y. Selective electro-thermolysis in aesthetic medicine: a review. Lasers Surg Med 2004; 34(2): 91–7.

7　The aging face in a multiethnic world

Stephen C Adler, Eric T Adler, and Paul J Carniol

The multiethnic population is one of the most rapidly growing demographic segments of North America. According to the 2000 United States Census, 29% of the population is non-Caucasian and by 2056, greater than 50% of the population in the United States will be of non-European descent.(1)

Beauty magazines and the fashion industry have helped us understand the evolution of beauty in our society. In the 1970s Caucasian men and women mostly dominated fashion runways, but today, these runways are shared with faces of individuals of multiethnic backgrounds. It is to no surprise that the face of the aesthetic patient is also changing. As surgeons, no longer are we only addressing patients from different ethnic backgrounds, but more importantly, patients, who share a mixture of different ethnic traits. Diversity of the ethnic traits can be seen through the ever-increasing melting pot in our society, which results from diversity within ethnic groups, industrialization, and migration and interethnic marriages.

Fanous and Yoskovitch have presented a new classification of races based on racial skin differences and features.(2) This new classification divides races into three founding races: Caucasoid, African, and Asian; and six subraces or categories: Nordics, Europeans, Mediterraneans, Indo-Pakistanis, Africans, and Asians. Patients of ethnic mixtures may exhibit both Caucasian and non-Caucasian facial features with regards to skin, soft tissue, cartilage, bone structure, and healing. Facial plastic surgeons, dermatologists, plastic surgeons, and other medical providers must understand the aesthetic variability among these diverse patients in our population.

The goal of facial plastic surgery is to achieve a natural result while maintaining a balance and harmony between facial features. During the Classical Greek Period (499–338 BC), Plato initiated the concept of defining beauty; he believed that the ideal human body had to have more than just perfect proportions. To be truly beautiful, he asserted, a figure must be balanced and posses the elusive quality of good taste.(3) During the Renaissance Period (late 14th century to mid-16th century), artists stressed the ideals of perfect human form, body proportions, and beauty. The main goal of the artist during this period was to mimic nature with the aid of science and mathematics. Leonardo DaVinci was known for his detailed study of human facial and body proportions. He defined the horizontal thirds off the face where the space from the chin to the beginning of the bottom of the nose is the third part of the face and equal to the nose to brow and the brow to the forehead hairline. He also divided the face into five equal parts as viewed from the front, each fifth equaling the distance from the medial canthus to the lateral canthus.(4)

It is well known that the pursuit of beauty has persisted through the ages and throughout all ethnic and cultural groups. As Aristotle described beauty, "something is considered beautiful if all parts are working together in harmony so that no one part draws unjust attention to itself". Aesthetic goals may vary widely among patients of both Caucasian and non-Caucasian origin as well as patients from different ethnic backgrounds. Cultural differences may influence not only the interaction with the physician, but also the way results are interpreted after the surgery. It is helpful to have some knowledge about the cultural differences between different ethnic groups during the cosmetic surgery process.

The preoperative discussion should focus on a realistic and a desired postoperative result that reshapes, and refines rather than distort and change the ethnicity of the patient. The attempt to change the ethnicity of a feature or a patient may be most difficult to achieve and will potentially result in an unhappy patient and surgeon. It is important that physicians spend time during the consultation period understanding the needs and expectations of the patients, and in addition, perform a detailed facial analysis and physical exam, and thoroughly explain the surgical procedure, anticipated results and variation of these results. The consultation should include addressing type of anesthesia, postoperative recovery process, limitations, risks, and postoperative instructions. The use of computer imaging may be helpful in communication, displaying potential outcomes, and presenting limitations of the treatment. Computer imaging although helpful in this process, should not be used to guarantee or assure a surgical result. Attempts to radically change ethnic features may result in a disruption of facial balance and symmetry. Regardless of ethnic or variety of multiethnic traits, the results of aging face surgery should focus on achieving a natural, refreshing, soft, and unaltered appearance, while refining the different facial features. The goals of the treatment must be understood and agreed between the surgeon and the patient before any treatment or surgery.

Understanding the aging process as it relates to the multiethnic face is the first step in patient evaluation. A detailed facial analysis and physical examination will help establish a basis of understanding and education for patients interested in cosmetic surgery. This phase is perhaps the most important in determining which features stand to benefit the most from any treatment or surgery. As always, concerns of healing and complications should be included in the pretreatment consultation. It should be noted that some complications may be more prevalent in patients with certain ethnic traits.

FACIAL AGING

Knowledge and understanding of the aging face has evolved in the past three decades. Aging is a complex, and constantly changing process, which affects the entire human body throughout life. The aging process is affected by both genetic and acquired factors. There exist many genetic aging theories, which include DNA mutations, decrease in hormone production, free radical damage, and autoimmune events among others. Diseases, nutritional deficiencies, smoking, and excessive sun exposure are well known to influence and accelerate the aging process. Although, the signs of aging such as wrinkles, skin dyschromia, sagging skin, loss of volume or fat atrophy vary among patients, these are applicable to all ethnic groups.

Aging is not limited to the skin, but also to its supporting structures. The paradigm shift in facial plastic surgery has changed from a two-dimensional perspective, where surgeons are mainly focused on lifting, pulling, and removing tissue, to a three- dimensional perspective, where in addition, bone structure and soft tissue atrophy is recognized and treated with volume enhancement procedures. During the past 5 years, the aesthetic field has witnessed an exponential growth in volume-enhancing agents and fillers. According to recent surveys, and trends, soft tissue augmentation is increasing in popularity to the point of revolutionized the cosmetic surgery market. The use of neurotoxins such as Botox® (Allergan, Irvine, California) continues to be an important option in the treatment of hyperactive muscle lines in patients of all ethnic and multiethnic backgrounds.

The skull and all bone structures become smaller, muscle tone and strength decreases, facial ligaments lengthen, subcutaneous fat atrophies, elasticity of skin decreases, and there is loss of water in the skin and underlying tissues. Gonzales-Ulloa has identified fat atrophy as one of the main components of aging.(5) These factors contribute to loss of structural mass while the skin envelope structures increase its relative surface area. The envelope becomes larger than the contents. Additionally, bone density and therefore bone loss occur during the aging process and as a result decrease the structural support for the more superficial soft tissue and skin. Coleman (6) has popularized and expanded the concepts of facial atrophy and the new model of aging with regards the loss of the third dimension of the face. He has been a strong advocate for the need to replenish soft tissue with techniques of autologous structural fat grafting. When analyzing the multiethnic face, understanding multiethnic features must include the evaluation of facial bone structure and soft tissue.

For example, a person with Native American or Asian heritage may exhibit high prominent cheek bones which project a fuller and more youthful look. Many ethnic groups consider these to be desirable facial characteristics. Alternatively, some Asians may have diminished nasal dorsal projection, along with flattening of midface and chin regions. While respecting the different multiethnic traits, the current trend is to consider volume enhancement as a primary option or as an adjunct to other facial rejuvenation procedures.

Clinically, loss of volume is responsible for descent of the brow-forehead and eyelid complex, descent of the lower lid-midface tissues and descent of the lower cheek, jowl and neck skin. As the periorbital soft tissue deteriorates, the upper and lower eyelid skin becomes redundant, and hollowing of the eyes is revealed. Thinning of the lip and collapse of the perioral and submalar structures contribute to the aggravation of nasal labial folds, marionette folds, and prejowl sulcus.

When inelastic skin looses the underlying support it tends to become redundant. Skin redundancy will fold and accentuate areas such as the nasal folds and prejowl sulcus. In the perioral and periorbital area the loss of soft tissue will cause the skin to come near the facial muscles and this results in the increased muscle effect on skin folding in areas such as the crows feet lines,

lower cheek lines, and lip lines. With increasing time, these lines, which originally are only seen with animation and smiling, will become permanently printed in the skin.

Skin aging is mostly caused by photo damage from ultraviolet light exposure.(7) Aged and photo-damaged skin displays disorganized collagen fibrils, elastin, and fibroblasts.(8) Clinically, the aging skin displays rhytids, discoloration or dyschromia, solar lentigos, coarseness, telengiactesias, and dryness. The presence and the production of melanin in the multiethnic skin protect the skin from photo damage caused by ultra-violet radiation. The increase melanin content in African Americans prevents them from displaying many of the typical signs of aging found in Caucasians.(9)

Histologically, aged skin reveals decrease loss of collagen and elastin in African American skin, to a lesser degree than Caucasian skin.(10) Signs of aging therefore present later in patients of Mediterranean, Hispanic, Asian, and African Americans than in Caucasian skin. Skin classifications have traditionally been determined by the skin complexion or color and the response to sunlight exposure.

The Fitzpatrick classification (11) originally developed in 1975 which groups different skin types by skin color and the reaction to sun exposure is still considered a major reference point in the evaluation of how patients will respond to facial treatments such as chemical peels, lasers, and other minimally invasive skin treatments. Neither Fitzpatrick nor Glogau skin classifications take into account the place of ethnic origin and possible multiethnic heritage of the patients.

As there are genetic variations beyond these broad classification systems, they should only be used as aids in predicting the reactions of patients to skin treatments. Examination of the skin must anticipate the variable potential responses to different treatments including hyperpigmentation, hypopigmentation, scar, keloids, and prolonged redness.

For example, although unlikely, it is possible for a faired skinned blue-eyed patient to develop hyperpigmentation or other dyschromia after laser or chemical peel. This patient may very well be genotypically Latin, Native Indian, African, or even Asian ancestry. During the medical evaluation, it is important to have some knowledge of the patient's heritage and ancestry to anticipate possible side effects of the treatment described.

FACIAL ANALYSIS IN A MULTIETHNIC PATIENT

Evaluation of any patient who presents with aging face changes is a complex process. It requires a detailed assessment of the face in conjunction with a methodical exam. This should include, as possible, consideration of potential genetic factors that can influence the result and affect the recovery process. The interview of the patient is a time of opportunity to learn about heritage, ancestry, and cultural background.

Perception of the face involves forming an initial impression of the affect and appearance of the face. Does the face portray someone who appears tired, sad, worried, happy, mad, older than stated age, age appropriate, younger than stated, or refreshed? Which ethnic features are dominant, such as color of skin, shape of the nose, height of the malar prominence, chin, eyes, and lips? Which features interrupt the flow of the face, or attract undue attention? For example is the nose too prominent or is there a problem with retrognathia, or even a hypoplasia of cheek bone/ soft tissue? Does the face appear to be deflated and hollow or have full and soft appearance?

Perception is an important part of the facial analysis because it helps prioritize the areas that, when addressed, will provide the highest benefit and improvement. Interestingly, a patient's perception may differ significantly from the aesthetic surgeon's. Many of the changes of the aging face will extend across all ethnic groups.

Extensive variability of features within ethnic groups should avert physicians from solely following anthropometric measurements when planning an operation. Anthropometric analysis may apply, but is less relied upon when attempting to formulate a sense of aesthetic balance and beauty in the ethnic and multiethnic patient.

The examination must include an assessment of static and dynamic anatomy; what problems or concerns are present at rest versus what is present during muscle movement of the face. Lines and folds that occur with muscle activity in the upper face are best addressed with the available neurotoxins and not necessarily a surgery that could distort an ethnic feature on the face. For example, lines that occur in the lower eyelids during smiling, which are not present at rest are best-treated conservative with neurotoxins and possibly resurfacing treatments. Surgery may prove to be excessive and result in ectropion and a change in the natural shape of the eyelid.

Treatment of aging changes involving the skin in multiethnic patients can be challenging. The evaluation of the skin must extend beyond Fitzpatrick skin type. It must be directed toward the treatment of the condition and the variable potential responses to treatment. The color of the eyes may also provide added information when planning a treatment protocol. A patient with Fitzpatrick type II or III skin and dark eyes may respond to skin treatment like a type IV skin with dyschromia or hyperpigmentation.

Interestingly some patients who appear to be Fitzpatrick III with hazel eyes, and some Mediterranean background frequently will react to cutaneous procerures as if they have Fitzpatrick type IV skin. A patient with relatively fair skin and some Asian heritage may also respond to skin peels or lasers with hyperpigmentation or other dyschromia.

The patient in Figure 7.1, who has Native American ancestry, underwent a TCA35% peel and responded with moderate hyperpigmentation. This was treated with Jessner's peels, topical retinoic acid and hydroquinone creams, with adequate resolution of the problem.(Figure 7.2) The scars in the preauricular area in the same patients following a facelift showed adequate healing and confined around the curvature of the ear (Figure 7.3, 7.4).

Combinations of varied level resurfacing, fractional resurfacing, or peels may be indicated in a patient with differing skin problems depending on the treated area of the face. An example is a patient with deep rhytids in the perioral and lower eyelid region and may have slight dyschromia and solar lentigos on the cheeks. He or she may benefit from a phenol peel in the periroral and periorbital area and a TCA35%/ Jessner's to complete the rest of the face.

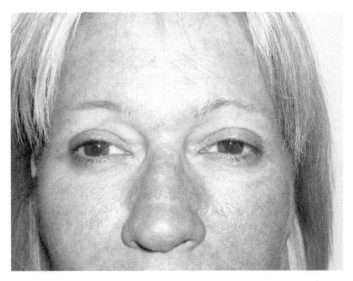

Figure 7.1 Caucasian Patient with Native American Indian ancestry and Type II Fitzpatrick skin following a Trichloroacetic Acid (TCA) 35% chemical peel resulting in skin hyperpigmentation.

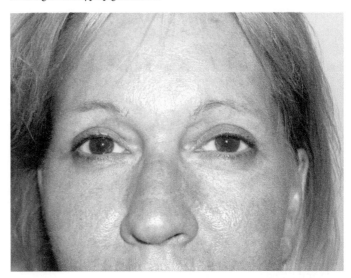

Figure 7.2 Same Patient with resolution of hyperpigmentation following the treatment with Jessner's chemical peel in combination with topical retinoic acid and hydroquinone treatment.

Soft tissue and structural examination may reveal the need for volumetric enhancement via fillers, fat transfer, and/or structural cheek and chin implants. Patients of Asian, American Indian, or Northern European may exhibit prominent cheek bones and soft tissue.

Aesthetic Nasal Surgery

The nose may be one the most ethnic appearing features of the face. When planning nasal surgery it is important to first discuss with the patient whether their goal is to maintain an ethnic appearance or to have a less ethnic appearing nose. Another issue to consider when planning the procedure is keeping the nose in harmony with the rest of the face.

The African-American nose can be highly variable. It can exhibit dark, thick skin, increased fatty content, short columella, wide dorsum, bulbous tip with ptosis, weak projection, diminished nasal height, and horizontal flared nostrils. The Asian nose may exhibit wide intercanthal distance, and thick skin, bulbous

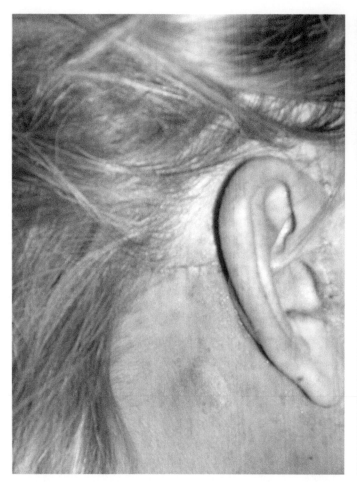

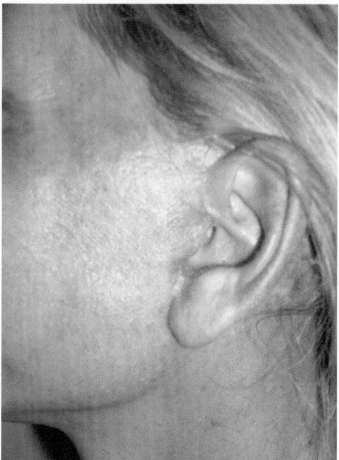

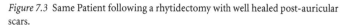

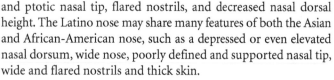

Figure 7.3 Same Patient following a rhytidectomy with well healed post-auricular scars.

Figure 7.4 Same Patient with well healed pre-auricular scars.

and ptotic nasal tip, flared nostrils, and decreased nasal dorsal height. The Latino nose may share many features of both the Asian and African-American nose, such as a depressed or even elevated nasal dorsum, wide nose, poorly defined and supported nasal tip, wide and flared nostrils and thick skin.

Patient in Figures 7.5, 7.6, with Brazilian ancestry presents with blue eyes, type III skin, a wide nasal bridge, moderate skin thickness, bulbous tip with moderate tip ptosis with midfacial hypoplasia. The patient underwent upper blepharoplasty, rhinoplasty, fat grafting midface with 2-year followup with good improvement. The patient in Figures 7.7, 7.8, 7.9, 7.10 has Chilean, South American Indian heritage presented for rhinoplasty and facial rejuvenation. Her evaluation revealed brow and facial ptosis, nasal dorsal prominence, and a wide bulbous nasal tip. She underwent a rhytidectomy, endoscopic browlift and rhinoplasty. (Figure 7.7, 7.8, 7.9, 7.10).

Rejuvenating The Periorbital Region
Many patients are interested in maintaining the ethnicity of their eyelids and periorbital region. This is important in planning aesthetic procedures in this region. The upper eyelid drapes from the supraorbital ridge to the lashes, and there is absence of the superior palpebral fold. Anatomic differences in the Asian eyelid include attachment of the levator fibers to the tarsal plate without making attachment to the orbicularis muscle and skin above the tarsal plate, the fat compartments because the lack of preseptal

attachments descend anterior to the tarsal plate, and the presence of the epicanthal fold. The goal is to create a palpebral line that divides the eyelid into pretarsal and preseptal components, lighten the eyes by removing some of the preseptal fatty tissue and possibly removing the epicanthal fold. The latter should be discussed and agreed upon with the patient before any surgery is performed.

Patients with Mediterranean ancestry usually do not have special anatomical considerations when planning eyelid rejuvenation procedures. However, they may be a greater risk of having noticeable scars, or developing hyperpigmentation after surgery. This patient of Mediterranean heritage presents with deep hollow lower eyelid groove and lower eyelid dermatochalasis with pseudoherniations of fat. The patient underwent lower eyelid blepharoplasty with fat repositioning and a lower eyelid phenol peel as a second stage procedure (Figure 7.11, 7.12).

The Lower Two-Thirds Of The Face
The midface and lower face in the multiethnic population will present a diversity of variables. The midfacial area may vary from a flattened or sunken look to the full, augmented high cheekbone appearance. The presence of high cheekbones and a full midface is a desired youthful feature coveted in patients of most ethnicities.

High cheekbones may be found in patients of Northern European, American and South American Indian and Asian

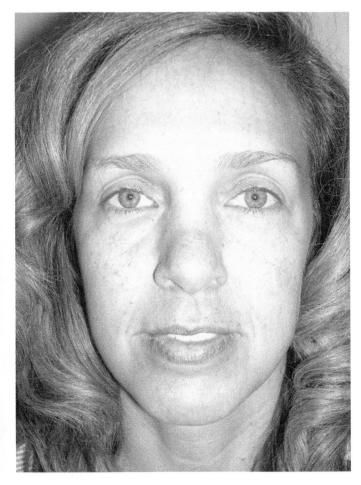

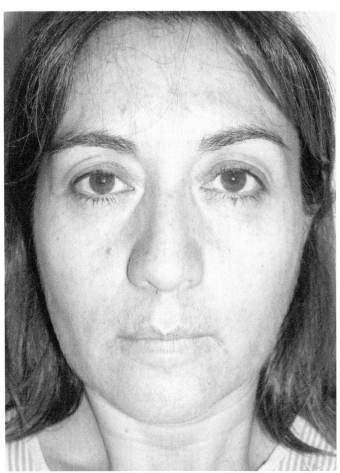

Figure 7.5 Patient of Brazilian ancestry with blue eyes, Type III Fitzpatrick skin, wide nasal bridge, upper eyelid dermatochalasis, moderate skin thickness, bulbous nasal tip, and midface hypoplasia and malar flattening.

Figure 7.7 Patient of Chilean and South American Indian heritage with strong facial bone features and midface with soft tissue collapse with brow and lower face ptosis. (Frontal view)

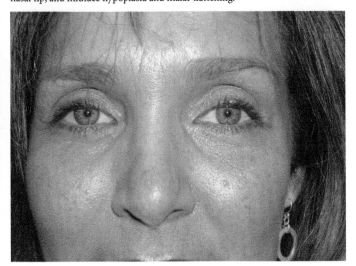

Figure 7.6 Same Patient 2 years after undergoing upper blepharoplasty, rhinoplasty, fat grafting to midface.

ancestry. Midface flattening may be from a combination of malar bone deficiency and/or loss soft tissue volume. Midfacial volume loss may present with a flattened, hollowed, tired appearance, a deep naso jugal trough, and/or ptotic nasal folds.

Midface lift has been advocated as a treatment for the ptosis of this area, but care should be taken in patient selection. Lifting soft

tissue over a flat malar eminence may lead to an over-pulled and distorted appearance, and it can exaggerate the flattening of the midface and alter normal facial contour.

The patient in Figure 7.13, 7.14 is of Hispanic heritage. She presented with cheek soft tissue hypoplasia, cheek and brow ptosis. She underwent rhytidectomy, endoscopic brow lift, and fat transfer to the midface with excellent improvement.

Rhytidectomy in African Americans, Asian, and Mediterranean patients with thick skin and loss of structural support are approached by standard incisions to allow adequate exposure and tissue mobilization. Often, this cannot be achieved with minimal incision surgery. The greater more traditional surgical exposure will more readily allow for adequate superficial musculoaponeurotic system (SMAS) suspension and anterior platysmal plication as needed.

As for all patients the skin flap advancement must be tailored to the shape of the face and oriented in the appropriate vectors. For patients that require more structural definition, treatment options may include chin, cheek, sub-malar and tear trough implants which provide a structural augmentation of bony regions and/or soft tissue augmentation with fat transfer.

When planning a rhytidectomy procedure the patient's medical problems should be considered. For example, hypertension, which is common in the general population and is more prevalent in the African Americans, predisposes the patients to hematoma formation and can increase incidence by 2.6 times.(15)

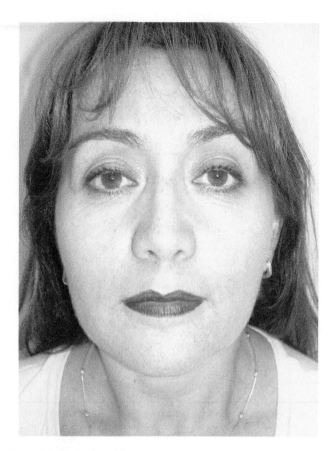

Figure 7.8 Same patient following a rhytidectomy, endoscopic browlift and rhinoplasty.

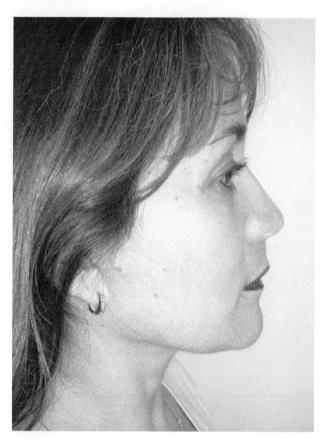

Figure 7.10 Same patient, post-operative lateral view following rhytidectomy, endoscopic browlift and rhinoplasty.

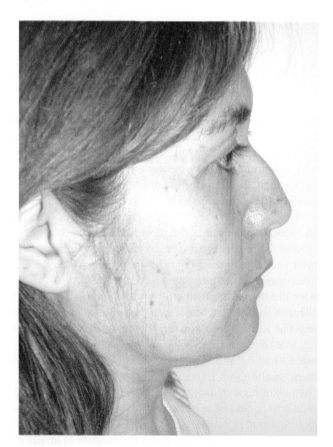

Figure 7.9 Same patient pre-operative lateral view.

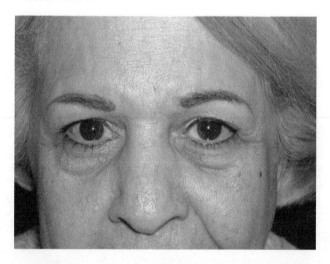

Figure 7.11 Patient of Mediterranean ancestry, Type III Fitzpatrick skin presenting with deep hollow lower eyelid groove, lower eyelid dermatochalasis and pseudohernias of fat.

The lips are considered an important focal point of the face. They also can vary in appearance between individuals as well as ethnic groups. Furthermore they are subjected to changes due to photoaging and underlying volume loss.

Full lips are considered attractive, sensuous, and project a youthful quality in the face. Full, prominent, youthful lips are frequently seen in patients with African American, non-white Hispanic, Indian, Mediterranean, and Asian ancestry. Aging causes degenerating changes in multiple levels of the lips. The upper lip becomes

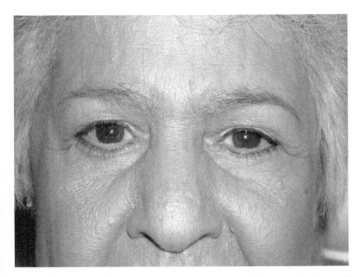

Figure 7.12 Patient following lower blepharoplasty with fat repositioning and second stage phenol chemical peel.

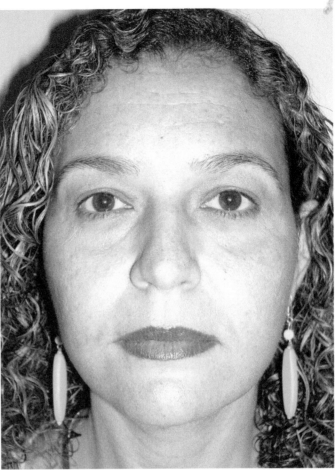

Figure 7.14 Same patient following rhytidectomy, endoscopic browlift and fat grafting to cheek and midface.

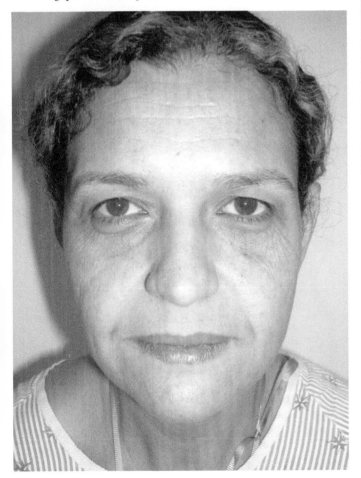

Figure 7.13 Patient of Hispanic, Caribbean ancestry presenting with brow ptosis, cheek soft tissue hypoplasia and ptosis with Type IV Fitzpatrick skin.

flatter and the phitrum ridges become less prominent. The prominence and outward projection of the vermilion border is lost and decreases in height. The volume of both the dry and wet lip decreases due to the loss of subcutaneous fat, thinning of the epidermis and the oral commissures drop giving the appearance sadness.

Full and prominent lips are coveted features in ethnic, multiethnic and Caucasian populations. Lip enhancement may incorporate lip lifting or vermilion advancement for patients with thin lip lines and minimal volume. Lip volume augmentation may involve fat grafting, dermal-fat grafting and hyaluronic acid fillers among other options. The goal of any lip rejuvenation must aim at maintaining a natural, soft and voluminous appearance. Any sign of alteration or unnatural appearance will result in a less than satisfactory outcome.

The Aging Neck

Cervical ptosis contributes to the aged, and tired appearance found in patients of all ethnicities. The underlying osseous support of the lower third of the face makes an important contribution to this process. A strong, prominent and square mandible in conjunction with a high placed hyoid bone may support the soft tissues and strengthen favorably the cervicomental angle. Patients with retrognathia and/or type II malocclusion will often have greater visible ptotic cervical changes.

A patient of Hispanic heritage presented with significant lipodystrophy of the neck, and with associated microgenia. She underwent submental, cheek liposuction and chin implant (Figure 7.15, 7.16).

CONCERNS AND COMPLICATIONS

Patients of African American, Mediterranean, and Asian ancestry may present with increased incidence of keloids, hypertrophic scarring and hyperpigmentation.

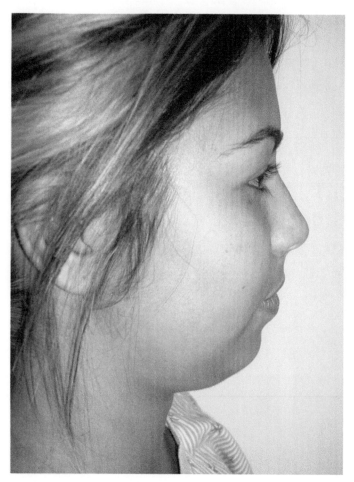

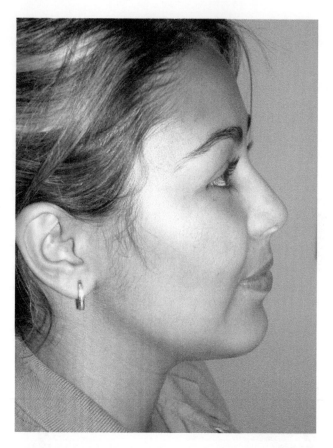

Figure 7.16 Same patient following a chin implant and cervicofacial liposuction.

Figure 7.15 Patient of Hispanic ancestry with significant lipodystrophy of the neck and microgenia.

Keloidal scars can occur in all skin types, but its rate has been shown to be 5–15 times higher in African Americans than in the Caucasian population (12), three times more common in Japanese population, and five times more common in Chinese population.(13)

Patients at risk for developing keloids are best followed closely after any procedures which might put them at risk. Many physicians will start these patients on topical silicone gels or sheeting early in the healing process prophylactically. If they still start to develop in some of the fairer patients, they can be treated with vasculars lasers, such as 532, 585, or 595 nm. Since these wavelengths are also absorbed by melanin, there is a risk of dyschromia and should not be used in patients with Fitzpatrick V or VI skin types. Keloids developing in surgical scars may be treated with serial injections with triamcinolone. These serial injections can cause hypopigmentation or atrophy of the underlying subcutaneous tissues.

Hypertrophic or keloid scarring in facelift scars is more common in African American, Asian, and Mediterranean ancestry patients, even though most will heal without any complications (Figure 7.17). The frequency of hypertrophic scars and keloids may be diminished by minimizing the tension on the skin flap closure.

Laser resurfacing and chemical exfoliation may be complicated by prolonged erythema, hyperpigmentation, dyschromia, infections, scarring, and dermatitis in the multiethnic patient.

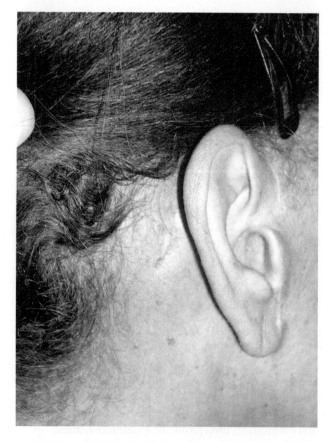

Figure 7.17 Patient of African American ancestry with well healed facelift scars and no evidence of hypertrophic scars or keloids.

Resurfacing in darker skin individuals may produce hyperpigmentation in 17–83% of the cases.(14) Most physicians will not perform traditional resurfacing in Fitzpatrick V and VI patients.

Hyperpigmentation may be treated with retinoic acid, glycolic acids, azelaic acid, hydroquinones, sun block, and possible Jessner's peels (lactic acid 14% and salicylic acid 14%).

Beauty exists in all ethnic and multiethnic faces. The goals of aging face surgery must be directed at refining ethnic features while attaining a natural, balanced, and harmonious result. Analysis of the multiethnic face continues to evolve and therefore cannot be defined with anthropometric analysis. The aging multiethnic face must be understood in three dimensions to assess structural and volumetric changes as well as skin redundancy. Perception of the face and its individual features is unique to each individual. It is important to determine areas of priority, and which procedures stand to be of most benefit. Communication is important in establishing an understanding of cultural differences, realistic expectations, risks and limitations of any treatment or surgery. Surgery may involve combining and incorporating both soft tissue and structural bone augmentation with other conventional surgical procedures such as blepharoplasty, rhytidectomy, and browlift among others.

REFERENCES

1   Projections of the resident population by race, Hispanic origin, and nativity: middle series, 2006-2010. Washington, DC: Population projections program, Population division, US census bureau; 2000.

2   Fanous N, Yoskovitch A. New classification scheme for laser resurfacing and chemical peels, Modification for the different ethnic groups. In: Facial Plastic Surgery Clinics of North America. (10) 2002: 405–13.

3   Romm S. The Search for Perfection. In: The Changing Face of Beauty. Mosby-Yearbook, Inc. 1992: 30.

4   McCurdy E. Human Proportions. In : The Notebooks of Leonardo DaVinci. Konecky & Konecky 207.

5   Gonzales-Ulloa M, Flores E. Senility of the face: Basic study to understand its causes and effects. Plast Reconstr Surg 1965; 36:239–46.

6   Coleman SR. Structural Fat Grafting.St. Louis, Missouri: Quality Medical Publishing, Inc. 2004.

7   Fisher GJ, Wang ZQ et al. Pathophysiology of premature skin aging induced by ultraviolet light. N Engl J Med1997; 337: 1419–428.

8   Kang S, Fisher GJ, Voorhees JJ. Photoaging: pathogenesis, prevention, and treatment. Clin Geriatr Med 2001; 17: 643–59.

9   Herzberg AJ, Dinehart SM. Chronologic aging in black skin. Am J Dermatopath 1989; 11: 319–28.

10 Taylor SC. Skin of color: biology, structure, function, and implications for dermatologic disease. Am J Acad Dermatol 2002; 46: 41–62.

11 FitzpatrickTB. The validity and practicality of sun-reactive skin types I through VI. Arch Dermatol 1988; 124: 869–71.

12 Kamer FM, Pieper PG. Surgical treatment of the aging neck. Facial Plast Surg 2001; 17: 123–28.

13 Levine VJ, Lee MS, Geronemus RG. Continuous wave and quasi continuous wave laser. In Lasers and cutaneous and aesthetic surgery. (Arndt KA, Geronemus RG, Dover JS, Olbrichtd SM, eds.) Lippincott-Raven, 1997: 67–107.

14 McBurneyEI. Clinical usefulness of the argon laser for the 1990's. J Dermatol Surg Oncol 1993; 18: 358–62.

15 Arnold HL, Franer FH. Keloids: Etiology and management by excision and intensive prophylactic radiation. Arch Dermatol 1959; 80: 772.

8 Hispanic facial plastic surgery
Eric T Adler, Stephen C Adler, and Paul J Carniol

As the landscape of North America changes, we are now faced with a growing Hispanic population which according to some is estimated to be 20% by the year 2010.(1) Additionally, Hispanic Beauty has been witnessed in the past 50 years in TV commercials, Soap operas, TV stars, and international beauty pageants (Figure 8.1).

In the past 10 years there are 5 Hispanic winners of the Miss Universe crown.(2) We can find that in its 55-year history over one-third of all winners had Hispanic heritage. There is no doubt that the concept of beauty in the Hispanic culture is seen as one of importance. Review of the medical literature reveals scant information pertaining to treatments and procedures that benefit Hispanic patients.

However, there is a written report of the Afro-American and Middle Eastern Nose (3), as well as laser resurfacing and other cutaneous treatments in the ethnic skin.(4) Much has also been devoted to surgery involving the Asian eyelid.(5) The importance of the Ethnic facial balance has also, in the past decade, been given the attention with aims of avoiding the improper assessment and unnatural appearing results of surgical interventions.(1)

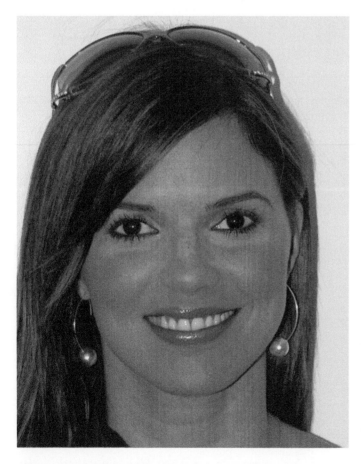

Figure 8.1 The top Cuban model and television show host Rashel Diaz was selected by People en Espanol magazine in 2001 as one of the '25 Most Beautiful Faces in TV'.

WHO IS A LATINO? WHO IS HISPANIC?

To some of us there is a clear distinction, to most, the words Latino and Hispanic have been used interchangeably to describe people who speak Spanish and come from Puerto Rico, Mexico, and Colombia, just to mention a few. The word Latin goes back to Italy, from a region called Latium, whose population spoke the 'Latin' language. With the spread of the Roman Empire, the language served as the base to forming other languages known as the Romance Languages. These include French, Italian, Portuguese, and Spanish. When listening to these languages, there are many similarities in the root of most words in which they differ only by one or two syllables. The term Hispanic is derived from Hispania, the ancient name of the city of Seville, back when the Roman Empire took over the Iberian Peninsula. The name of Hispania later on went to be applied to the peninsula as a whole. After several centuries of living there, the Romans acquired many of the traditions and values that still today characterize this growing sector of our society in America today. The Hispanic society's culture and social ways had definitely been impregnated in this conquering group, originally known as the Latin. Not only was the Spanish language adopted, but also other important things such as family traditions, religion, customs, and even their cooking. The word Hispano is then the name given to the people of the New World countries who got conquered by Spain. This name was then popularized by the US Government and the census to describe the people of Spanish descent. So in summary, a Hispano is a person whose culture, traditions, religion, and language has ties to Spanish influence and comes from the New World.(6)

In essence, Hispanics are an ethnic distinction that may include different races as well as physical traits. Latin America is a place composed of Latin Americans. Not necessarily all Latin are Hispanic like is the case of the people from Brazil were Portuguese, not Spanish is the official language. The bottom line is that it really doesn't matter for the purpose of having success as physicians when dealing with this population, as long as we recognize the culture, their traditions, mannerisms, and that the communication barrier of a different language must not be an excuse in not providing them state-of-the-art assessment and care.

US HISPANICS: WHITE AND NONWHITE HISPANICS

As of 2006, there were close to 44 million Hispanics in the United States. It is estimated that by 2050 there will be more than 100 million Hispanics living in the United States. According to demographic data, the Hispanic population of the United States is mainly concentrated along the Southwest states, Florida, Chicago, and New York. A little more than 50% were considered White Hispanics (Figure 8.2) while less than half are Nonwhite Hispanics (Figure 8.3). 64% of all Hispanics in the United States are Mexicans followed by Puerto Ricans and then Cubans. According to the United States Census Bureau, the concept of breeding between a Meztizo and a White Hispanic/Caucasian or between two Meztizos. Of the three leading groups of Hispanics, Cubans are the largest when it comes to White Hispanics followed by South Americans and then Puerto Ricans.

Hispanic Language: Bridging the Gap

Patient trust and confidence with a physician is an important issue. For the Hispanic patient this is closely linked to optimizing communication. This can be particularly important for the Hispanic patient who may not be fluent in English. It is not only the verbal but also the nonverbal language component that the physician should understand.

Hispanic patients appreciate a physician who is closer in proximity at the time of consultation. Many times the first author sits on the same side of the desk for meeting this requirement. An immediate comfort zone emerges when the patient feels a caring and not distant, easy to talk to and get to physician.

It is important to be tuned to other cues; a period of silence on the patient's part could mean not understanding or even frustration. It is of huge importance to pay attention to the patient's eye contact as well as general body language to be closer in tune with the patient's needs.

As with Caucasian patients the first author suggests avoiding technical talk as well as giving the patient a feeling of baby talk. In verbal communication you must as a provider make an effort to have tools implemented to improve the language barrier such as translators, bilingual staff, internal language banks, phone-based interpreter services or written translators. A cutting-edge national effort by the Robert Wood Johnson foundation is now looking at developing language technology for use in health-care system in emerging Spanish-speaking markets across the country. By bridging the language barrier, the provider will for sure minimize making misdiagnoses and committing medical errors, avoid faults in your informed consents, avoid overusing and/or underusing testing and referrals, minimize patient poor compliance, possibly reduce your patient dissatisfaction rate and mistrust, and overall improve your outcomes as well as minimize malpractice claims. Finally it is wise to recognize differences and similarities from your own culture. For example, Caucasians and/or Americans tend to be more informal but reserved in their initial contacts and relationships in general. On the other hand, Hispanics tend to be more formal on first encounters and usually call people by their last names. In relationships, Hispanics share more about their personal lives and are not afraid to talk about their children, husbands, and family. Anglo-Saxons usually are more reserved regarding their personal lives. Thus with Hispanic patients it is important to bridge any language and cultural gaps.

Hispanic Skin

The type of skin found in the Hispanic patient will vary according to the racial mix of each individual. We can find anywhere from a patient with light skin as is in the European descent Hispanic, or a darker skin complexion Meztizo patient to the darkest of Hispanics which represents the patients with mostly African-Indigenous heritage. By far the most common in Latin America is the Mestizo skin type. This type of skin has a higher melanin content and is thicker than Caucasian skin. Typically, it is more

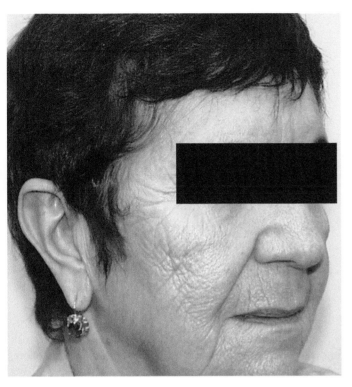

Figure 8.2 Severe elastosis in a White Hispanic, demonstrating problems similar to those seen in White Americans through lifelong sunlight over-exposure.

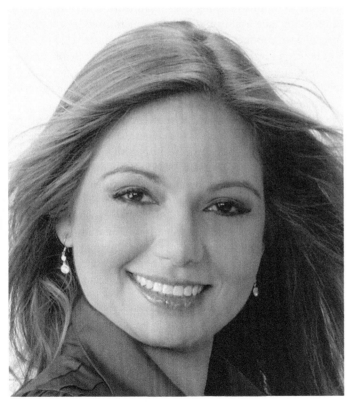

Figure 8.3 A darker complexioned non-white Hispanic.

race and ethnicity are mutually independent. When it comes to White Hispanics, the government agencies consider these as White with ancestries of Spain or any other Spanish-speaking Latin American. Non-white Hispanics are the result of interracial

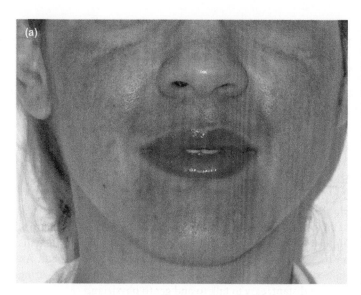
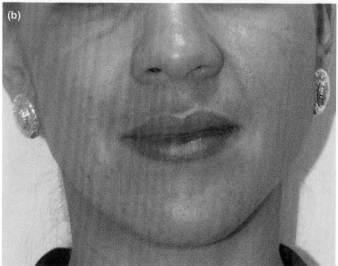

Figure 8.4 Typical Hispanic dyschromia in Type IV Fitzpatrick skin (A) before and (B) after treatment with topical retinoids and glycolic acid formulations.

resistant to photoaging effects. According to comparative studies, darker skin is protected from the environment by its melanin content and therefore visible aging effects are diminished.(7) These patients typically do not present to consultation for Botox and rhytid laser treatments with the frequency as patients with fairer skin.

However, these patients present more frequently for skin care treatments to improve pigmentary disorders such as melasma and postinflammatory hyperpigmentation as well as conditions such as Pseudofolliculitis barbae.

These patients can improve their dyschromias using cautious skin care regimens containing hydroquinone, tretinoin, as well as light chemical peeling such as Jessners or orglycolic peels (Figure 8.4). It is also important to emphasize sun avoidance in combination with strict sun protection.(8)

Another commonly seen condition in the Hispanic patient is hirsutism. When considering all the possible causes, most of them are patients who have no hormonal imbalance Since the advent of hair removal technology from electrolysis to laser, the one that the first author finds most versatile in view of the combination of dark skin with very thick coarse hair is the Diode Laser light technology, which can increase its pulse from 5 to 400 ms. As patients with higher Fitzpatrick skin types are at greater risk for complications and dyschromia with laser treatments, it is important to use test spots before starting treatment.(9) The first author titrates the energy in each and every treatment session, reminding the patient that the goal is reduction and not necessarily full elimination of their unwanted body and/or facial hair.

Pseudofolliculitis is also effectively treated with laser technology. When compared to Caucasian skin, Meztizo Hispanic skin is usually oilier, making this patient more prone to disorders such as acne. Skin care regimens recommended for these patients need to be adjusted to avoid an exacerbation due to creamy, thick topical preparations found in emollients and moisturizers. Frequently, patients present seeking to improve the late sequelae of acne, the varied type of acne scars. Acne scars can be divided into three categories: ice pick, boxcar, and rolling.

Hispanic patients with darker pigmentation are at greater risk for dyschromia with deeper resurfacing procedures.(10) Therefore, the resurfacing treatments of preference to improve these patients include superficial to deep skin abrasion utilizing crystal microdermabrasion, nitrogen plasma resurfacing, and limited old-fashioned diamond fraise dermabrasion. Broader depressed acne scars can be improved using filler treatments. Fillers which may be useful include hyaluronic acid gels, micronized hydroxyappatite, collagen products, and autologous fat transfer (Figure 8.5). Scar revision surgery is reserved for the worst scars. Before undertaking treatment, it is important to bring out early in the consultation period that the goal is to improve and not necessarily eliminate the scar.

Another skin condition that seems to be on the rise in the Hispanic population is skin cancer (Figure 8.6). When compared to Caucasian white, the Hispanic white patient had lower incidence of skin cancer, however the latter group being diagnosed at more advanced stages. According to the study at University of Miami published in *Archives of Dermatology* August 2007 (11), this finding had to do with the decreased awareness of white Hispanics on skin cancer and self skin examinations. The study also showed that white Hispanics are twice as likely not to use sunscreen when compared to Caucasians. In contrast to Caucasian patients, the non-white Hispanic usually presents with more advanced staged skin cancers including Melanoma.

Other skin diseases that affect the Hispanic population more often are actinic prurigo, Hermansky-Pudlak Syndrome and Kindler's syndrome, balanitis xerotic obliterans, and acanthosis nigricans.(1, 2) Further discussion of the treatment of these conditions is beyond the scope of this text.

Hispanic Eyes/Eyebrows

If there is anything about the Hispanic people that is really different, it is their ability to communicate just with their eyes. The expression of the Hispanic eye is not only part of the body language, but is also part of the culture. When it comes to Hispanic

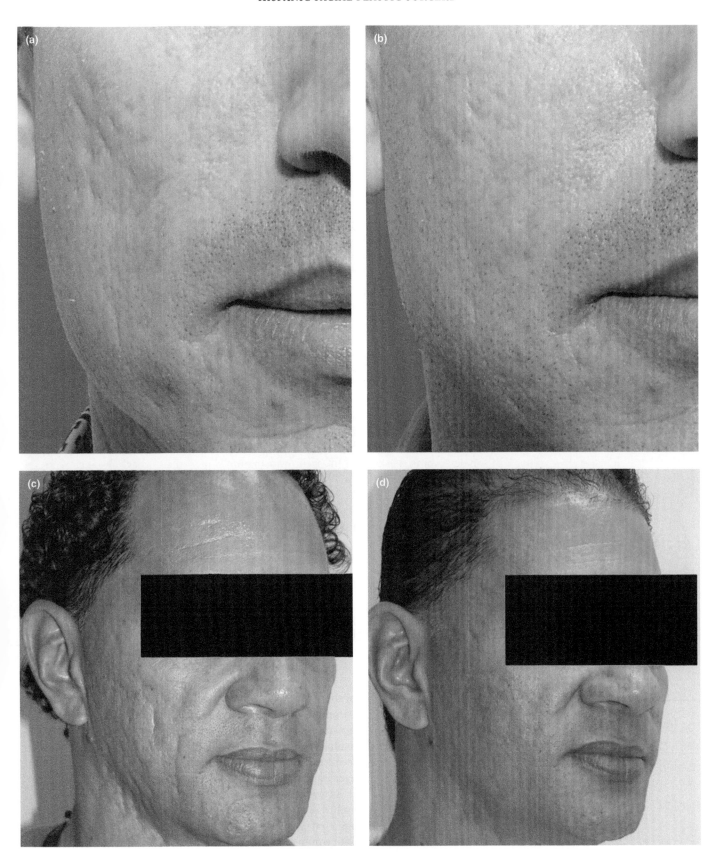

Figure 8.5 (A)Severe acne scarring as a result of nodular/cystic acne commonly seen in highly sebaceous Hispanic skin. (B) Treatment result using micronized hydroxiapatite filler (C) Ice pick acne scar (D) Ice pick acne scar treatment result using hyaluronic acid based filler and skin resurfacing.

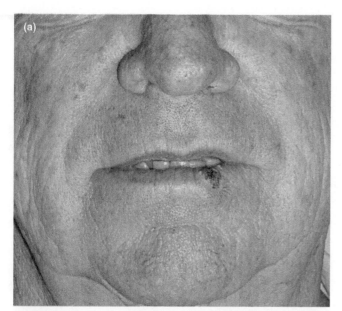

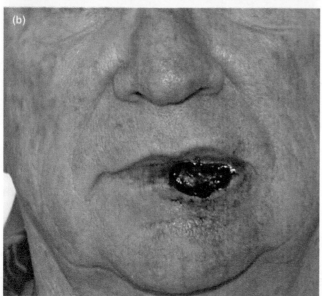

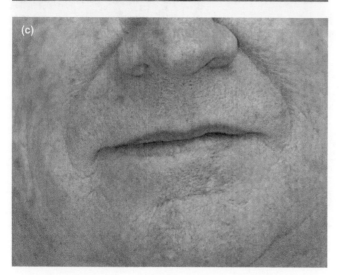

Figure 8.6 Skin cancer is increasing in incidence in Hispanics mostly of whiter skin. This case demonstrates (A) lower lip squamous cell carcinoma, (B) treated with Moh's excision and M plasty reconstruction.

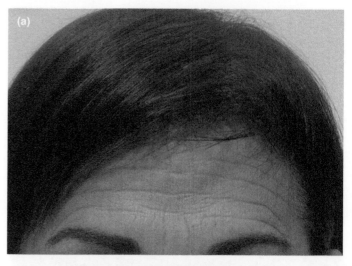

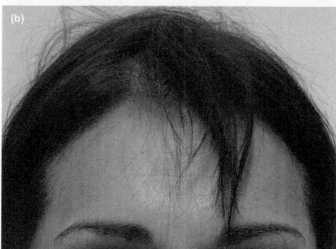

Figure 8.7 Neuromodulators are commonly used in cosmetic surgery practices to improve facial animation rhytids, as seen in the forehead of this dark skin Hispanic (A) before and (B) after treatment.

patients presenting for the evaluation of their aging face, the eyelids and brows are an important concern. Most Hispanics have darker and thicker skin including the eyelids.

In patients of Hispanic heritage who have lived in the tropics with extensive sun exposure, you can begin to see a descent of the eyebrow as early as 30 years of age. These patients usually present also with the classic glabellar rhytids from the constant frowning with hyperactive corrugator, procerus and orbicularis oculi muscles. Botulinum toxin (Botox® Allergan)-assisted upper face rejuvenation is a very popular procedure in young to middle-aged patients in my practice (Figure 8.7).

As with other ethnic groups, Hispanic patients can have ptotic eyebrows and thick infrabrow skin with a classical hooding and aging effect. This type of pseudodermatochalasis is best treated with combined brow and eyelifting.

The desired brow position is usually obtained by manually elevating the fallen brow and obtaining the highest point of the arch at the lateral limbus. Photographs of patients at earlier age can assist in deciding the level of elevation for each patient.

The first author prefers endoscopic brow lift for both males and females (Figure 8.8). In the evaluation it is also important to

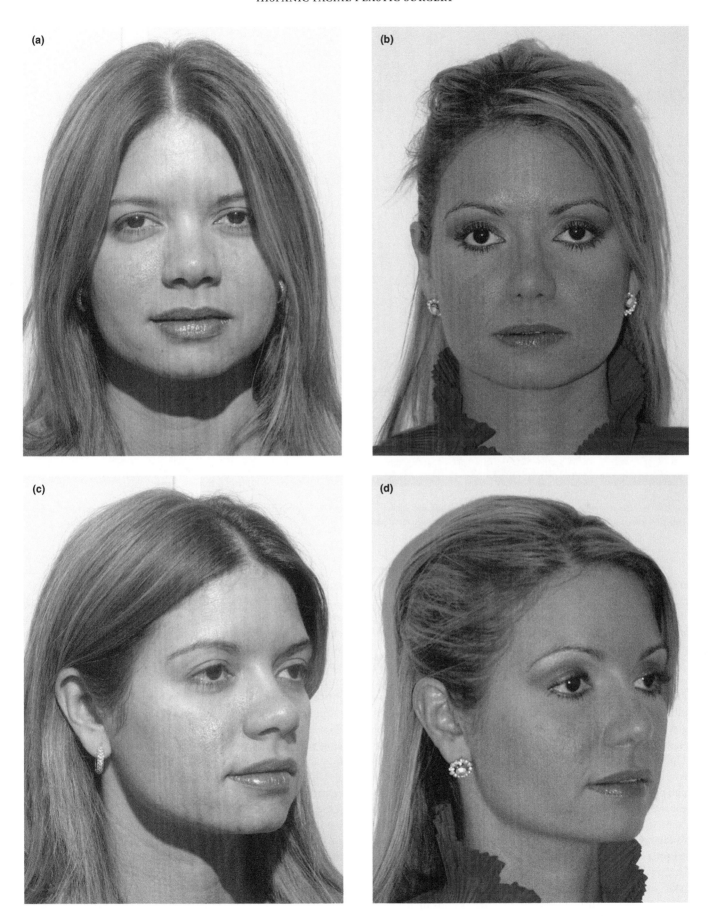

Figure 8.8 (A) Brow ptosis in 35-year-old Hispanic patient. (B) Endoscopic brow lift improving mild pseudo upper eyelid laxity. Simultaneous Latino rhinoplasty result. (C) Preoperative oblique view. (D) Postoperative oblique view: result of endoscopic brow lift and rhinoplasty.

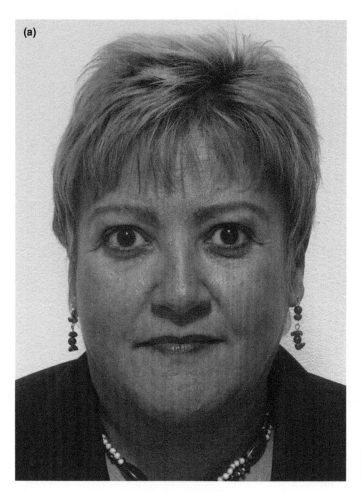
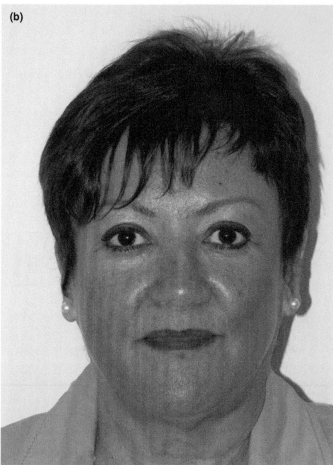

Figure 8.9 (A) Hispanic patient demonstrating severe brow ptosis and upper eyelid laxity. (B) Postoperative result after endoscopic brow lift and upper blepharoplasty. Of benefit is also the 35-lb weight loss postoperatively in a highly motivated patient.

note any lost volume at the level of the eyebrow. In this situation you may successfully rejuvenate mild brow laxity, and ptosis using facial fillers. This is currently an FDA off label use of fillers and as for all procedures the associated risks should be considered. Combined soft tissue augmentation with brow lifting is reserved for the most severe cases.

For males with high hair line and/or alopecia the first author prefers to utilize indirect forehead skin excisions placed on marked rhytids (see Figure 8.10) It is important to perform meticulous multilayer minimal tension closure to try to minimize the resulting scar. However, even with this there may still be a noticeable scar.

Upper eyelid laxity and/or redundant skin is treated with the classic blepharoplasty (Figure 8.9). The first author has found that a high percentage of Hispanic middle-aged patients due to excessive eyebrow plucking are left with no brow hair. Many of these patients present with improper tattoo brows, in unusually high position. This can create a deceptive impression of what appears to be excessive upper eyelid skin to be resected. Care should be taken to consider this when planning upper eyelid blepharoplasty. The degree of skin excision will determine the end result upper blepharoplasty scar which is usually poor in the event of advancing thick infrabrow skin to the eyelid itself. The improperly positioned tattooed brow may appear exaggeratedly elevated if routine brow

lifting is performed. Tattoo removal and repositioning is one recommendation for this selected group of patients.

Lower eyelid fat pseudoherniation with dermatochalasis can be treated with transconjunctival blepharoplasty and skin resurfacing. If orbicularis oculi muscle hypertrophy and/or severe laxity are noted, it is best to perform a subciliary lower blepharoplasty with or without lateral canthal tightening for best results. In cases of eyelid dyschromia, fractionated lasers or light resurfacing may be helpful in lightening the discoloration to some extent.(11)

However, it should be remembered that with healing, resurfacing patients can develop hyperpigmentation. In general this tendency increases with higher Fitzpatrick skin type (8A-D). (10) This pigmentation may also benefit from fractionated laser treatments.

One final note that must be considered is that many Hispanics are not aware of eye conditions that could affect them. A study by the American Academy of Ophthalmology has noted that Hispanics and blacks carry a threefold risk of developing glaucoma. The study also revealed that more than two-thirds of these patients are unaware of having an eye condition. Another study published in July 2008 from the Wilmer Eye Institute at Johns Hopkins University demonstrated diminished eye care and examinations in the Hispanic diabetic patient.(12) The main reason was

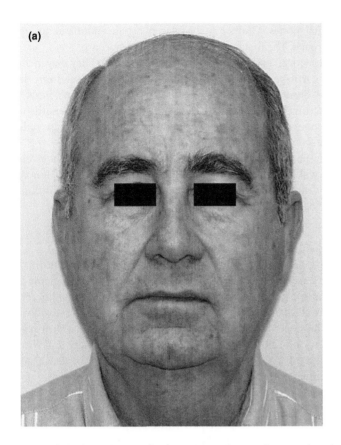 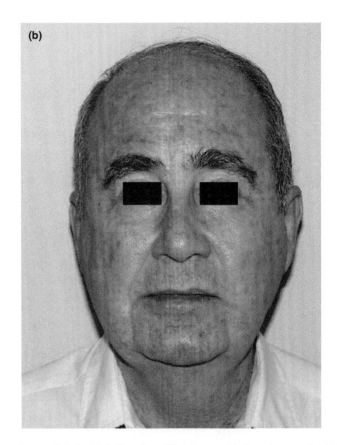

Figure 8.10 (A) White Hispanic of Cuban origin with severe brow ptosis and upper dermatochalasis. (B) Indirect brow lift and upper blepharoplasty result with excellent forehead scar result. White type of skin is ideal in the selection for indirect and direct brow lifting skin excisions.

attributed to a lack of education as well as a cultural-language communication gap. Other conditions such as heart disease, diabetes, and hypertension are also noted to affect these populations at higher rates. The reason the majority of Hispanics are unaware of being affected by any disease is that many of them have no medical insurance and thus unlikely to have routine preventive medicine checkups.

Hispanic Nose

In a 2002 study by the American Society of Plastic Surgery, 7% of all cosmetic surgeries involved members of the American Hispanic community. Rhinoplasty was the number one procedure performed in this growing group.

The concept of the ethnic nose goes back to the beginning of the century. In 1913, Schultz first described ethnic rhinoplasty when referring to the African-American patients undergoing surgery to change one or more aspects of their nose.

Although all of these may have similarities, most are considered different due to the large genetic pool from which they derive. In review of the literature, JP Porter (12) describes the Hispanic nose as one of soft tissue excess, shortened columella with poor tip projection, short middle third due to vertically oriented lower lateral cartilages, and an obtuse nasal root slope, thus requiring dorsal augmentation rather than osteotomizing to refine a somewhat acute nasolabial angle.

In the non-Caucasian hispanic nose, there are frequent variations of broad, flattened dorsum with poorly defined, wide and projected nasal tips with abundant and thick skin. The extent in

the expression of these traits will vary from one patient to the other, even among siblings. In 2003 a simplified classification system of the Hispanic nose by Rollin Daniel described three types of noses (13).

Type I, the Castilian nose consists of a high bridge and dorsal hump with normal tip projection. Type II or the Mexican American was seen as a low radix, normal bridge with poorly defined nasal tip. Type III is the Meztizo nose which has a low bridge, low radix, and a poorly projected broad nasal tip. This type of nose shares many features with the African-American noses.

Before examining each patient it is important to have them express their motivation and expectations before undergoing any type of procedure. Many of these patients will have inadequate tip support. As such it is important to carefully evaluate this region. The first author has found that observation at rest and during inhalation is helpful with assessing the strength of the underlying cartilage. Palpation of the nose is also helpful in determining cartilage integrity as well as soft tissue thickness. Many rhinoplasty surgeons have found that the maneuver of gently depressing the nasal tip is helpful in assessing tip support. Furthermore it is important to evaluate changes in the nasal tip with smiling.

The goals of surgery should be discussed and agreed to by the patient before undertaking the procedure. Many patients will want to preserve their ethnic heritage characteristics while refining some of the features. As many of the patients will have thicker skin, soft tissue surgery frequently involves the use of cartilage grafts. Limited soft tissue resection under open approach with care to preserve the

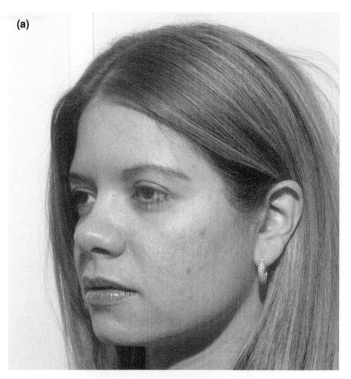

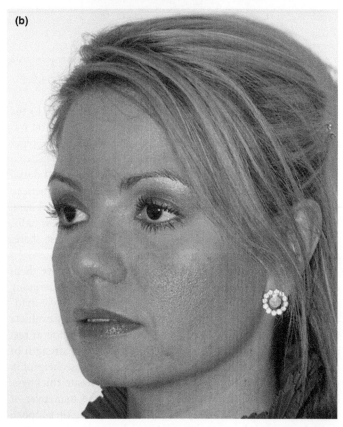

Figure 8.11 (A) A typical Hispanic nose reveals a bulbous tip with thick skin and low radix. (B) Postoperative Latino rhinoplasty with tip refinement and dorsal augmentation/refinement to create a balanced nose.

subdermal plexus can also benefit these patients in obtaining Nasal Tip/alar refinement. For most patients these grafts can be obtained from the nasal septum or conchal region of the ear. If larger dorsal grafts are needed these can be fashioned from rib cartilage or

cranial bones. Grafts can be placed by an endonasal or open approach. The first author favors an open approach.

As with all patients, nasal tip procedures vary. They may include alar cartilage reduction, tip grafts, struts, and vertical dome division. Some patients will benefit from subcutaneous nasal tip "defatting." Other patients will benefit from nasal lengthening procedures including oversized spreader grafts. Alar base reduction is reserved for extreme cases of wide nasal base.

As patients who present with thick or poorly defined nasal tips will only obtain limited improvement with surgery, it is very important to downplay the potential for nasal tip definition as part of the preoperative discussions. See Figures 8.11–14.

Hispanic Lips

Hispanic people are frequently characterized for having normal to above average sized lips. From Hollywood stars to the patients that come into our practices, we can see the contribution of voluminous and well-defined lips that makes them look sensual and exotic.

The singer Shakira and actress Jennifer Lopez are a clear representation of how important lips are in the sensuality and youthfulness of a face. The actor Antonio Banderas is also a good example of the Hispanic male's average lip form and size.

When it comes to lips, the non-white Hispanic patient usually has more than adequate red lip volume with all different shapes. The aging of the typical non-white Hispanic lips and perioral region includes most of the features noted in the white Hispanic. Thinning and elongation of the upper lip and vermillion, flattening of the philtral architecture, and ptosis of the lower lip are accompanied by the effects of aging dentition. Ultimately these changes are responsible for the aged smile with decreased upper incisor show and lateral commisure downturning. In addition in the fairer skinned patient, more so than in the non-white hispanic, we can see vertical rhytids adjacent to both the upper and lower lips which are exacerbated by pursing of the lips.

In non-white Hispanics who present with oversized lips, reduction cheiloplasties are most commonly requested. Conservative reduction of red lip volume can safely be accomplished through wet line hidden incisions with a slight overcorrection in the reduction excision of the lip skin and subcutaneous tissue. Limited flaps are developed internally as well as externally before the removal of excess lip tissue. Careful tissue approximation using buried fast-absorbing vicryl, or monocyl suture (Ethicon, Sommerville, New Jersey) and 6.0 silk, or monofilament suture to evert the skin are in most cases going to result in excellent scar result.

Fairer skinned Hispanics present for consultation with similar complaints to other Caucasians. As these patients usually have thinner lips in contrast to many of the people in Latin America, they frequently seek lip enhancement and/or enlargement procedures (Figures 8.15–17). Injectable fillers, autologous fat transfer as well as lip lift/advancement procedures can be considered. For any lip lift/advancement procedures the possibility of visible scarring should be considered and discussed.

Additionally, procedures including lasers, dermabrasion, and chemical peels have been helpful in this population seeking to improve the aging signs of the perioral region. Selective injection of fillers can be used to elevate the lateral commisures. In patients with severe lateral oral commisure downturning, commisure

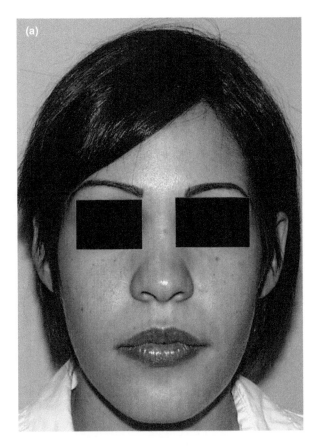

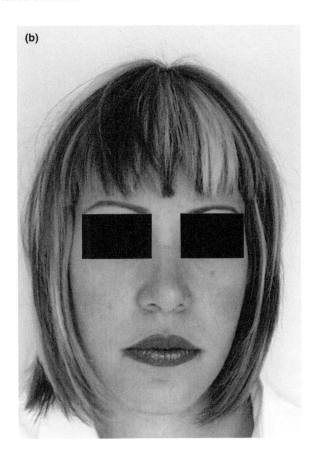

Figure 8.12 (A) Hispanic nose with bulbous and wide nasal tip. (B) Postoperative Latino rhinoplasty with tip refinement-skin thinning/alar base reduction/dorsal augmentation.

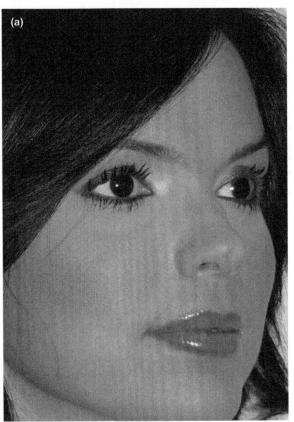

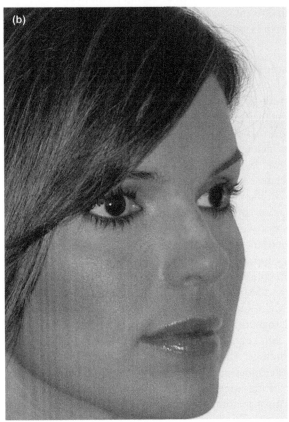

Figure 8.13 (A) Hispanic nose revealing flat dorsal irregularity and bifid asymmetric nasal tip. (B) Latino rhinoplasty to smoothen dorsum and soften sharp irregular nasal tip.

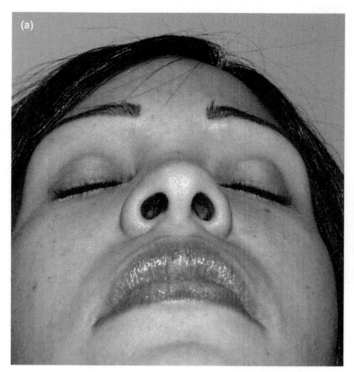
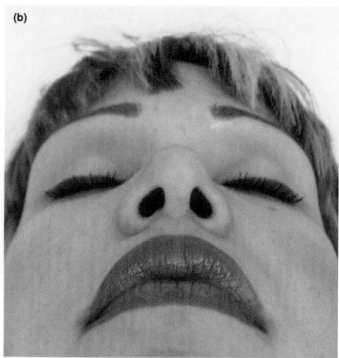

Figure 8.14 (A) The nose basal view demonstrates a classic Hispanic bulbous, ill-defined and broad nasal tip. (B) Postoperative photograph after open rhinoplasty to define, project, and narrow the nasal tip.

surgical commisure lifts with vermillion and lip skin excisions can be performed. Limited Botox injections to address Depressor Anguli Oris muscle are also commonly used to minimize melolabial grooves as well as enhance the patients' smile.

Hispanic Face/Neck

When looking at the non-white Hispanic face and neck laxity, there are several considerations that must be taken into consideration. Many of these patients have in the first place thicker oilier skin with minimal rhytids. The subcutaneous fatty layer varies with multiple factors including weight, body fat content, and individual genetics. The lower face can demonstrate prominent nasolabial fold due to excess fatty subcutaneous tissue and cheek ptosis.

According to comparative cephalometric analysis of Hispanics and Caucasians(15) we can see a higher incidence of bimaxillary protrusion which tends to exacerbate the nasolabial fold. Maximal benefit of the nasolabial folds may be accomplished if multidisciplinary approach takes place. Example includes premolar extraction in combination with orthodontics, nasolabial conservative filler, and SMAS or deep plane facelifting. There is also a prominent Melolabial fold that may be accompanied by some degree of micrognathia. These patients if properly selected will benefit from chin augmentation procedures according to the preoperative findings. Alloplastic implants, mandibular and/or imabxillary ostetomies in combination with sliding genioplasty, as well as facelifting surgery may all be considered to correct the patient in the most anatomic and natural way (Figure 8.18). Hispanics can also present with short neck and low and an anteriorly lying hyoid bone. It is important to discuss with the patients first the limitations of obtaining neck definition. Aggressive neck liposuction and

or lipectomy as well as platysmaplasty is going to produce the best results for these difficult neck patients.

Gore-Tex® sling-assisted neck lifting has been used in our practices with limited success (Figure 8.19). Complications of this procedure include neck discomfort, skin retraction, and implant marking, and need to re-suspend in touch-up procedures due to the elastic properties of the implant. It is important when discussing facelifting surgery with the Hispanic patient to include the motivation and realistic expectations of the procedure, the recovery, the likely need for tuck-ups due to the thicker tissues and/or excessive laxity in the case of an older patient more or less >60 years of age. Preoperative and postoperative standardized photography will be the best tool to demonstrate the level of improvement obtained. Hispanic patients tend to be overly sensitive to external comments and opinions. In many cases, this can have a negative effect on the level of satisfaction by the patient from the procedure's results.

Hispanic Noninvasive Trends

A remarkable trend that has not spared the Hispanic population seeking to improve their appearance is the increase in the injectable procedures being done to them. They too have discovered the powerful and simplified way of rejuvenation through the noninvasive ways of fillers and Botox®. There has been on average a 300% increase in these procedures in the past 2 years in the author's experience. Even though this practice is located in San Juan, PR, there is vast information in recent surveys attesting to the high numbers of Hispanics seeking to improve their appearance in the mainland. According to AAFPRS 2007 survey, Hispanics are the highest minority group undergoing plastic surgery procedures. In my opinion, non-white Hispanics benefit more from resistant

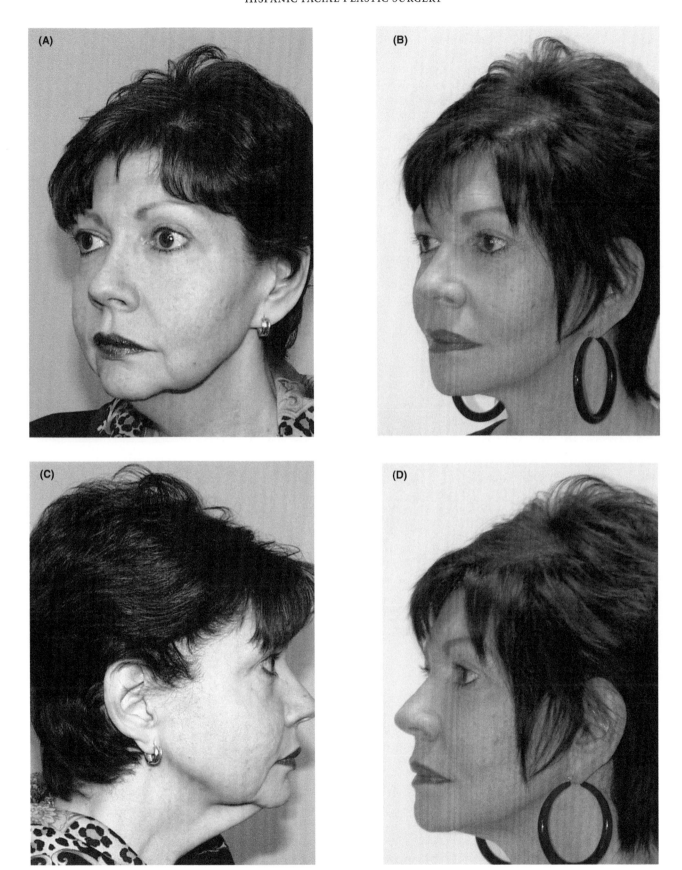

Figure 8.15 (A) Moderate to severe Cervicofacial Ptosis in 60 year old Hispanic female. (B) 5 year Postoperative result after Rhytidoplasty and Chin Augmentation and Goretex Sling Assited Neck Lift. (C) Severe Neck Laxity in same patient. (D) Marked improvement in Cervicofacial Angle.

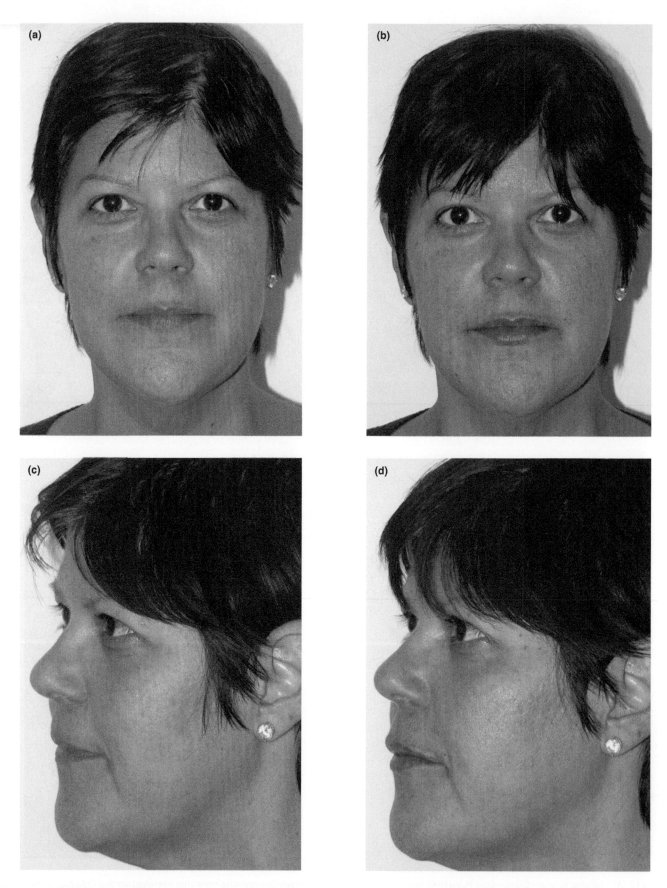

Figure 8.16 (A) Middle-aged Hispanic female patient requested lip enhancement. (B) Postinjection of upper and lower lips with 1.0 ml hyaluronic acid-based filler. (C) Preinjection lateral view. (D) Postinjection lateral view demonstrates improved definition and projection of vermillion and body of both lips.

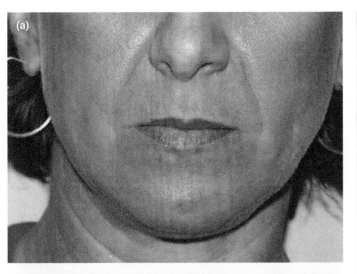

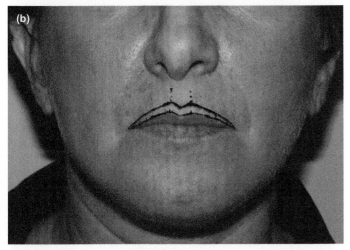

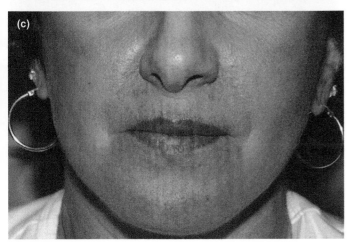

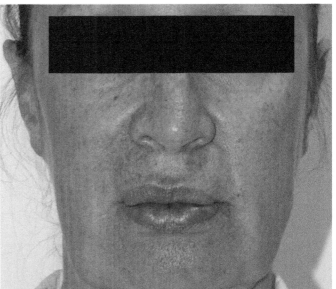

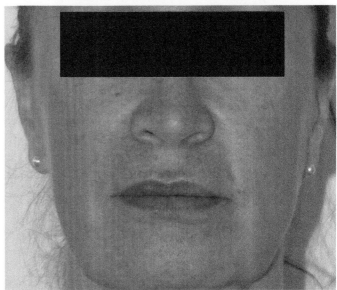

Figure 8.18 (A) Biopoyimer/silicone filler with unpleasant lip morphology (B) Postoperative: lip filler was removed and lips reconstructed through wet line incisions.

Examples of Botox® and filler treatments are illustrated above. On the other hand, these patients who present with their thicker skin and moderate to severe rhytids do require on the average 10-20% more Botox® than if treating a fair-skinned individual to obtain satisfactory results. The thicker skin and probably somewhat hypertrophic muscles are the main reason for this.

HISPANIC FACIAL PLASTIC SURGERY CONCLUSIONS

The Hispanic population is presently the biggest minority group in the United States as of now. By 2050, some experts attest that 50% of the US population will be Spanish speaking. Hispanics are likely to become an important demographic in the patients that solicit plastic surgery in our offices. In a study conducted by the American Society of Plastic Surgeons, there were more than half a million plastic surgery procedures in Hispanics in 2004. According to this

Figure 8.17 (A) Hispanic female with thin upper lip and marked nasolabial creases (B) Prelip advancement upper lip outline, approximately 4-5 mm in width. (C) Postlip advancement result.

fillers consisting of calcium hydroxyapatite microspheres due to their thicker and oilier skin. Their skin in particular allows for the material to be injected in a more superficial fashion, thus imparting superior correction for a variety of rhytids. Other fillers composed of hyaluronic acid are also deemed helpful as part of the overall filler needs of white and non-white Hispanics.

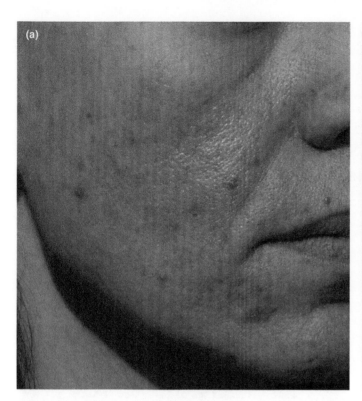
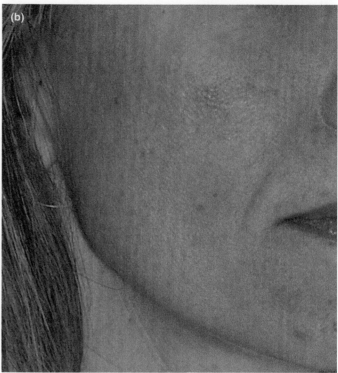

Figure 8.19 (A) Hispanic female seeking improvement of cheek ptosis and associated nasolabial fold/crease. (B) Notice the cheek-lifting effect as well as the nasolabial fold correction achieved by the use of Radiesse® filler.

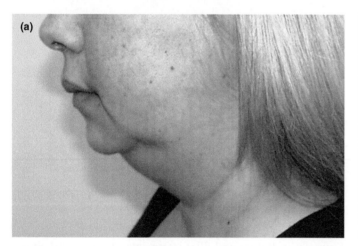
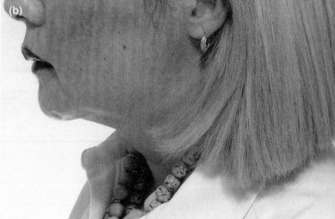

Figure 8.20 (A) Micrognathia in a 38-year-old Hispanic female. (B) Postoperative photograph after neck liposuction and assisted Gore-tex sling suspension in addition to alloplastic chin augmentation.

study, this number represents a 50% increase from 2000 as well as 6% of all plastic surgery procedures practiced in the United States. The number one procedure in the Hispanic as well as the African-American patient was rhinoplasty. Botox and the wrinkle-fighting fillers were among the most common noninvasive procedures performed. In a recent survey by the American Academy of Facial Plastic & Reconstructive surgery, 89% of the surgeons predict cosmetic surgery will increase for ethnic populations. Understanding their motivations, their mentality, their culture, knowing proficiently their language, their driving internal forces and what procedures are likely to help them is a must if a physician wants to be involved with this growing sector of our patient population. While

many differences exist in this varied ethnic race, the Hispanic patient will most likely also benefit from the same procedures that Caucasians do. With an understanding of some of the differences when it comes to their physical findings, knowing important information about their culture, and attempting to minimize any communication gap, you as a physician are likely going to be seeing and treating a large number of Hispanics in the years to come.

REFERENCES

1. Balanitis Xerotica Obliterans: Epidemiologic Distribution in an Equal Access Health Care System. Kizer WS, Prarie T, Morey AF. South Med J. 2003;96(1):9-11.

2. Acanthosis Nigricans and Insulin Resistance. www.infocusonline.org/acanthosis

3. J. Porter. Non-Caucasian rhinoplasty: preoperative analysis. Facial Plast Surg Clin North Am 2003; 11(3): 327–33.

4. Jackson BA; Facial Plast Surg Clin N Am 2002; 10: 397–404.

5. McCurdy JA; Facial Plast Surg Clin N Am 2002; 10: 351–68.

6. Logan John, R., How Race Counts for Hispanic Americans., Lewis Mumford Center for Comparative Urban and Regional Research, University at Albany, Business Administration B-10, Albany, NY, Non-Journal, 2003-07-14.

7. Kaidbe KH, Agin PP, Sayre RM et al. Photoprotection by melanin- a comparison of black and Caucasian skin. Am J Acad Dermatol 1979; 1: 249–60.

8. West TB, Alster TS. Effect of pretreatment on the incidence of hyperpigmentation following cutaneous CO2 laser resurfacing. Dermatol Surg 1999; 25(1): 15–7.

9. Fitzpatrick TB. The validity and practicality of sun-reactive skin types I through VI. Arch Dermatol 1988; 124(6): 869–71.

10. Fitzpatrick RA. Facial resurfacing with the pulsed carbon dioxide laser. A review. Facial Plast Surg Clin North Am 1996; 4(2): 236.

11. West TB, Alster TS. Improvement of infraorbital hyperpigmentation following carbon dioxide laser resurfacing. Dermatol Surg 1998; 24(6): 615–6.

12. Munoz B, O'Leary M, Fonseca-Becker F et al. Knowledge of diabetic eye disease and vision care guidelines among Hispanic individuals in Baltimore with and without diabetes. Arch Ophth 2008; 126(7): 968–74.

13. Daniel R. Hispanic rhinoplasty in the United States, with emphasis on the Mexican American nose. Plastic and Reconstructive Surg 2003; 112: 244–56.

14. Hispanics-Latinos, diverse people in a multicultural society : a special report.,Washington, DC : National Association of Hispanic Publications : U.S. Bureau of the Census, Periodical.

15. Milgrim LM, Larson W, Cohen AF. Anthropometric analysis of the female latino nose: revised aesthetic concepts and their surgical implications. Arch Otolaryngol Head & Neck Surg 1996; 122: 1079–86.

9 Aesthetic rejuvenation for Asian patients
Samuel M Lam

INTRODUCTION

Rejuvenation of the aging Asian face mandates a unique set of strategies that include understanding the cultural aspects of the Asian patient, the anatomy of the Asian patient, and the techniques that would be appropriate based on these cultural and anatomic considerations. Oftentimes, the Western surgeon becomes easily frustrated by the perceived enigma of the Asian patient because the surgeon applies the same aesthetic standards as for a Western patient or, alternatively, the surgeon is relatively indifferent/ignorant to the cultural biases that may inform a patient's decision to undergo cosmetic enhancement. These issues will be explored in depth in this chapter and hopefully the reader will thereby gain better insight and sensitivity.

The specific surgical strategies will be divided into the management of the aging Asian eyelid and then the broader subject of the Asian face. The reason for this division is that the aging Asian eyelid is one of the most complicated topics that require both mastery of a unique surgical technique (supratarsal crease formation) and cultural sensitivity to the proper upper eyelid crease shape and height. This chapter will focus primarily on surgical but also mention dermatological intervention for the aging Asian face. Furthermore, although surgical technique will be briefly discussed, this chapter primarily attempts to outline a philosophical strategy toward management of the aging Asian face.

CULTURAL ISSUES

Oftentimes, the Asian patient seeking cosmetic facial enhancement has a separate layered agenda beyond simply desiring aesthetic improvement. Cultural and folkloric beliefs may not be overtly expressed but should be gently investigated to ensure patient satisfaction following a procedure. For example, Asians at times desire creation of a dimple on their face because it may be thought to increase fertility or the prospect of marriage. A larger nose through augmentation rhinoplasty may only be desired because of its association with greater wealth or the chance of obtaining it. That is also why reduction otoplasty may be less common in the Far East, as large ears are thought to be a sign of wealth and wisdom. Asian patients can be very obsessed with unblemished skin, as a sign of beauty and also of good fortune. Whereas freckles may be deemed attractive in the West, Asians in general want porcelain, untainted skin. Fortunately for many Asians, besides a predisposition toward less aging than their Caucasian counterpart, they actively avoid the sun to maintain their spotless skin, which in turn helps to limit photoaging.

Asians can also be much more secretive about undergoing plastic surgery than Caucasians, especially if the Asian has only recently immigrated to the West. Although HIPAA (Health Insurance Portability and Accountability Act) rules apply universally, the surgeon should be particularly circumspect when talking with any family member or friend regarding an Asian patient's surgery. Asian patients can also tend to be more negative of each other following cosmetic surgery, and the surgeon should prepare one's patient for this possibility. Certain negative remarks by family members or social peers may be made to the patient due to the less socially acceptable nature of plastic surgery as compared to its more recently accepted position in the reality-television-dominated West.

Another trend to consider is an increasing convergence of standards of beauty today given the global images of Western beauty that permeate Asia as well as the ubiquitous use of models of mixed racial heritage. Despite these trends, Asians who live abroad or even those who reside in the West are primarily concerned about preservation of ethnicity following cosmetic facial surgery. Eyelid creases that appear too high or noses that are raised to a profile equal to a Caucasian nose may not only be unacceptable to the Asian patient but also to the surgeon striving to achieve ethnically appropriate and natural appearing results. Although augmentation rhinoplasty falls beyond the scope of this chapter, maintaining a natural eyelid crease following rejuvenative blepharoplasty lies at the core of this chapter and will be discussed in the following section.

Despite some of these cultural similarities among Asians, there are also very distinct differences that exist between nationalities. For example, the Vietnamese and Koreans are more predisposed toward having cosmetic enhancement. The Chinese are only now becoming enamored with cosmetic surgery given their recent newfound wealth in a surging Chinese economy (and given its illegal status before 1979 in China). Even Asians who have immigrated from the Far East carry these cultural biases for or against plastic surgery from their native country. Second- or third-generation Asian Americans may begin to shake some of these longstanding cultural biases as they assume more of a Western perception toward plastic surgery and toward life in general.

Also, some of these second- or third-generation Asian Americans who are more likely inclined toward marrying someone of a different race may desire cosmetic enhancement for an entirely different reason: to look more like their spouse. Interestingly, many Caucasians who wed Asians choose Asians who look more ethnic because they are attracted to those ethnic features, whereas Asians who marry Caucasians may want to blunt those features to be more accepted into their spouse's culture.

Delving into the underlying motivation for cosmetic surgery beyond merely improving one's aesthetic appearance can be a fundamental aspect to dealing with the Asian patient. Cultural biases may be overt or unspoken but should be investigated as appropriate during cosmetic consultation with a prospective Asian patient.

STRATEGIES FOR THE AGING ASIAN EYELID

In general, with the advent of fat grafting for periorbital rejuvenation, a trend of using a person's old photographs as a blueprint for rejuvenation has become in vogue. Oftentimes, brows that appear to have fallen and extra skin (dermatochalasis) that develops may in large part be due to volumetric loss of fat and soft tissue around the eyes. According to this author, traditional eyelid and brow surgery performed in isolation can alter a person's identity in a fundamental and irrevocable manner. Most young women (not all) have a very low eyelid crease and relatively low brow position but the shape and contour of that brow and eyelid are typically very full. Traditional brow and eyelid surgery—which are at heart reductive in nature—both serve to rejuvenate by cutting or lifting, which in turn ultimately increases the distance between the ciliary margin and the supratarsal crease. What's interesting is that a high-arched supratarsal crease *can* exist in the Caucasian race but generally is quite rare to find in the Asian race. This author believes that converting a Caucasian woman from a low crease to a high crease through browlift and eyelid surgery without fat grafting still unfavorably alters a white woman from her true identity in youth. However, like Nicole Kidman, some white women can be born with a high eyelid crease. Therefore, the result of reductive periorbital surgery can still look natural. This is not the case when it comes to Asians or how Asians perceive their own face after cosmetic surgery. One of the most important attributes of the Asian eyelid is the relatively low crease structure that exists in almost all Asians of any age. The alternative to this shape would obviously be an Asian who does not possess an eyelid crease at all. It is the contention then that simply cutting away skin and performing a browlift can adversely lift an eyelid crease in an Asian until it looks glaringly unnatural. Other considerations are also important. How do you manage an Asian without a natural crease who wants to have eyelid and brow rejuvenation? Or, how do you manage an Asian patient who already had previous eyelid crease formation? Is there a different strategy? This section will elaborate a strategy that combines both cultural sensitivity and surgical judgment to approach an Asian patient for eyelid rejuvenation by classifying that individual into one of three categories: Asians with a natural eyelid crease, Asians without a crease, Asians who have had an eyelid crease surgically fashioned in the past.

Asians with a natural crease

Perhaps this category seems unnecessary to deal with since the surgical technique is exactly the same as that for an occidental patient. However, as indicated in the opening remarks, raising an eyelid crease beyond 1–2 mm above the ciliary margin through reductive eyelid and brow surgery ultimately can render an Asian face unnatural in appearance. Maintaining eyelid crease position should be underscored as a fundamentally important objective with every endeavor. The way that this author maintains eyelid crease position is to avoid browlifts in almost every case and to maintain or decrease eyelid position by using fat grafting in the upper eyelid and along the brow. Fat transfer to the upper eyelid/brow complex will actually reduce the height of the eyelid crease rather than raise the eyelid crease, as traditional blepharoplasty would do (Figure 9.1). If the eyelid skin rests along the ciliary margin, it is recommended to remove a little bit of skin (but typically no fat) from the upper eyelid, usually about 2–3 mm in height of skin removal along with fat grafting to reduce and thereby maintain eyelid crease position. If the eyelid crease

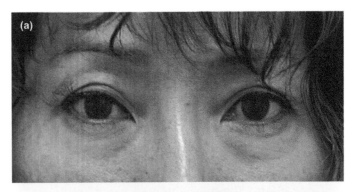
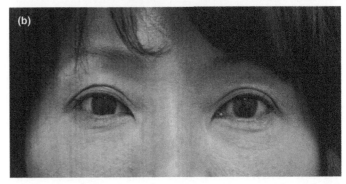

Figure 9.1 This Korean patient underwent periorbital fat transfer to the brow, upper eyelid, and lower eyelid and is shown before (A) and after (B) this procedure. As can be noted, this individual was born with an upper eyelid crease that would have looked worse if raised through traditional blepharoplasty and browlift procedure. Instead, fat transfer has maintained if not slightly decreased her eyelid crease height.

is 1 mm or greater above the ciliary margin, removal of skin is unnecessary (and counterproductive) and fat transfer alone is used. If the crease is much higher than 1–2 mm, additional fat can be used to lower the crease further. Traditionally, 1–2 mm of fat is transferred to the brow and upper eyelid depending on the degree of brow and upper eyelid deflation as well as crease position. Looking at a patient's old photographs and discussing in detail with a patient his or her desired changes should frame each aesthetic consultation as it pertains to upper eyelid rejuvenation in the Asian patient.

Asians without a crease

The patient who does not have a natural crease presents a much more complicated topic. Oftentimes, the absence of a fold already makes the eyes look narrower so any brow and upper eyelid deflation can lead to a very narrow palpebral fissure that is both aging and unaesthetic. Many surgeons simply decide an arbitrary height at which to remove skin without reference to thinking about the crease. This is problematic for two reasons. First, arbitrary removal of skin without crease fixation can leave behind a visible scar (even if placed right above the ciliary margin) since there is no crease to hide it. Second, the already narrow palpebral fissure will not be significantly altered by skin removal without attention to the postseptal fat. Even if the patient has been used to a narrow palpebral fissure all of his or her life, the patient expects a sufficient opening of the eyelid to have made the cosmetic endeavor worthwhile. This is difficult to achieve with simple skin removal. The temptation then is to open the orbital septum and to remove

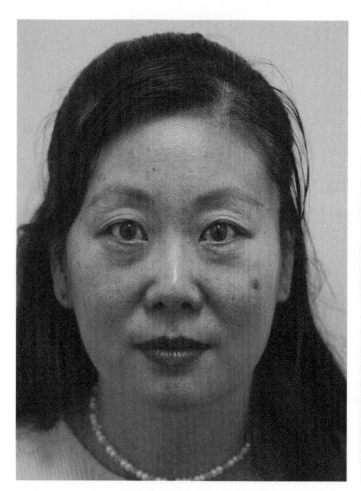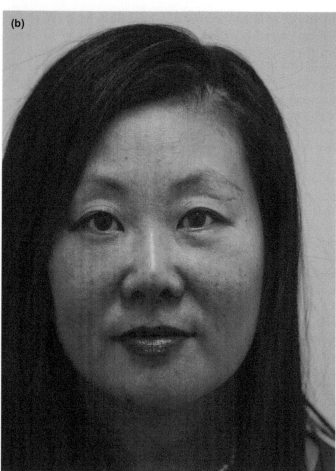

Figure 9.2 This Chinese patient demonstrates multiple incomplete, or partial, creases—which as the text states should be treated as if she has no crease at all. In addition, she has a relatively negative vector eye shape. She was rejuvenated with only full facial fat transfer and is shown before (A) and after (B) the procedure.

some fat in the postseptal plane without crease fixation with the thought that doing so will open the palpebral fissure somewhat. Although removal of postseptal fat can help, there are now two problems with this maneuver. First, variable crease fixation can occur inadvertently which if complete can be disconcerting to a patient who did not consent to it, unusual looking if only partial fixation is achieved, and perhaps fortunate if no fixation occurs at all. Variable crease fixation can occur due to unpredictable scarring between the preseptal and postseptal tissues.

Instead, two options should be presented to the patient according to this author's opinion when it comes to treating the Asian patient without a defined crease. One option is to create a crease. Making a crease opens up the eyelid shape enough to make an individual appear more awake or open-eyed. Using the full-incision method is ideal so that some dermatochalasis can be removed as need be. However, creating a crease requires that the surgeon know how to perform this procedure well, which if not performed frequently, can be technically difficult to achieve consistently superlative results. Second, the patient must assent to wanting to change his or her "look" since the eyelid will per force appear rounder in configuration. Third, the long recovery time with a full-incision "double eyelid" procedure must be carefully elaborated, involving an artificial look that can persist even for several months and ultimately only look completely natural after a year. This issue is particularly important to discuss with the male patient for two

reasons. First, the Asian male patient looks bizarre with too high a crease (just like Caucasian male patients), and it takes a while for the crease to assume a natural height. In addition, men have a more difficult time adjusting to a change in their look, especially after the adolescent years. This well-known psychological fact has been established in the rhinoplasty literature.

If the patient does not want a crease but still wants eyelid rejuvenation, then fat grafting to the upper eyelid and brow alone without skin removal can be the ideal way to improve the look without changing one's identity. Although the pretarsal tissue is already full in both youth and maturity in the Asian patient without a crease, converting an eyelid contour that is slightly concave in aging to more convex can bring back the look of a youthful eye. The patient must understand the limitations (if there are any) in simply adding fat to the brow and upper eyelid in the individual with an already narrow palpebral fissure born without a suprartarsal crease.

One more point to make: many Asians are born with a partially fixated crease on one or both eyelids. They mention that the crease appears sometimes and disappears at other times. Or, when the surgeon examines the patient, the crease appears barely visible and very low almost at the ciliary margin. Also, the Asian patient could have a well-defined crease on one side and an absent or partial crease on the other side. For any of these combinations, the patient should be classified and therefore treated as a patient without a crease at all (Figure 9.2).

Asians with prior surgery for supratarsal crease formation

Asian patients who have a natural appearing but surgically created crease that is not too high or over-resected can be easily treated as a patient who has a natural crease. Unfortunately, for many Asians today who are aging, their crease was surgically created during a time in which "Westernization" procedures were in vogue, i.e., when overzealous fat and skin removal were in fashion along with very high creases. These patients offer a uniquely difficult situation to address. Removing any more skin or lifting their brows can make their crease appear even more unnatural and should be avoided. Interestingly, 20 years later following a Westernization procedure, the eyelid crease height can approximate a "normal" or low position of about 1 or 2 mm with ongoing brow deflation. These individuals can be identified in that their crease appears to be of a normal, low height but there is something unmistakably unnatural appearing about their eyelids. The reason for this unnatural appearance is that the thick brow skin (all that remains after excessive eyelid skin removal) falls over the eyelid crease and the appearance of the crease appears too thick. Removing more skin or lifting the brow can literally unmask a bad prior result. If the surgeon is uncertain whether the crease is too high, he or she can simply lift up the brow skin to reveal how high the crease position is. For these Asian patients who have had a "Westernized" eyelid, adding some fat along the brow and upper eyelid complex may be about the only course of action that can be the remaining lesser of all evils. Even though it was mentioned that the appearance of the upper eyelid appears unnatural because it is thick, adding fat to the brow complex can actually make the appearance more natural in that it converts a thick concave structure (which is unnatural) to a thick, convex structure, which can actually partially camouflage the thick skin appearance.

STRATEGIES FOR THE AGING ASIAN SKIN

Asian skin is remarkably different from white skin and responds quite differently when being treated for age-related skin conditions. Asian skin can be more impervious to rhytids than in whites even in fairer-complected Asians. The mistake is to treat a fair skinned Asian like a Fizpatrick III when the skin in all Far East Asians acts like a Fizpatrick IV (or above) despite skin coloration (or absence of it). This fact predisposes Far East Asians to a higher incidence of pigmentary problems following resurfacing as well as unique problems of prolonged erythema and thicker scarring in nonfacial regions (the neck and postauricular regions and at times the medial eyelid canthus). Besides exuberant responses to healing, Asian skin is also plagued by pigmentary problems that are hormonal and solar related even more so than in whites. In addition, Asians can be even more sensitive to skin dyschromias that can be interpreted as being culturally unaesthetic and can also be viewed as harbingers of bad fortune. The surgeon should not underestimate the influence of cultural-related opinions and should delve into those matters preoperatively.

Treating Asian skin should always be more conservative than in whites and proper preoperative counseling should be undertaken to make an Asian patient aware of the potentially protracted recovery period that lies ahead after any skin treatment, especially ablative in nature. In general, most nonablative or fractionated treatments are safe in Asians who do not exceed

a Fitzpatrick IV. Superficial to medium-depth ablative treatments such as Jessner's /35% tricholoroacetic acid and even carbon-dioxide laser can be undertaken in Asian patients. Again, preoperative counseling must be established. It is of equivocal benefit whether pretreatment with hydroquinone can consistently and effectively diminish postinflammatory hyperpigmentation (PIH). However, PIH that does arise can last months and at times past a year following ablative resurfacing even with the use of 4% hydroquinone as a postprocedure treatment. Conservative treatments, expectations, and counseling should inform every skin treatment on an Asian patient whether nonablative or ablative in nature.

STRATEGIES FOR THE AGING ASIAN FACE

Besides the Asian eyelid, the Asian face can be quite different from the Caucasian face in many respects. The Asian face can be perceived as wider and flatter than that of the white individual. The skin and the soft-tissue envelope can also be thicker and heavier. The bone structure can be weaker especially in the lower region of the face. For all of these reasons, the Asian face should be evaluated for improved balance that can yield an aesthetically more appealing result. Interestingly, fat grafting can be used successfully to offset the apparent width of the Asian face by placing fat along the anterior jawline and upper cheek to make the lower cheek and outer jawline appear less heavy (Figure 9.3). Simply put, the relative size of an object appears smaller when placed adjacent to an object that is larger. This optical illusion works very well when shaping an Asian face to create a more three-dimensionally structured face. If the patient has a relatively retruded jawline, then just adding fat to the chin may not be ideal, as the chin can simply look fatter in appearance. A chin implant is preferred in this situation. However, mildly retrusive microgenia can be offset simply with fat transfer, especially in the female patient.

The neck of the Asian tends not to age as prematurely or as significantly as in the Caucasian counterpart. However, when the neck does begin to fall, rhytidectomy results can be less stellar than in whites for several reasons. First, the neck tends not to descend as much so the difference between the before and the after result can be less noticeable. Second, as mentioned, the soft tissue is heavier and the bone architecture is less prominent, which predispose toward a less than ideal result. For these reasons, the surgeon should only perform a lower facelift in the Asian patient who truly needs that procedure and, moreover, for the patient who has been presented realistic outcomes given the anatomic limitations of the Asian neck.

STRATEGIES FOR HAIR LOSS IN THE ASIAN PATIENT

Hair restoration in the Asian patient can present unique challenges to the surgeon. Caucasian hair tends to be finer, curlier, and lighter color as well as have less color contrast with the scalp skin. Asian hairs tend to be coarser, straighter, and darker with relatively higher color contrast between the hair shaft and the scalp. For these reasons, a grafty and artificial appearance can develop in the surgeon unaccustomed to transplanting Asian hair. The low anterior angles of the recipient sites and smaller graft sizes along the frontal hairline can be extremely important to

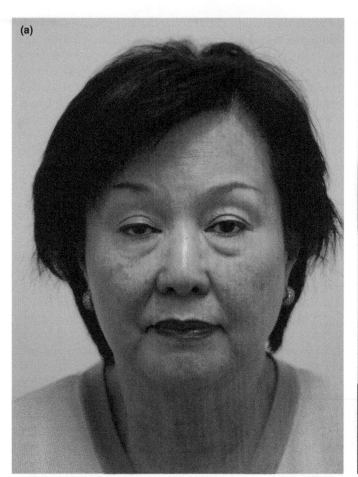
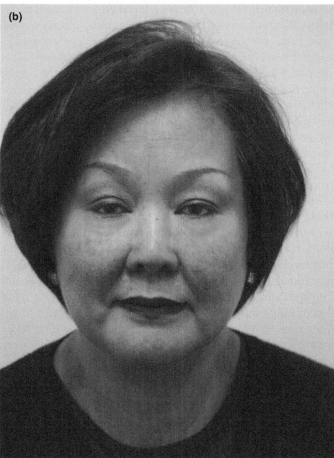

Figure 9.3 This Chinese patient (my mother, actually) shows a more prominent steatoblepharon and a relatively high crease height due to fat involution. She would have had a terrible result with any kind of browlift and/or skin removal from the upper eyelid. Instead, she underwent a concurrent transconjunctival blepharoplasty and full facial fat transfer including to the inferior orbital rim, brow, and upper eyelid region. Of note, she also has a wider, heavier lower face. By filling fat into the periorbital region, anterior cheek, and anterior chin, the face can ultimately look more dimensional (less flat) and less wide. She also underwent a corset platysmaplasty to improve her neck contour.

avoid a transplanted look. An exposed graft that is placed almost perpendicularly to the scalp can draw attention to the graft to scalp interface and thereby look artificial, especially given the constraints enumerated above. Another important consideration is evaluating the normal density of hair in nonreceding portions of the scalp. Oftentimes, the regular nonbalding density of the Asian scalp can be on the lower end of the spectrum with an average of 70–80 follicular units (FU) per cm² as opposed to 90–100 FU/cm² in a white individual in the donor region. Therefore, dense packing the recipient sites may overkill and cause undue depletion of precious donor hair. Fortunately, the graft dissection team generally loves working with Asian hair because it is so easy to dissect large caliber, straight black hair with paler surrounding skin as opposed to white hairs with little to no color contrast or African hair that can have low color contrast as well as also be very curly. Experienced graft cutters can even do an excellent job without microscopic magnification in the Asian patient. Like the other sections in this chapter, this text is not intended to teach how to do hair restoration or a facelift but to offer guidelines that inform decision-making and technique when addressing the Asian patient.

CONCLUSIONS

The Asian patient differs radically from the Caucasian patient in both anatomy and in cultural perspective. Keeping in mind these differences can help a surgeon stay clear of surgical misadventures and the ramifications of poor communication. Today, cultural sensitivity when performing aesthetic surgery in any ethnic patient is no longer optional. It is the key to a successful surgical outcome and maintaining a proper relationship with every patient.

BIBLIOGRAPHY

1. Lam SM, Glasgold MJ, Glasgold RA. Complementary Fat Grafting, Lippincott, Williams, & Wilkins, Philadelphia, PA, 2006.
2. McCurdy JA Jr, Lam SM. Cosmetic surgery of the Asian face. 2nd edition. Thieme Medical Publishers, New York, NY, 2005.
3. Lam SM. Aesthetic facial surgery for the Asian male. Facial Plast Surg 2005; 21: 317–23.
4. Lam SM. Aesthetic strategies for the aging Asian face. Facial Plast Surg Clin North Am 2007; 15(3): 283–91.
5. Shirakabe Y, Suzuki Y, Lam SM. A new paradigm for the aging Asian face. Aesthetic Plast Surg 2003; 27: 397–402.
6. Shu T, Lam SM. Liposuction and lipotransfer for facial rejuvenation in the Asian patient. International J Cosmetic Surg Aesthetic Dermatol 2003; 5: 165–73.

10 Aesthetic rejuvenation in Indian or Pakistani patients

Rashmi Sarkar, Vijay Kumar Garg, Munish Paul, and Amit Luthra

The aging face is affected both by intrinsic as well as extrinsic aging. Extrinsic aging is primarily related to the quantitative effect of sun exposure with resultant ultraviolet damage to structural exponents such as collagen and elastic fibers. On the other hand, intrinsic aging is genetically determined and includes volumetric loss due to fat atrophy and also gravitational soft tissue movement.

The signs of photodamaged skin are coarse and fine wrinkles, dyspigmentation, textural roughness, prominent pores, and telangiectasias. Intrinsic aging results in thin skin with reduced elasticity that retains normal skin pigmentation and texture. (1) An active lifestyle and a greater preoccupation with retaining a youthful appearance have ushered in an increased demand for rejuvenation techniques. An approach to facial rejuvenation incorporates both medical and surgical approaches. Medical approaches include the combined use of topical and systemic pharmaceuticals, neutraceuticals and cosmeceuticals, whereas surgical methods include nonablative rejuvenating devices, dermal fillers and injectable collagen stimulation, as well as botulinum toxin, which work at altering the three-dimensional frame work of the aging face to create a youthful appearance.(2) However, most of the aesthetic rejuvenation techniques address the extrinsic aging of the face.

CLINICAL FEATURES OF PHOTOAGING IN PATIENTS OF THE INDIAN SUBCONTINENT

The clinical manifestation of photoaging may differ in Caucasian skin as compared to darker skin types. South Asians (Indians, Pakistanis, Sri Lankans, and Bangladeshis) are of Caucasian ethnic background but have brown to dark brown skin.(3) In patients of Indian origin, photodamage is characterized by fine wrinkles, texturally rough skin, and pigmentation changes including mottled facial pigmentation, lentigines, actinic keratosis as well as larger pores.

Advanced and severe photodamage is less common in Indians. (4) Skin cancers and telangiectasias are also less frequent. They also develop thicker, deeper wrinkled on the forehead, periorbital and crow's feet area when compared with finer wrinkles in these regions in fair skinned patients. Moreover as Indian and Pakistanis patients have Fitzpatrick's skin photo-types IV to V, overall photo-aging is delayed and less severe. It may not be apparent till the fifth or sixth decade of life.(3)

Antiaging therapies can be divided into medical and surgical approaches.

MEDICAL APPROACH

- Cosmetological care
- Topical agents
- Systemic agents

SURGICAL PROCEDURES

Medical therapies

Medical therapies for aesthetic rejuvenation include the use of pharmaceuticals, neutraceuticals, and cosmeceuticals. These are combined with surgical procedures to get good results.

Cosmetological care

Good sun-protection is one of the key therapies for antiaging. Proper selection and usage of both UVA and UVB protective sunscreen is advised as ultraviolet irradiation reduces production of type 1 procollagen, which is the major structural protein in human skin.(5) Various cosmeceuticals including estrogen creams to reduce cutaneous atrophy and collagen loss, creams containing collagen, elastin and essential fatty acids are available, but there is insufficient scientific data to support their usage.

Topical therapies

Topical therapies such as tretinoin cream, Vitamin C, alpha hydroxy acid creams, idebenone, N-furfuryladenine 0.1%, chlorella and copper peptide complex have the advantage of being noninvasive but require a prolonged period of application of 3–6 months before any visible change can be observed.(6) They are also expensive and have the potential of causing contact irritancy or allergy.

Systemic agents

Currently, antioxidants are considered as one of the premier antiaging substance for scavenging of free oxygen radicals and other harmful agents that have deleterious effects in the body and on the skin. These includes vitamin C and E, glutathione, alpha lipoic acid, coenzyme Q10, green tea polyphenols, super-oxide dismutase, alpha lipoic acid, melatonin, selenium soy isoflavone, and zinc. Bone loss can be prevented by estrogen hormone replacement, biphosphenates vitamin D and calcium carbonate supplements.

SURGICAL TECHNIQUES

These are office-based surgical procedures which are performed by the dermatosurgeons. The bone and subcutaneous fat compartment also require attention. Microdemabrasion and superficial chemical peels can improve the appearance of the stratum corneum by exfoliation. Fillers, deep chemical peeling, and ablative laser resurfacing are used to replace or regenerate lost dermal collagen. Botulinim toxin is used to minimize the effect of hyperkinetic facial muscles on the thinning skin. Pigmentation can be improved with medium depth chemical peeling and intense pulsed light laser.(7) In Indian patients, a combination of superficial and medium depth chemical peels, fillers, botulinum toxin

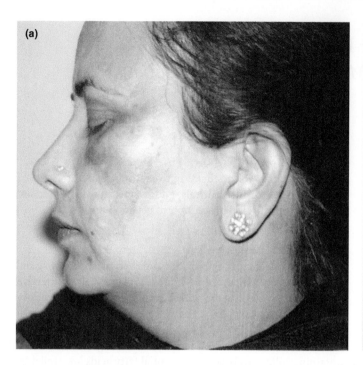
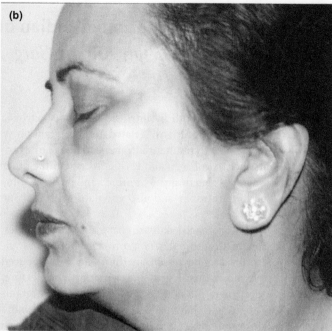

Figure 10.1 (A) Patient with melasma. (B) Clearing of pigmentation after 6 serial salicylic acid peels.

and intense-pulsed light laser are the most frequently used techniques for aesthetic rejuvenation.

Microdermabrasion

This is a simple and safe technique in which the skin surface is abraded with rough aluminum oxide or sodium chloride crystals. This procedure is based on the principle of superficial trauma, which damages the skin barrier which regenerates within a day and also stimulates the fibroblasts to produce collagen. With each pass, 15 um of skin is removed.(8) The treatment is repeated weekly and has an effect in improving fine lines, skin texture, and pore size. Although the risks of side effects are low, as Indian patients are dark skinned, one has to be cautious of bleeding and infection, which could lead to postinflammatory hyperpigmentation and scarring.

Chemical peels

These are important aesthetic rejuvenation techniques, which are commonly used in Indian patients. These are also less expensive as compared to nonablative lasers, hence more popular in India. The clinical features of photoaging, which can be addressed with clinical peels in dark skinned Indian patients are fine wrinkling, pigmentation, rough skin texture and pores. The major concern in Indian patients when they approach a dermatologist for aesthetic rejuvenation is the pigmentary dyschromias, which are more common due to the labile response of cutaneous melanocytes in dark skinned patients. This can be well addressed with superficial chemical peels such as glycolic acid, trichloroacetic acid and salicylic acid peels. Most superficial chemical peels especially glycolic acid peels are tolerated well in Indian and Pakistani patients.(10) On the other hand, a medium- depth chemical peel refers to a peel or a combination of peels, which can cause destruction of the epidermis and the papillary dermis and also the upper

reticular dermis. Medium depth peels are used less commonly in Indian patients because of a greater risk of postinflammatory hyperpigmentation. On the other hand, in our setup, deep chemical peels are best avoided due to severe complications such as hypo- pigmentation, hyperpigmentation, uneven skin pigmentation and scarring which could cause more emotional distress than the original condition.(11) Medium depth peels should only be performed by experienced dermatosurgeons who have a sound knowledge of the peeling agents, in only highly motivated dark-skinned patients, using a good prepeel and postpeel maintenance regimen to minimize the postpeel complications.

Prepeel evaluation

At the initial consultation, a detailed history and cutaneous examination should be performed. A history of abnormal scarring, use of medications such as isotretinoin in last 6 months, amount of sun exposure, immunosuppression and history of herpes simplex should be taken. The potential complications are explained to the patient. A written consent and prepeel photographs are taken of the patient.

PREPEEL PRIMING of the skin must be done for 2–4 weeks before the procedure to allow more rapid penetration of the peel, accelerate re-epithilialization, cause skin lightening due to dispersion of melanin granules. The agents used as priming agents are: hydroquinone 2–4%, broad spectrum sunscreens, tretinion 0.025–0.05%, glycolic acid 8–12%, salicylic acid and lactic acid.

Peeling technique

Mild sedation may be offered preoperatively with short acting sedation (Diazepam 5–10 mg orally) and mild analgesia with oral nonsteroidal antiinflammatory agents. The patient is requested to repeatedly wash the face with soap and water. The patient wears

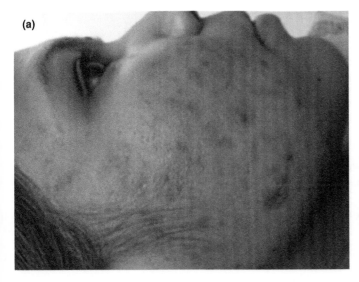

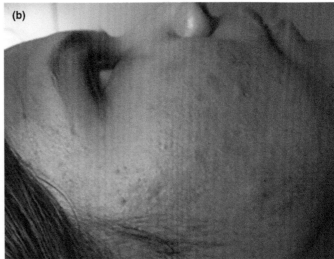

Figure 10.2 (A) Patient of acne (prepeel). (B) Same patient with clearing of acne and postacne pigmentation after serial glycolic acid peels.

a surgical cap and lies down with the head elevated. The eyes are kept closed or covered with gauze pieces. Vigorous cleaning of the face is done with methyl alcohol using 2 × 2inch gauze pieces followed by degreasing the skin with a cotton ball soaked with acetone. The chemical peel is applied with cotton- tipped applicators, cotton balls, 2 × 2 inch gauze pieces or sable brush until the end point is reached which is intolerable stinging and burning or uniform frosting in case of trichloroacetic acid peel (15–25%) eythema in the case of 20–70% glycolic acid peel and pseudofrosting in the case of 20–30% salicylic acid peels. The chemical peel is terminated by washing with cold water sponges for 5–10 minutes. In the postpeel period, the patient uses only broad spectrum sunscreens and moisturizers. She is informed about the postpeel reaction which is in the form of erythema and burning followed by exfoliation or vesiculation in the following week. Of the superficial chemical peels, glycolic acid peels 20–70%, and salicylic acid peels 20–30% are well tolerated in patients of Indian origin(Figures 10.1a,b, 10.2a,b) especially as several studies indicate that they provide benefit when combined with a topical regimen, such as hydroquinone, tretinoin or topical steroids. (10, 12) A recent study from Pakistan has demonstrated the safely and efficacy of serial salicylic acid peels in various dermatoses in Pakistani patients including photoaging.(13) Although TCA may be used in Indian/ Pakistani patients there is definitely a smaller margin of safety as compared with glycolic acid and salicylic acid or Jessner's peels.(14)

In our experience, in the medium- depth peels, 70% glycolic acid peels as well as Jessner's +35% TCA peels are best tolerated in Indian patients.

Combination procedures

For aesthetic rejuvenation procedures, the cosmetic units of the face are blended together. Laser resurfacing can be applied to the perioral and periorbital areas whereas the forehead, cheeks and chin are treated with a medium- depth peel. A superficial chemical peel can be used for the neck region. Such a blending technique avoids demarcation lines and shortens the postoperative healing period.

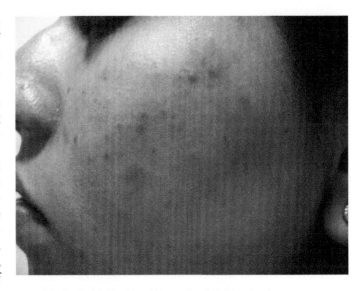

Figure 10.3 Post glycolic acid peel hyperpigmentation.

COMPLICATIONS

The complication of superficial and medium depth chemical peels are postinflammatory hyperpigmentation (Figure 10.3), persistent erythema, infections, scarring, atrophy of the skin, textural changes, milia, allergic reaction to the chemicals. Medium depth chemical peels carry the additional risks of postinflammatory hypopigmentation, scarring, accentuation of telangiectasias, enlargement of pilosebaceous pores and increased sensitivity to wind, sunlight and changes in temperature.

Botulinum toxin injections

These are considered as an effective treatment for dynamic wrinkles. In dark skinned Indian patients, the areas targeted include forehead, glabellar region, crow's feet and fuller upper and lower lips (Figure 10.4a,b). The main purpose of the treatment should be to soften the facial lines, not cause paralysis. The main inhibiting factor is the cost of the treatment.

Botulinum toxin can also be combined with dermal fillers and resurfacing techniques to optimize patient satisfaction.(15) There

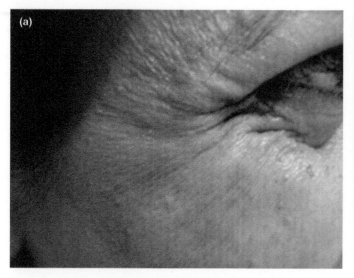
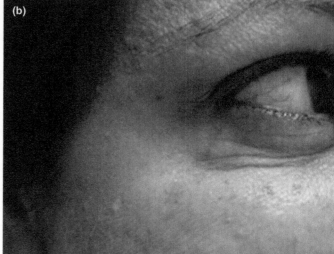

Figure 10.4 (A) Crow's feet before Botox. (B) Crow's feet after Botox.

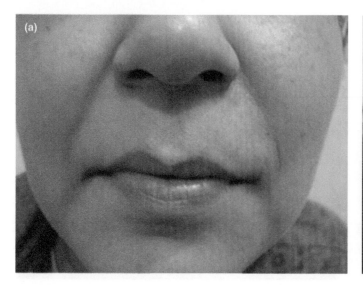
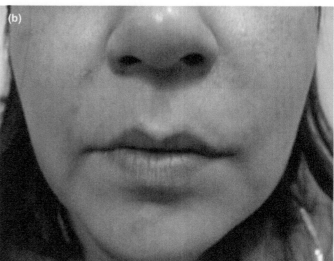

Figure 10.5 (A) Nasolabial fold before Hyaluronic acid filler. (B) Nasolabial fold after Hyaluronic acid filler.

is a low incidence of side effects in the cosmetic use of botox. There are excessive weakness of the injected muscles mild pain, bruising and parasthesia at the injection sites during or immediately after the injection. Burning can occur in the crow's feet area because of thinner skin and the presence of superficial blood vessels in that area. Headache, nausea and injection related post inflammatory hyperpigmentation and hypopigmentation may occur. Although Indian patients age slower than Caucasians, dynamic wrinkles, especially in the glabellar area, can be successfully treated by botulinum toxin injection.

Dermal fillers

Aesthetic volume rejuvenation with dermal fillers is a popular procedure which is sought by an increased number of patients who seek the rounder softer appearance of the face which gives them a more youthful appearance, including fuller curves of the cheeks, lips and temples. The procedure also has the advantage of offering less downtime or surgical intervention. While botulinum toxin eliminates only dynamic wrinkles, dermal fillers are the choice for static wrinkles.

Indications for fillers include facial static wrinkles, lip enhancement, facial deformities including depressed nasolabial folds, depressed scars periocular melanoses, sunken eyes, angular cheilitis, scleroderma, AIDS lipoatrophy, earlobe plumping, earlobe ptosis, hand, neck, décolleté rejuvenation.(16)

Due to the longer duration of action and good safety record, hyaluronic acid fillers have become one of the most common filler injectables in patients of Indian origin (Figures 10.5a,b, 10.6a,b). At present fillers from different countries are available in India and many of these may not have received approval from the drug authorities. However, one may have to use such fillers after gathering full information about its approval status from the distributer.

At preoperative evaluation of the patient, a history of anticoagulant therapy should be taken to avoid bruising in patient. In the postprocedure period, avoidance of extra cold or heat, massaging treatment areas for 6 hours, avoiding strenuous physical exercise for 6 hours, sleeping with the head elevated, taking medication to relieve pain and resuming skin care with products such

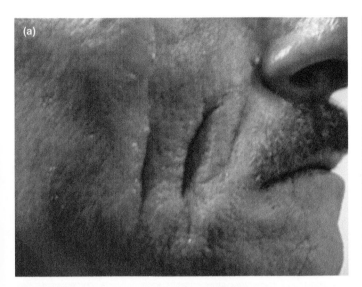
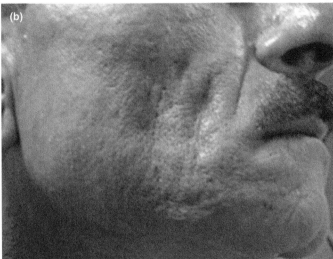

Figure 10.6 (A) Cheek grooves before polyacrylamide filler. (B) Cheek grooves after polyacrylamide filler.

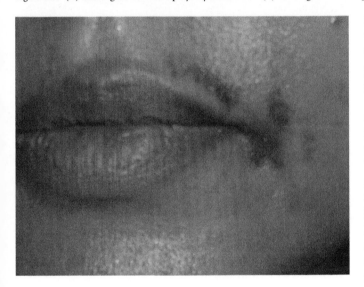

Figure 10.7 Ecchymoses post aquamid.

as retinoids, alphahydroxy acid the day after the procedure are necessary.

It is better for the dermatologist to use a temporary filler, at least initially as a first injection. Semipermanent or permanent fillers are administered for longevity of results after explaining all aspects of their potential complications to the patient.

The complications are minor. The immediate complications are pain, bruising (Figure 10.7), erythema, anaphylaxis, edema, acneiform eruptions, asymmetry, bumpiness. The late complications are inflammatory nodules, Tyndall effect, vascular occlusion, allergic reactions and granulomas.(16)

LASERS

Photorejuvenation consists of the use of visible or infrared light energy sources to reverse the process of sun induced or environmental damage to the skin. Ablative processes consist of visible disruption of the overlying epidermis while visible disruption of the overlying epidermis should not occur while trying to accomplish this is a nonablative manner. Ablative skin resurfacing can

be accomplished by the use of pulsed carbon dioxide and erbium YAG laser while nonablative dermal remodeling can be achieved by nonablative neodymium: YAG system, radiofrequency, intense pulsed light, fractional photothermolysis or light emitting diode photomodulation.

In the Indian setup, the dermatologist uses more of the chemical peels for aesthetic rejuvenation in combination with dermal fillers and botulinum toxin as compared to nonablative lasers due to less expertise in the latter technique and also due to higher costs. The primary objective of nonablative rejuvenation is to correct dyspigmentation, static fine wrinkles, course texture, telangiectasias and prominent pores while the secondary objective is recontouring of mild surface irregularities via dermal collagen remodeling. Nonablative facial rejuvenation (NAFR) finds its place between aggressive ablative laser resurfacing and the chemical peels and microdermabrasion which address only the epidermal component. NAFR works on ephelides lentigines, telangiectasia and deeper cosmetic concerns such as wrinkle reduction, pore size reduction and skin tightening.(17)

Intense pulsed light laser (IPL)

Intense pulsed light (IPL) is preferred in Indian patients due to better tolerability, lesser complication and no downtime. Studies also observe that the results are maintained over a long period of time.(18) In a patient, complete treatment is broken down into approximately 6–8 sessions at an interval of 3–4 weeks with each session lasting 30 minutes. IPL is produced by a noncoherent flashlamp-pumped light source that is capable of emitting light from 500 to 1200 mm. Due to the use of cutoff filters, it is possible to eliminate some of the shorter wavelengths of the visible light spectrum in order to limit melanin absorption. VPL (variable pulse light, Energist, UK) is used which is a system that limits a broad spectrum of wavelength of light from 530 nm to 950 nm. With the VPL, each macro pulse can be further broken down in micro pulses and the machine permits the operator to control the number of micropulses. The energy can also be varied according to the requirement. These advantages make the VPL system rather versatile in the Indian setup.

Table 10.1 Some commonly used parameters in Indian patients treated with IPL laser.

Indication	No of Pulses	On Time (ms)	Off Time (ms)	Energy
Pigmentation	4	3	1	22–25 J/cm^2
Telangiectasia	5	5	1	28–30 J/cm^2
Collagen	5	3	5	28–30 J/cm^2
Hair	5	5	5	30–34 J/cm^2

Table 10.2 Response to treatment of Indian patients treated with IPL laser.

Cutaneous Pathology	Average No. of Sessions	Interval Between Sessions	Grading of Results
Freckles	2–4	2–3 weeks	Excellent
Lentigines	2–4	2–3 weeks	Good
Melasma	2–4	3–4 weeks	Poor
Telangiectasia	2–4	3 weeks	Good
Rosacea	2–4	3 weeks	Good
Wrinkles	6–8	3–4 weeks	Average
Pore size	6–8	3–4 weeks	Average
Acne scars	6–8	3–4 weeks	Average
Unwanted facial hair	4–6, maintainance	6–8 weeks	Excellent

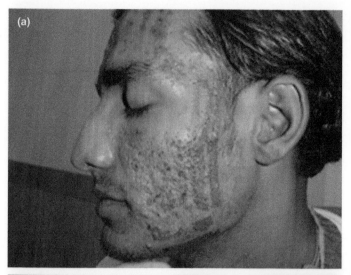

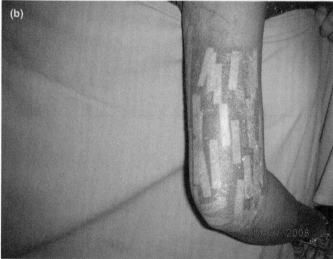

Figure 10.9 (A) Post IPL burn indication of IPL treatment active acne & acne scars. (B) Post IPL burn hypopigmentation.

The procedure involves the following steps. The commonly used parameters and response to treatment in Indian patients are given in Tables 10.1 and 10.2. In addition to the above mentioned conditions there is an improvement in the skin texture, smoothening of skin and glow (Figure 10.8a,b). These are the most frequent demands from the patient however they are most difficult to evaluate and quantify and improvement achieved is very subjective. Photorejuvenation can also be used in conjunction with other procedures to enhance results, such as laser resurfacing, chemical peeling, and microdermabrasion.

Containdications to photorejuvenation are photosensitizing disorders, photosensitizing medication, patients on isotretinoin, recently tanned patients, or patients with unrealistic expectations, the last two being the most common reason to deny treatment to a patient. IPL treatment with the correct parameters and good case selection is a very safe procedure with minimum adverse effects. Most common side-effects include temporary mild crusting, erythema which usually subsides without any residual hyper- or hypopigmentation however if very aggressive parameters are used in Fitzpatrick's type 5 or 6 skin or a person who is highly tanned, it can result in burns and scarring (Figure 10.9). Photorejuvenation

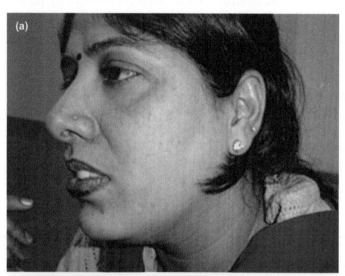

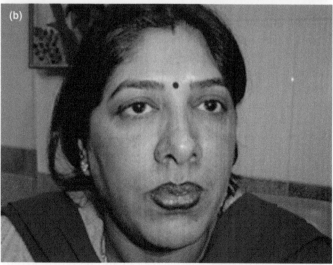

Figure 10.8 (A) Before IPL laser at baseline. (B) Post 4 sessions of IPL given at intervals of 3 weeks clearance of pigmentation, skin lightening, improved texture.

is a nonablative treatment that works simultaneously to repair collagen in the dermis, while gently erasing signs of aging in the epidermis, with minimal side effects and no downtime.

NONABLATIVE RADIOFREQUENCY

This has a two fold mechanism of action: immediate contraction of existing collagen fibrils and a delayed wound healing response resulting in neocollagen production by stimulated fibroblasts. As radiofrequency energy is not dependent on specific chromophore interaction, epidermal melanin is not at risk of destruction and treatment of all skin types is possible. The disadvantage is the high cost of the procedure and need for annual maintenance treatments.

Nonablative radiofrequency has been used in a series of 85 Asian patients who were dark skinned and it was concluded that RF treatment was well tolerated for skin tightening in Asian facial skin.(19) The complications are transient skin numbness and subcutaneous fat atrophy. Nonablative radiofrequency can also be combined with diode laser for greater efficacy and lesser side effects.

In the Indian setup, other methods of photorejuvenation such as fractional photothermolysis (Fraxel), Nd-Yag laser and infrared tightening are also used but less commonly. Expertise with some of the newer devices is still in its infancy and they are greatly limited by their high costs of treatment. Scientific data on their use is still lacking in the Indian setup and they do not seem to be well tolerated in Indian patients.

CONCLUSIONS

There is a renewed interest in the cosmetic treatment of aging skin in the Indian patients in spite of the constraints of high costs of most treatment modalities. Medical therapies including topical and systemic drugs and moisturizers are popularly used. Microdermabrasion and superficial chemical peels are used most frequently for the epidermal changes of aging of the face. Medium depth chemical peels and nonablative skin rejuvenation technique such as IPL and nonablative radiofrequency appear to be promising in selected patients if performed by dermatologists with good expertise. Botox and dermal fillers are used in combination with these techniques to address the facial wrinkles but are limited by cost constraints. Overall scientific literature on use of aesthetic rejuvenation technique in Indian patients is still lacking and more experience is required regarding their use.

REFERENCES

1. Kim KH, Geronemus RG. Nonablative laser and light therapies for skin rejuvenation. Arch Facial Plast Surg 2004; 26: 186–95.
2. Ruiz –Esparza J, Gomez JB. The medical face –lift: a noninvasive, nonsurgical approach to tissue tightening in facial skin using nonablative RF. Dermatol Surg 2003; 29: 325–32.
3. Elsaie ML, Lloyd HW. Latest laser and light based advances for ethic skin rejuvenation. Indian J Dermatol Venereol Leprol 2008; 23(3): 49–53.
4. Grimes PE, Hexsel DM, Rutowitsch M. The aging face in darker racial ethnic groups. In: Grimes PE, ed. Aesthetics and cosmetic surgery for darker skin types. Philadelphia: Lippincott William and Wilkins, 2008: 27–36.
5. Gordon ML. A conservative approach to the nonsurgical rejuvenation of the face. Dermatol Clin 2005; 23: 365–71.
6. Vedamurthy M. Antiaging therapies. Indian J Dermatol Venereol Leprol 2006; 72: 183–6.
7. Draelos ZD. The facial rejuvenation algorithm. J Cosmetic Dermatol 2006; 5: 195.
8. Fields KA. Skin breakthroughs in the year 2000. Int J Fertil Women's Med 2000; 45: 175–81.
9. Bhalla M, Thami GP. Microdermabrasion: Reappraisal and brief review of literature. Dermatol Surg 2006; 32(6): 809–14.
10. Sarkar R, Kaur C, Bhalla M, Kanwar AJ. The combination of glycolic acid peels with topical regimen in the treatment of melasma in dark skinned patients. Dermatol Surg 2002; 28(9): 828–32.
11. Sarkar R. Medium depth chemical peels and deep chemical peels. In: Grimes PE, ed. Aesthetics and cosmetic surgery for darker skin types. Philadelphia: Lippincott Williams and Wilkins, 2008: 170–8.
12. Javaheri SM, Handa S, Kaur I, Kumar B. Safety and efficacy of glycolic acid facial peel in Indian women with melasma. Int J Dermatol 2001; 40: 354–7.
13. Bari AU, Iqbal Z, Rahman SB. Tolerance and safety of superficial chemical peeling with salicylic acid in various facial dermatoses. Indian J Dermatol Venereol Leprol 2005; 71(2): 87–90.
14. Grimes PE, Rendon MI, Pallano J. Supervicial chemical peels. In: Gimmes PE, ed. Aesthetics and cosmetic surgery for darker skin types. Philadelphia. Lippincott Williams and Wilkins, 2008: 170–8.
15. Trasi SS. Botulinum. In: Sehgal VN, ed. Dermatologic Surgery Made Easy. New Delhi: Jaypee Publishers, 2006: 119–40.
16. Vedamurthy M, Vedamurthy D. Dermal fillers. In: Sehgal VN, ed. Dermatologic Surgery Made Easy. New Delhi: Jaypee Publishers, 2006: 109–18.
17. Goldberg DJ, Cutler KB. Nonablative treatment of rhytides with intense pulsed light lasers surg Med 2002; 26: 196–200.
18. Weiss RA, Weiss MA, Beasley KL. Rejuvenaton of photo aged skin: 5 years result with intense pulsed light of the face, neck, and chest. Dermatol Surg 2002; 28: 1115–9.
19. Kushikata N, Negishi K, Tezuka Y, Takeuchi K, Wakamatsu S. Non-ablative skin tightening with radiofrequency in Asian skin. Lasers Surg Med 2005; 36: 92–7.

11   Aesthetic rejuvenation for patients of Middle Eastern descent
Issam R Hamadah, Natalie A Kim, and Murad Alam

INTRODUCTION

The Middle Eastern population in the United States is projected to be 3.4 million by 2010.(1) These patients represent a rapidly growing, ethnically diverse population who are presenting to dermatologists and plastic surgeons for various cosmetic procedures. When treating ethnic populations, physicians must take into account not only the structural and functional differences of the skin, but also the diverse cultural backgrounds including unique skin and hair practices and varying standards of beauty. These nuances must be taken into consideration to avoid potentially disfiguring complications from cosmetic procedures.

Patients of Middle Eastern descent have a range of skin types; the lightest of which is no different from Caucasian complexions and the darkest of which is type VI. The most common, however, is the olive complexion. While the risk of keloid formation is not increased in these patients, postinflammatory and post-traumatic dyschromia is quite concerning. Particular attention must be paid to patients with a history of vitiligo and physicians should practice caution with procedures associated with potential Koebnerization, as hypo- and depigmentation are more evident in darker skin types. Finally, patient expectations can be very high in the Middle East and extra time should be spent to ensure that the patient understands the results, limitations, and shortcomings of any procedure.

CULTURAL CONSIDERATIONS

Individuals of ethnic skin commonly have traditional practices to attain culturally specific ideals of beauty. Some of these practices can lead to several adverse events that are relevant to dermatologists.

Skin Bleaching (Table 11.1)

Many Middle Eastern individuals regard fair skin as a source of beauty and prestige. According to a self-administered questionnaire study of Arab Americans from community health centers, mosques, and churches, more than 50% reported that they viewed very fair and fair skin visually pleasing in comparison to olive and dark skin.(2) This same survey reported that the most annoying skin concerns were uneven skin tone, skin discoloration, dry skin, acne, and facial hair.(2) To treat these subjective concerns, many individuals use commercially available, nonprescription topical bleaching agents in hopes of lightening their complexions or correcting dyschromias.(3) Active ingredients commonly in these products include 2–10% hydroquinone, phenolics, and corticosteroids.(4) Also, a study that analyzed 38 skin-lightening creams found about 45% contained mercury at levels well over the US Food and Drug Administration's limit of 1 ppm.(5)

Individuals who use these agents can develop dermatologic or medical complications, and therefore should be monitored by

Table 11.1 Potential complications associated with common ingredients in nonprescription skin-bleaching products.

Ingredient	Potential Clinical Implications
Hydroquinone	Dermatitis
	Exogenous ochronosis
	Pigmented colloid milia
	Patchy depigmentation
Corticosteroids	Skin atrophy
	Hypopigmentation
	Erythema
	Telangiectasia
Mercury	Pneumonitis
	Gastric discomfort
	Neurological manifestations
	Nephrotoxcity

dermatologists. Common adverse events include skin atrophy, hypopigmentation, erythema, and telangiectasia from the chronic use of steroids.(3) Reported complications of hydroquinone are dermatitis, exogenous ochronosis, pigmented colloid milia, and patchy depigmentation.(6–8) Acute mercury toxicity may present as pneumonitis and gastric discomfort, whereas chronic toxicity may present with neurological manifestations and nephrotic syndrome.(9–11)

Threading

Threading, or Khite in Arabic, is an ancient method of manual hair removal in parts of India and the Middle East. Unwanted hair is removed from the root by passing twisted cotton thread over the skin.(12) A service initially offered at ethnic beauty salons, threading is now gaining popularity and becoming increasingly available all over the United States. The purported advantages of this practice include minimal cutaneous irritation and fast hair removal. Common side effects include pain, folliculitis, and temporary erythema, edema, pruritus, and pigment alterations. Case reports of complications include bullous impetigo (13) and warts (14) from external exposure to infected materials following the procedure.

Henna

Several countries in the Middle East, Northern Africa, and India commonly use natural henna for skin adornment. A solution made from crushed dried leaves of the shrub, *Lawsonia inermis*, henna is used worldwide for a variety of cosmetic applications such as temporary tattooing, marriage adornment, and dyeing hair. There has also been an increase in the number of reports of allergic contact dermatitis (Figure 11.1), although natural

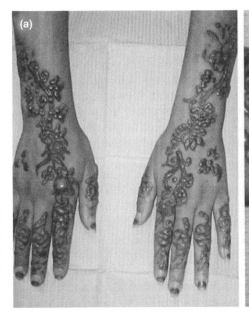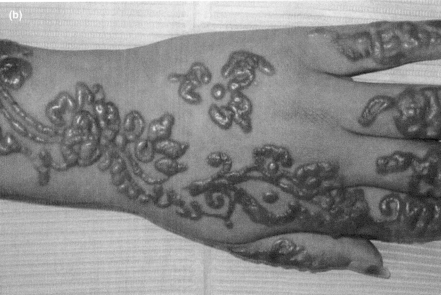

Figure 11.1 (A) A 19-year-old woman after the application of temporary henna tattoo exhibiting burning, itching, and vigorous blistering. (B) Examination revealed tense bullae without surrounding inflammation in a pattern that mirrored the sites of application.(19)

henna is reported to have a low potential for allergic reactions. (15) Common additives like chemical-coloring agents such as phenylenediamine, diminotoulene, and diaminobenzene may be the cause for these complications.(16–18)

Temporary henna tattoos fade over a period of days to weeks, and associated contact dermatitis is avoidable by refraining from future henna use. However, there are reports of residual postinflammatory hyper- and hypo- pigmentation following lesion resolution. (19–21)

DISORDERS

Melasma and melasma-like conditions

Classical melasma need not be defined, but melasma-like conditions include diffuse pigmentation of the temples, lateral cheeks, and forehead as well as constitutional facial hyperpigmentation (Figure 11.2). The former is considered as melasma-like for the lack of better classification. Characteristically, the pigmentation is diffuse with no speckling, quite dark, and presents more commonly in men than women. There is no history of drug intake and the pigmentation pattern definitely corresponds to photodamaged areas. The involvement worsens with time and is quite difficult to treat. The etiology remains unknown and treatment is the same as that for melasma. This condition should not be confused with actinic lichen planus, and when in doubt, a biopsy should be performed.

A misleading condition is the pigmentary demarcation line (Figure 11.3). The patient complains of having two colors and mostly asks to change the darker to the lighter tone. If not properly examined, the physician can mistake this for melasma-like conditions and manage accordingly. The condition does not respond to any treatment modality including lasers. Any attempt

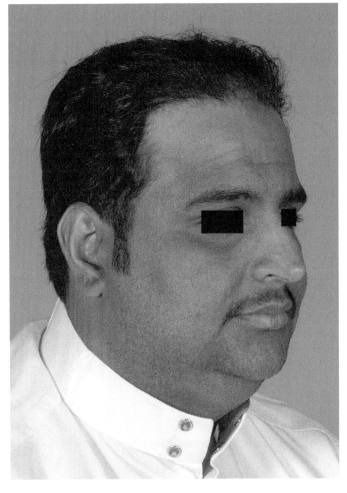

Figure 11.2 Diffuse pigmentation of the forehead, temples, and infraorbital cheeks, in melasma-like condition.

81

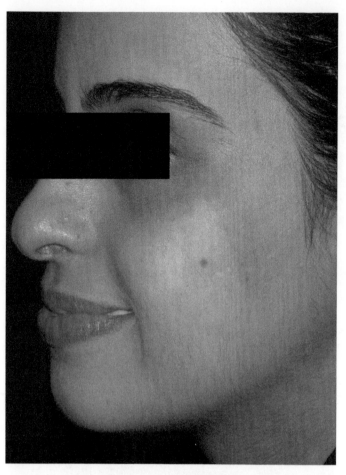

Figure 11.3 Pigmentary demarcation line of the cheeks in melasma-like condition, wherein the skin has two pigmentations. Photo courtesy of Dr. Abdullah Alsamary, Derma Clinics, Riyadh, KSA.

with bleaching agents or lasers results in accentuating the demarcation, hence aesthetically worse.

Another type of facial pigmentation of the temples is constitutional, appears early in adulthood, and has no relation to sun exposure. This condition does not respond to any topical therapy or peel. Response to lasers has not yet been reported and is not recommended. Patients with melasma and melasma-like conditions should be made aware that by and large, only partial clearance can be achieved with treatment and continuous maintenance therapy is necessary.

Of the topical treatment modalities for melasma, the modified Kligman formula has stood the test of time. This formula is a combination of tretinoin 0.1%, hydroquinone 4%, and vitamin C 1% in Synalar cream. Rather than applying each cream separately to the skin, patients should be instructed to combine the creams in the hands before application for best results. The reason for this may be simply due to increased patient compliance. Most patients, however, discontinue treatment because of irritation. To minimize this, do not begin with a full strength formula. Instead, instruct patients to apply a formula with tretinoin 0.01% 2–3 times a week and increase frequency to daily application. Then, gradually escalate the concentration of tretinoin to 0.1%. Adequate facial moisturization is necessary to combat the dryness and irritation induced by treatment.

For recalcitrant melasma, trichloroacetic acid (TCA) peels in carefully selected patients can yield excellent and long-lasting results (Figure 11.4). Dermamelan and Cosmelan mask peels clear the superficial component of melasma. The deeper component, though markedly lightened, does not disappear completely and becomes visible after maintenance therapy is halted. Glycolic acid peels give unsatisfactory results and can produce significant and chronic postinflammatory hyperpigmentation.

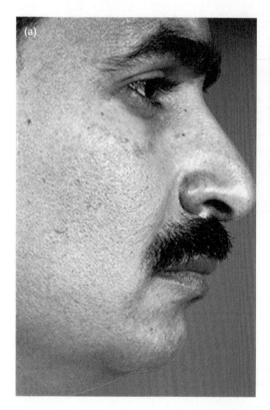
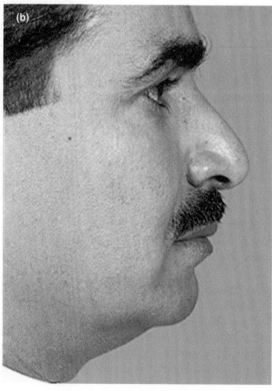

Figure 11.4 Before (A) and after (B) treatment of infraorbital melasma with trichloroacetic acid peel.

The Q-switched alexandrite laser can be entertained for deep melasma if the patient understands the risk of worsening melasma, and accepts the need for multiple sessions and combination therapy with topical treatments.(22, 23) The Q-switched Nd:Yag laser has been studied in the Far East with promising results, but with the risk of postinflammatory hyperpigmentation.(24) As for fractionated laser resurfacing, the results, so far, are mixed, with some investigators reporting significant and persistent remission and others noting little efficacy with risk of additional postinflammatory hyperpigmentation.

Dark circles

Only a minority of patients have genuine periorbital hyperpigmentation; the majority has pseudo-hyperpigmentation due to the vessels, underlying tissues, and hollow nature of the anatomic area (Figure 11.5). To treat genuine hyperpigmentation, only limited lightening can be achieved with bleaching agents and mild peels. Additionally, maintenance therapy for an indefinite period is required. Pseudo-hyperpigmentation, however, will improve with fillers. Hyaluronic acids are safe, biodegradable, and can be dissolved with hyaluronidase if overcorrection results, which makes them particularly useful in this anatomic area.(25, 26)

Lentigines/freckles

Lentigines/freckles can be quite difficult to eradicate with lasers. Laser treatment can be complicated and potentially result in lesion hyper- or hypo- pigmentation. Moreover, the results are temporary and range from a few months to 1–3 years. Another option is to simply offer the patient chemical peels followed by maintenance therapy to lighten lesions.

Solar lentigines

These respond very well to Q-switched 532 nm Nd:Yag and alexandrite lasers.

Dermatosis papulosa nigra

While mild electrocautery results in excellent clearing with no residual dyschromia or scarring, new lesions will reappear after 2–3 years, as this is a constitutional condition.

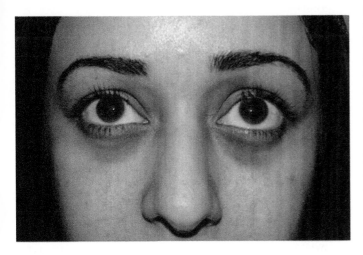

Figure 11.5 Characteristic periorbital gray-brown pigmentation at baseline in a young Middle Eastern female. Note especially the infraorbital crescentic pigmented patches.

PROCEDURES

Fractional Resurfacing

The light complexioned Middle Eastern patient will have the same indications and expected results as patients of European descent. Fractional resurfacing procedures in those with darker complexions will result in some lightening and a "glow."

Acne scarring is the most common indication for fractional resurfacing, with limited results in superficial scars.

Ablative Resurfacing

Patients with an olive complexion can benefit from ablative resurfacing for treatment of acne scars. However, the risk for permanent hypopigmentation is a serious limitation.

Laser-assisted Hair Removal

Carefully avoid treating vellus or thin hair to prevent paradoxical hair thickening especially on the face and anterior neck, which will necessitate multiple, and sometimes endless, sessions to achieve acceptable results. Moreover, caution must be practiced with every treatment session for dyschromia. Although the patient may not present with discoloration from previous sessions, the future may still bear some risk. This is especially true when the hair density is markedly reduced and the chromophore becomes the melanin in the epidermis and dermis rather than that of the hair. The laser light, then, is mostly absorbed by the skin and not the hairs.

Facial Fillers and Facial Lipoaugmentation

In general, many women in the Gulf region deem full, round faces as cosmetically appealing and as a sign of youth. Hence, contouring with liposculpture and fillers should be tailored to the patient's wish. Prominent cheek bones may not be desired by some women, and it is crucial that before the procedure is done, these expectations are addressed and taken into account.

Fillers can also be used as an alternative or compliment to rhinoplasty (Figure 11.6). While not ideal for those who want to eliminate all ethnic characteristics of their natural nose, fillers may be effective in sculpting a smoother nasal contour while preserving the natural ethnic features. This procedure is ideal for patients hesitant to undergo surgery or patients with postrhinoplasty asymmetries. Calcium hydroxylapatite can successfully augment the contour of the nasal dorsum through injections into the nasion, rhinion, supratip, ala, and tip.(27, 28, 29) Common adverse events include transient edema, erythema, and bruising.

Botulinum toxin

Cosmetic tattoos were worn traditionally in North Africa and the Middle East as far back as the Bronze Age. A lasting common practice, cosmetic tattoos are frequently used to create or enhance existing eyebrows. Eyebrow elevation is frequently requested even by young females in their 20s with no apparent wrinkles. Achieving a natural look can be difficult in those with eyebrow tattoos since elevating the tattoo line, which often is unnatural in its arch and position, can further enhance the unnatural appearance.

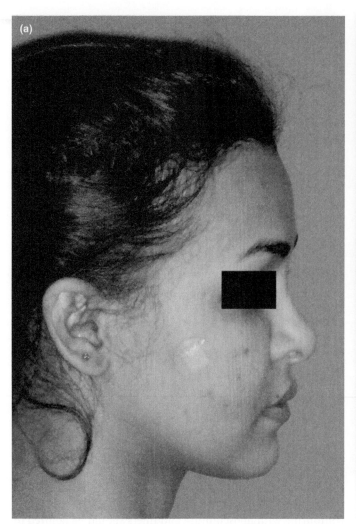

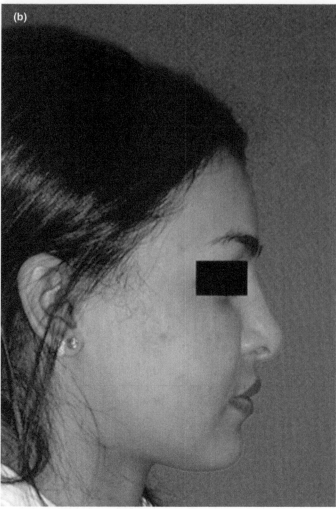

Figure 11.6 (A) Preoperative lateral view of a 23-year-old patient and (B) postoperative view 6 months after injection of 0.5 mL Radiesse.(27)

SUMMARY

Not only have countless laser technologies recently been developed for patients with ethnic skin, but cosmetic and skin care industries have also begun formulating products for, and marketing to, people of color. Still, it remains important for cosmetic dermatologists and surgeons to tailor procedures and topical regimens for each patient to minimize adverse events like postinflammatory and posttraumatic dyschromia or hypertrophic scar development. Integrating the understanding of cultural nuances into clinical practice is paramount in providing safe and effective cosmetic services to these patients.

REFERENCES

1. Camarota SA. Immigrants from the Middle East. Center for Immigration Studies [document on the Internet]. 2002. Available from: http://www.cis. org/articles/2002/back902.html.

2. El-Essawi D, Musial JL, Hammad A, Lim HW. A survey of skin disease and skin-related issues in Arab Americans. J Am Acad Dermatol 2007; 56: 933–8.

3. Taylor SC. Skin of color: biology, structure, function, and implications for dermatologic disease. J Am Acad Dermatol 2002; 46: S41–62.

4. Olumide YM, Akinkugbe AO, Altraide D et al. Complications of chronic use of skin lightening cosmetics. Int J Dermatol 2008; 47: 344–53.

5. Al-Saleh I, al-Doush I. Mercury content in ski-lightening creams and potential hazards to the health of Saudi Women. J Toxicol Environ Health 1997; 51: 123–30.

6. Findlay GH, Morrison JG, Simson IW. Exogenous ochronosis and pigmented colloid milium from hydroquinone bleaching creams. Br J Dermatol 1975; 93: 613–22.

7. Lawrence N, Bligard CA, Reed R, Perret WJ. Exogenous ochronosis in the United States. J Am Acad Dermatol 1988; 18: 1207–11.

8. Hull PR, Procter PR. The melanocyte: an essential link in hydroquinone induced ochronosis. J Am Acad Dermatol 1990; 22: 529–31.

9. Barr RD, Rees PH, Cordy PE et al. Nephrotic syndrome in adult Africans in Nairobi. Br Med J 1972; 2: 131–4.

10. Oliveira DB, Foster G, Savill J, Syme PD, Taylor A. Membranous Nephropathy caused by mercury-containing skin lightening cream. Postgrad Med J 1989; 63: 303–4.

11. Silverberg DS, McCall JT, Hunt JC. Nephrotic syndrome with use of ammoniated mercury. Arch Intern Med 1967; 120: 583–5.

12. Abdel-Gawad MM, Abdel-Hamid IA, Wagner RF Jr. Khite: a non-Western technique for temporary hair removal. Int J Dermatol 1997; 36: 217.

13. Bloom MW, Carter EL. Bullous impetigo of the face after epilation by threading. Arch Dermatol 2005; 141: 1174–5.

14. Kumar R, Zawar V. Threading warts: a beauty parlor dermatosis. J Cosmet dermatol 2007; 6: 279–82.

15. Wohrl S, Hemmer W, Focke M, Gotz M, Jarisch R. Hypopigmentation after non-permanent henna tattoo. J Eur Acad Dermatol Venereol 2001; **15:** 470–2.

16. Chung W, Chang Y, Yang L et al. Clinicopathologic features of skin reactions to temporary tattoos and analysis of possible causes. Arch Dermatol 2002; 138: 88–91.

17. Le Coz CJ, Lefebvre C, Keller F, Gosshans E. Allergic contact dermatitis caused by skin painting (pseudotattooing) with black henna, a mixture of henna and p-Phenylenediamine and its derivatives. Arch Dermatol 2000; 136: 1515–7.

18. Kazandijeva J, Grozdev I, Tsankov N. Temporary henna tattoos. Clin Dermatol 2007; 25: 383–7.

19. Evans CC, Fleming JD. Allergic contact dermatitis from a henna tattoo. N Engl J Med 2008; 359: 6.

20. Tomlinson JE, Winterton RIS, Liddington MI. Henna reaction. J Plast Reconstr Aesthet Surg 2007; 60: 1164–5.

21. Jovanovic DL, Slavkovic-Jovanovic MR. Allergic contact dermatitis from temporary henna tattoo. J Dermatol 2009; 36: 63–5.

22. Lee GY, Kim HJ, Whang KK. The effect of combination treatment of the recalcitrant pigmentary disorders with pigmented laser and chemical peeling. Dermatol Surg 2002; 28: 1120–3.

23. Rusciani A, Motta A, Rusciani L, Alfano C. Q-switched alexandrite laser-assisted treatment of melasma: 2-year follow-up monitoring. J Drugs Dermatol 2005; 4: 770–4.

24. Ho SG, Chan HH. The Asian dermatologic patient: review of common pigmentary disorders and cutaneous diseases. Am J Clin Dermatol 2009; 10: 153–68.

25. Fedok FG. Advances in minimally invasive facial rejuvenation. Curr Opin Otolaryngol Head Neck Surg 2008; 16: 359–68.

26. Goldberg RA, Fiaschetti D. Filling the periorbital hollows with hyaluronic acid gel: initial experience with 244 injections. Ophthal Plast Reconstr Surg 2006; 22: 335–41.

27. Siclovan HR, Jomah JA. Injectable calcium hydroxylapatite for correction of nasal bridge deformities. Aesth Plast Surg 2008 [Epub ahead of print].

28. Rokhsar C, Ciocon DH. Nonsurgical rhinoplasty: an evaluation of injectable calcium hydroxylapatite filler for nasal contouring. Derm Surg 2008; 34: 944–6.

29. Stupak HD, Moulthrop TH, Wheatley P, Tauman A, Johnson CM Jr. Calcium hydroxylapatite gel (Radiesse) injection for the correction of postrhinoplasty contour deficiencies and asymmetries. Arch Facial Plast Surg 2007; 9: 130–6.

12 Blepharoplasty for Asian patients
Jung I Park and Edward S Kwak

INTRODUCTION

Double eyelid surgery is the cosmetic procedure performed most frequently in East Asian countries. *Double eyelid* is the term used to define an upper eyelid appearance with a supratarsal crease. The term *single eyelid* is used to describe the appearance of an eyelid lacking a supratarsal crease. The double eyelid operation is designed to convert a single eyelid to a double eyelid. When applied to East Asians, the term *upper eyelid blepharoplasty* refers almost exclusively to double eyelid surgery. The ethnic description of the Asian eyelid connotes an eyelid shape without a supratarsal crease, while the Caucasian eyelid typically has a supratarsal fold. It should be noted, however, that the presence of the supratarsal crease is present in many other non-Caucasian races, e.g., African descendants. Furthermore, there are many regions in Asia where people have natural double eyelids, such as India and Middle Eastern countries. Approximately 40% of Koreans have natural double eyelids. But because of the high number of people with single eyelids in this region, it is generally regarded as an East Asian trait, concentrated in China, Japan, and Korea—as well as in the Southeast Asian countries to which many Chinese migrate.

Principles for Asian aging eyelid surgery differ from other ethnic groups. Factors such as maintaining a single crease, creating a double fold, and differences in eyelid skin thickness are factors unique to the Asian eyelid. Besides addressing skin redundancy, Asian aging eyelid surgery frequently requires concurrent implementation of double eyelid surgical techniques and forehead lift surgery.

Among younger East Asian patients, there is little difference between the double eyelid surgery procedure for males and females. Among older East Asian patients, however, males express much greater reluctance in accepting the surgery than their female counterparts. The need for subtlety in double eyelid surgery and blepharoplasty for elder male patients remains a challenging issue.

ANATOMY

There are several differences between the anatomy of the eyes of East Asian and non-Asian populations. East Asian eyelids are characterized by 1) a lack of a supratarsal crease, thus a lack of double eyelid folds; 2) thicker eyelid skin and muscle; 3) an abundance of fat tissue distributed in various layers of the eyelid as well as subcutaneous tissue between the orbicularis oculi and levator aponeurosis and possibly more fat in the preaponeurotic area; 4) a smaller orbital cavity in relation to the size of the globe and as a result more anterior placement of the eye in relation to the orbital rim; 5) the presence of the epicanthal fold and a partially or totally obliterated lacrimal lake; 6) shorter and less abundant eyelashes; 7) a narrower tarsal plate; and 8) a smaller palpabral fissure.(1–3)

The most significant difference, and therefore the one that prompted the popularity of double eyelid cosmetic surgery in Asian countries, is the lack of supratarsal creases in Asian eyelids. The supratarsal crease is formed only when the eyelid is opened by the contraction of the levator muscle. Fibrous extensions of the levator aponeurosis attach to the pretarsal skin. As the tarsal plate is retracted by the action of the levator muscle, the pretarsal skin is also retracted, causing invagination of the skin, which produces the creases. The terms *crease* and *fold* are often used interchangeably in the literature. In order to avoid confusion in this text, the authors use the term *crease* to refer to the supratarsal fixation where the incision or suture was made and *fold* for the double eyelid fold which is a folding of the supratarsal skin on its own. The supratarsal crease is hidden, whereas the double eyelid fold is what the patient sees and therefore uses to gauge the surgery's outcome.

Conventional knowledge based on Doxanas and Anderson's study is that the preaponeurotic fat compartment in the Asian eyelid, which lacks double fold, extends down over the tarsal plate.(4) This extension of the preaponeurotic fat inferiorly prevents the levator aponeurosis from extending its fibrous attachments to the eyelid skin, thereby prohibiting a supratarsal crease from forming. Contrary to this principle, the senior author has observed though his career; patients without a congenital supratarsal crease generally did not have preaponeurotic fat compartments, which extended down to the tarsal plate. Anatomically, the preaponeurotic fat lies superficial to the levator aponeurosis and deep to the orbital septum. The inferior extension of this fat compartment is limited by the fusion of the orbital septum and levator aponeurosis. This fusion point is generally superior to the superior tarsal margin. According to the senior author's observations, the average distance of the attachment of the orbital septum to the levator aponeurosis from the lower tarsal margin generally is 10.6 cm on the right and 10.8 cm on the left. Based on this observation along with the fact that the average width of the Asian tarsal plate ranges from 6.5 to 7.5 cm (5), the preaponeurotic fat is unlikely to be the only anatomic barrier preventing attachment of the levator aponeurosis to the eyelid skin.

The levator muscle has two major functions: (1) Its major role is to elevate the tarsal plate, thus opening the eye. (2) While the fibrous extension of this muscle to this skin tightens the pretarsal skin during muscle contraction.

The lack of anchorage by fibrous extensions of the levator in Asian upper eyelids causes the upper eyelid skin to droop over the inferior tarsal margin when the eyes are open, covering portions of the palpebral fissure and reducing the true size of the palpebral fissure. The redundant eyelid without a supratarsal fold also covers portions of the upper eyelashes, reducing the amount of eyelash show. By excising the redundant eyelid skin and creating a supratarsal fold, the amount of eyelash show increases, which is often an aesthetically favorable outcome for many patients.

For clarification on terminology, the region of the eyelid above the supratarsal crease is referred as the *supratarsal eyelid* while the lid below the crease is the *pretarsal eyelid*. When the eyes are closed, the supratarsal crease appears as a barely visible faint line.

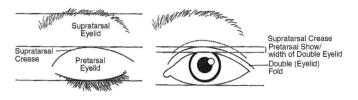

Figure 12.1 For clarification on terminology, the region of the eyelid above the supratarsal crease is referred as the supratarsal eyelid while the lid below the crease is the pretarsal eyelid. When the eyes are closed, the supratarsal crease appears as a barely visible faint line. As the eye opens, the eyelid skin begins to fold on its own at the supratarsal crease. The supratarsal skin then folds again on its own to create a double eyelid fold. The pretarsal skin is then partially covered by the folded supratarsal skin. Only the lower portion of the pretarsal skin becomes visible. The part of the pretarsal skin that is visible is defined as a pretarsal show.

As the eye opens, the eyelid skin begins to fold on its own at the supratarsal crease. The supratarsal skin then folds again on its own to create a double eyelid fold. The pretarsal skin is then partially covered by the folded supratarsal skin. Only the lower portion of the pretarsal skin becomes visible. The part of the pretarsal skin that is visible is defined as a *pretarsal show* (Figure 12.1). This has an anatomical significance because the shape of this portion of the eyelid determines the beauty of the eyelid along with the shape of the double fold.

HISTORY OF SURGICAL TECHNIQUES

Despite the numerous techniques that have been published on double eyelid surgery each technique is based on one key principle, which is establishing an adhesion, either directly or indirectly, between the skin and the levator aponeurosis. The earliest described double eyelid technique was in 1896 by Mikamo.(6) He described a suture technique intended to fix the pretarsal skin to the levator aponeurosis. Although early results were acceptable, long-term follow up demonstrated frequent loss of the supratarsal fold. This loss of fold was associated with the dynamic nature of the eyelid and the constant force applied to the suture material. With time the suture was found to either cut through tissue or accommodate and relax, resulting in loss of attachment between the levator and the skin. Later suture techniques where developed to promote more scar tissue formation to permanently fix the skin to the levator. Although some studies published favorable outcomes using various novel suture techniques, (such as interlocking sutures, increasing the number of sutures) no technique has reliably resulted in predictable long-term results.(7–9)

Incisional techniques have been developed to provide increased longevity and more reliable results than the suture techniques. (10) The fundamental principle for each of the myriad of incision techniques described is direct suture fixation of the skin to the levator aponeurosis. Although the suture material can still weaken or shear through the targeted tissues, substantial scar tissue develops using direct fixation via the incisional technique, thus binding the other two tissues more effectively.

FACTORS IN ASIAN DOUBLE EYELID SURGERY

When a patient describes how high he or she wishes his or her fold to be, this tells the surgeon the desired amount of pretarsal show. The amount of pretarsal show varies depending on two factors: the placement of the supratarsal crease and the skin laxity of the supratarsal eyelid skin. The implantation of suture material or placement of the incision does not necessarily dictate the ultimate height of the supratarsal crease.

A solid fixation of the supratarsal skin to the levator will result in a higher fold, as the fixation from the skin to the levator becomes more lax; the crease height tends to migrate downward. In younger patients with minimal dermatochalasia, placement of a high crease results in an increased amount of pretarsal show. Older patients with more dermatochalasia, the same placement of the crease results in less pretarsal show, as the redundant skin folds over the pretarsal skin.

The thickness of the eyelid skin also influences the outcome of the fold. Asian upper eyelid skin becomes thicker as it approaches the eyebrow area. Higher placement of the supratarsal crease recruits thicker skin to fold over. Incorporating this thicker skin, in addition to factoring in skin redundancy, results in a well-defined supratarsal crease with a bulky appearing double fold.

The placement of suture material or an incision varies greatly among surgeons. Generally most surgeons make the crease on average distance of 7–10 mm from the ciliary margin. However as mentioned earlier, placement of the crease does not determine the final height of the pretarsal show, and the surgeon must account for several factors when determining the final outcome. Typically the desired amount of pretarsal show for most Asians is generally 2–3 mm. To achieve the desired amount of pretarsal show and eyelid symmetry, several variable factors must be considered by the surgeon. Each surgeon may have his/her own technique to achieve the desired amount of pretarsal show. One surgeon may place a supratarsal crease fixation at 7 mm, while using multiple fixation sutures to the levator to establish a stronger fixation. Another surgeon may choose to place the supratarsal crease fixation at 10mm while incorporating fewer fixation points and accounting for relaxation of the fixation points over time. Both outcomes can result in the desired 2–3 mm range of pretarsal show.

For individuals with a strong fixation at the supratarsal crease, the pretarsal eyelid skin is tightly stretched. As a result, when the eyelid opens and closes, the pretarsal eyelid skin moves in parallel to the tarsal plate (Figure 12.2A). In an eyelid without a firm supratarsal fixation, the pretarsal eyelid skin slides toward the inferior tarsal margin as the eye opens (Figure 12.2B). In some patients (including younger patients) lacking a supratarsal fold, the upper eyelid skin can significantly extend below the inferior tarsal margin, narrowing the appearance of the palpebral fissure (pseudoptosis). To address this, a conservative amount of skin can be excised. As mentioned earlier, the amount of skin excision also has significant impact on pretarsal show. The Asian eyelid surgeon must account for a certain amount of upper eyelid skin that overhangs the pretarsal skin to achieve the desired amount of pretarsal show. Excising too much skin can result in a larger amount of pretarsal show, which may result in an unnatural look to the eye. This philosophy on conservative skin excision is one of the major differences between Asian and Caucasian blepharoplasty.

The approach for upper eyelid fat excision also differs between the Asian and Caucasian blepharoplasty surgery. Eliminated fat is often necessary in Caucasian blepharoplasty to address fat

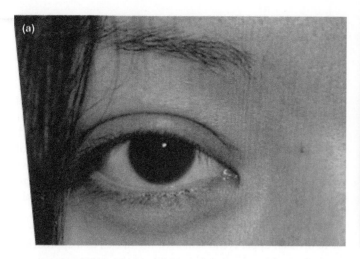
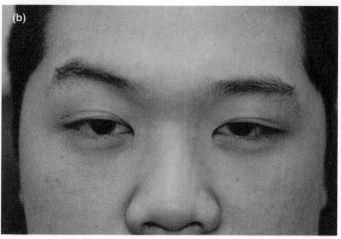

Figure 12.2 (A) For individuals with a strong fixation at the supratarsal crease, the pretarsal eyelid skin is tightly stretched. (B) As a result, when the eyelid opens and closes, the pretarsal eyelid skin moves in parallel to the tarsal plate. In an eyelid without a firm supratarsal fixation, the pretarsal eyelid skin slides toward the inferior tarsal margin as the eye opens.

pseudoherniation, especially medially. However, fat removal in Asian patients is commonly performed to address the overall full appearance of the upper eyelid. We do not recommend aggressive removal of fat during Asian blepharoplasty surgery. Besides having minimal effect on reducing the full appearance to the upper eyelid, several unwanted effects were frequently observed such as: hollowness, multiple creases, and an overly done appearance to the eye.

ORBICULARIS OCULI-LEVATOR FIXATION TECHNIQUE AND ORBICULARIS OCULI-LEVATOR APONEUROSIS FIXATION TECHNIQUE

The orbicularis oculi-levator aponeurosis fixation (OOLA) technique is based on two principles.(11–13) The first principle is that there is an inherently strong adhesion between the eyelid skin and the underlying orbicularis oculi muscle. There are prominent fibrous attachments between these structures, (as often verified when attempting to establish a surgical plane between these structures) as such, tension applied to the obicularis muscle is equally applied to the overlying pretarsal skin. The second principle of the OOLA technique is that a larger surface contact creates a more solid and permanent fixation. Both suture and incision techniques rely on fixation along the two-dimensional plane of scar formation. The pretarsal skin's thin edge is sutured to the surface of the levator aponeurosis. Orbicularis oculi-levator fixation technique, however, relies on a three-dimensional fixation. The OOLA technique fixates the two structures broadly, allowing a larger area of scar formation to occur (Figure 12.3). As the levator muscle contracts, the orbicularis oculi muscle is pulled up, which then pulls the firmly attached overlying eyelid skin and forming a crease.

Use of the OOLA technique affects the overlying pretarsal skin in two ways. First the pretarsal skin and subcutaneous tissue stretches as the levator retracts. This thinning of the pretarsal region prevents excessive bulk, thereby reducing the chance of a "sausage deformity." The second effect of the OOLA technique is that as the levator retracts, the pretarsal skin becomes more

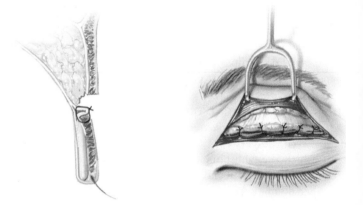

Figure 12.3 The obicularis oculi-levator aponeurosis fixation. A broad effacement of these to structures is evident. (PARK STUDY)

taut. This prevents unwanted wrinkling of the pretarsal skin or an "accordion deformity". The OOLA technique creates a dynamic supratarsal crease formation, which ultimately results in a pretarsal region that is thinner, tighter, and more delicate.

Consultation and preoperative care

Patients are instructed to wash their face with antiseptic soap both the night before and the morning of the surgery. Patients should also not apply facial cosmetics or other facial health products. Disregard to these instructions will result in difficulty in applying the necessary surgical markings. An alcohol pad can be used, to remove excess makeup or oil.

Markings

The eyelid is marked with the patient in a sitting position. This is done in the preoperative holding room and prior to local anesthetic infiltration. (Local anesthetic infiltration significantly distorts the skin, causing inaccurate surgical markings.) A fine point-marking instrument is used, such as a fine tip felt-tipped pen or a sharpened

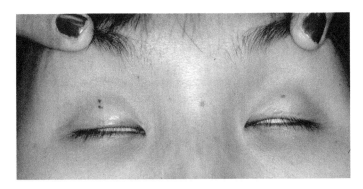

Figure 12.4 Measurement and markings are made with the eyelids stretched, just to the point of eyelash eversion.

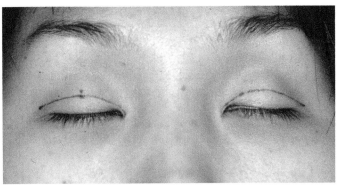

Figure 12.6 The incision line should be made parallel to the ciliary margin.

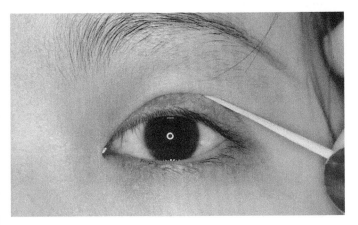

Figure 12.5 A cotton tip applicator or a lacrimal probe may be used to evaluate surgical markings.

end of a wooden cotton tip applicator and methylene blue dye. The tip of the marking instrument must be extremely fine, as a 1-mm difference in the height of the left and right double eyelid can result in significant asymmetry. Use of surgical eye magnifying loops during the marking process is helpful. The eyebrow is gently lifted to stretch the eyelid skin while the eye is closed (Figure 12.4). *(Each surgeon should develop his/her own approach to the amount of tension applied to the eyebrow. The senior author applies tension to the eye brow to a point when the eyelashes start to evert.)* The same tension should be applied on both eyes. The height of the first mark placed is generally placed about 7 mm from the ciliary margin. This distance may vary, depending on both the patient's desire as to how much pretarsal show is wanted and the extent of skin redundancy in the eyelid. To evaluate the marked position, the broken end of a cotton tip applicator or a lacrimal probe is placed at the marked position and gently pushed upward, creating a double fold (Figure 12.5). The fold is assessed by both the surgeon and the patient and adjusted as necessary to the desired outcome. For a patient wanting a low fold and narrow pretarsal show, a 6 mm mark is typically made, while for those wanting a high fold and wide pretarsal show an 8 mm mark may be used. For tighter pretarsal skin the marking is made slightly lower, while for looser pretarsal skin, the marking is generally made slightly higher. Redundant pretarsal skin may result in a narrow pretarsal show after OOLA fixation because more skin folds over the supratarsal crease

and causes a larger area of the pretarsal skin to drape downward. Three marks at equal distance apart are marked on the eyelid at the mid-pupillary, medially, and laterally. A line is drawn parallel to the tarsal margin by connecting these markings. In the region of the medial canthus, the fold tapers inferiorly even when the fixation is made at the same height as the mid-pupillary region (Figure 12.6). The surgeon should avoid the natural tendency to place the medial fixation lower than the mid-pupillary fixation in order to create a medial tapering eyelid fold, doing so may cause an absent medial fold.

After the marking is complete, the surgeon can release pressure on the eyebrow. When the patient opens his/her eyes the surgical markings tend to settle at or slightly above the level of the tarsal margin. For patients in their late teens and early twenties, with minimal dermatochalasia, no skin is required for excision and a horizontal incision is used. For patients in whom the excessive skin redundancy must be addressed a conservative amount of skin is excised. The design of the incision is similar to Caucasian blepharoplasty surgery.

Anesthesia

Anesthesia is administered both with use of oral and locally injected medications. *(Early in the senior author's career, versed injection were used for premedication, however use of oral premedications has been found to be just as effective. Although intravenous access is not routinely performed, it can be useful to maintain constant analgesia during the procedure.)* This surgery necessitates that the patient is completely responsive throughout the procedure. 30 minutes prior to the start of surgery, patients are premedicated with 1–1.5 mg of alprazolam (Xanax; Upjohn Inc, Kalamazoo, MI), 100 mg of propoxyphene napsylate, 650 mg of acetaminophen (Darvoct N-100; Purepac Pharmaceutical Co, Elizabeth, NJ), and 500 mg of cephalexin, provided the patient is not allergic to any of these medications.

The patient is brought to the operating room and placed in a supine position. Cardiac and oxygen monitoring devices are applied to the patient prior to administering local anesthetics. 2% lidocaine hydrochloride with 1:100,000 epinephrine solution buffered with sodium bicarbonate in a 1:10 ratio is injected through a 30-gauge, 1-inch-long needle. *(It is important to consider that the felt-tip marking can blur or erase if the anesthetic solution is applied to the skin and remarking on damp skin or after injection is difficult and inaccurate.)* The local anesthetic is injected in two layers: one just under the dermis and the second under the orbicularis oculi muscle.

A web of capillaries, venules, and arterioles are encountered during eyelid surgical procedures. Puncturing one of these small vessels can lead to a hematoma and subsequent tissue distortion. Hematoma formation significantly increases the risk of eyelid asymmetry and prolongs postoperative healing time. To avoid hematoma formation, the surgeon must inject into the proper plane and minimize the number of needle passes. If bleeding is noted, the area should be compressed immediately for about three minutes. Infiltrating too much local anesthetic will distort the anatomy potentially leading to eyelid asymmetry. To avoid this, an amount only required to achieve adequate analgesia and vasoconstriction is initially injected. As the procedure progresses additional local anesthetics can be used. It is also critical for the surgeon to avoid injecting anesthetics to the levator muscle. The slightest amount of anesthetics injected into the levator muscle can cause an asymmetric contraction of the muscle during the fixation stage, resulting in eyelid asymmetry. The asymmetrical appearance will reveal itself only after the patient has been sent home and the residual anesthetic effect has abated.

Instruments

A caliper is used to measure the distance from the ciliary margin to the proposed incision site. Also required are: a wide and sharp two-prong skin hook, a pair of iris scissors and a fine-toothed iris forcep, a bipolar cautery for hemostasis and a needle tip cautery for muscle incision, a fine-tipped curved hemostat clamps, and two eye shields.

Operative procedure

An incision is made through the skin layer only with a #15 Bard-Parker blade. The skin edge is spread apart to expose the underlying orbicularis oculi muscle (Figure 12.7A). The skin is tightly bound to this muscle. The incision must be made shallow enough that the muscle's fine capillaries can be preserved thus avoiding a subcutaneous hematoma. Capillaries may be coagulated with a fine bipolar cautery. The incision through the underlying muscle may be made with either a CO2 laser or a fine needle-tipped cautery. The incision through the obicularis should be made closer to the upper margin of the skin incision so as to ensure that muscle remains attached to the pretarsal tissue. Spreading the divided muscles apart reveals underlying loose areolar tissue. These two muscles are separated using two-pronged sharp skin hooks under tension while the septum is tented up. The orbital septum is also lifted from the underlying preaponeurotic fat compartment. *(Distinguishing factors the help identify the orbital septum from the levator aponeurosis is that the orbital septum has a dull, white, and somewhat fibrous texture, while the levator has a pearly-white glistening appearance. Superiorly, the orbital septum may be naturally fused with the levator aponeurosis. When encountered, the surgeon would see the levator aponeurosis just deep to the orbicularis oculi muscle. An inexperienced operator might cut the levator aponeurosis, thinking it is in fact the orbital septum.)* With the orbital septum tented up, a small portion of the orbital septum is divided (Figure 12.7B). Dissection is performed

deep to the divided septum, to develop a plane between the orbital septum and preaponeurotic fat (Figure 12.7C). Once established, the septum is opened widely (Figure 12.7D). The preaponeurotic fat is contained within a thin capsule. When the capsule is divided, fat easily herniates out, obstructing the surgical field and becoming difficult to manage. If fat excision is not necessary, the fat capsule should be preserved so as to avoid the nuisance of the obstructing fat hernation. The levator aponeurosis is located deep to the preaponeurotic fat compartment. A distinct plane exists between the fat compartment and levator, allowing for relatively easy blunt dissection between the two layers (Figure 12.7E). *Earlier in his career, the senior author would aggressively dissect the fat compartment from the levator aponeurosis, widely exposing the muscle. However, altering this anatomic relationship impacts the shape of the fold resulting potential asymmetric results. As such we currently recommend a limited dissection between these two structures.* Unless the fusion point is too low to expose the levator aponeurosis, the sac containing the fat should remain attached to the levator aponeurosis and fixation should be applied to the exposed portion of the levator aponeurosis.

The first fixation suture is placed along the mid-pupillary line (Figure 12.8A). To determine the proper fixation point on the levator, the exposed strip of pretarsal orbicularis oculi muscle is grasped and gently pulled superiorly, approximating the orbicularis directly to the levator. The appropriate height is determined when the pretarsal skin is stretched taut without everting the eyelashes. Fixation is made to the levator aponeurosis just above this point to the orbicularis (Figure 12.8B). A simple buried suture using a 6–0 or 7–0 nylon is used. The suture should be tied with just enough tension as to approximate the two tissues together with maximum contact surface. Suture tails should be cut to an appropriate length, if left too long a suture granuloma may develop.

At this point, the first operative field is temporarily covered and attention turned to the opposite side. The same technique is applied to each eye with the first fixation along the mid-pupillary plane. Once the midpupillary fixation suture is place bilaterally, the patient is then asked to open his or her eyes to compare the fixation and symmetry. If an asymmetry is noted this suture is adjusted accordingly. Once the desired fixation is achieved and symmetry is assured, a second suture fixation is placed in the region close to the lateral orbital rim. Patients frequently complain that the eyelid fold sags laterally. To prevent this, higher fixation to the levator along the region of the lateral canthus may be required. The levator aponeurosis is most well defined laterally, and becomes ill-defined or even absent along the medial canthal region. In the region of the medial canthus, an abundant amount of fibro-fatty tissue is found overlying the ill-defined levator aponeurosis. In addition, a small arteriole is frequently found in this area and can potential cause a significant hematoma. The medial suture fixation is frequently performed to the fibrofatty tissue and the pretarsal obicularis muscle (Figure 12.8C). Since this medial suture does not fixate to the levator, it does not demonstrate the dynamic properties as the lateral fixation sutures, which are fixated to the levator. Typically, a three-suture fixation is adequate, however for a more prominent fold or in revision cases, further fixation sutures can be placed between these three sutures. After placement of the fixation sutures, the skin edges are reapproximated, and the patient is reevaluated in

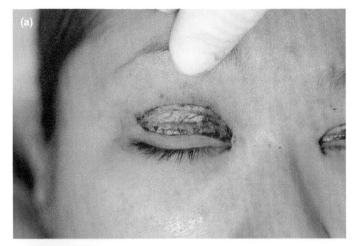

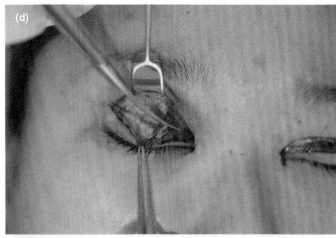

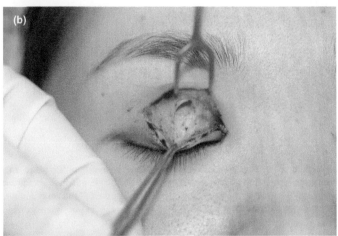

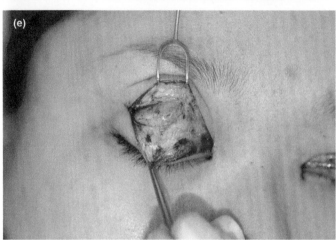

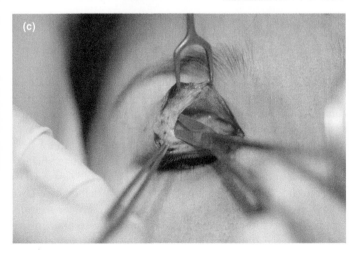

Figure 12.7 (A) Skin incision is made, exposing the underlying obicularis oris muscle. The obicularis muscle is divided. The muscle is retracted and the orbital septum is exposed. The orbital septum is distinguished from the levator aponeurosis by its adherence to the orbicularis oculi muscle and the lack of glistening surface of the levator aponeurosis. (B) The orbital septum is incised. (During this maneuver, the upper eyelid should be retracted tightly anteriorly and slightly downward while forceps apply a countertraction to tense the orbital septum.) (C) A pocket is created deep to the septum to help delineate the orbital septum. The preaponeurotic pocket is developed medially and laterally. (D) The orbital septum is devided, medially and laterally. (E) The levator aponeurosis (shiny white in appearance) and the preaponeurotic fat (within a thin, transparent capsule) are exposed.

the upright position for symmetry. Once the desired changes are confirmed, the skin is closed using a continuous absorbable 6–0 fast-absorbing gut sutures.

Recovery

Sterile wet gauzes are then placed over the eyes with the patient in a semi-reclining position. Ice bags are then placed over the gauze pads. Patients are asked to keep the ice packs on for 30-minutes then off for 30-minutes alternating this process for the following three days. Although absorbable sutures were used, sutures are

removed on one week after the primary procedure. In the immediate postoperative period, a high double eyelid fold is expected and the patients frequently require reassurance that the height of the fold will decrease. (The pretarsal show height is at least 50% higher in the first few weeks than it will be 2–3 years later). Mild eyelash eversion can be frequently seen and typically resolves with time. However severe ectropion should be identified and corrected in a timely manner. Patients are advised not to rub their eyes during the early stages of healing so as to prevent possible suture disruption.

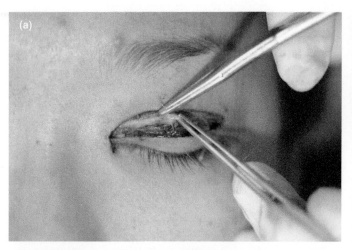

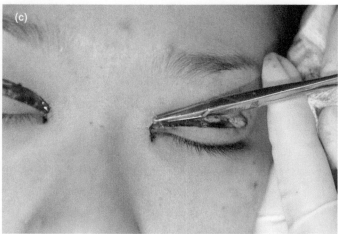

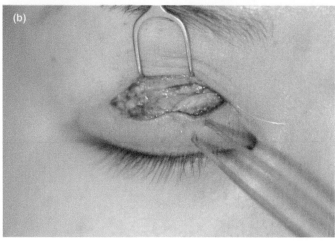

Figure 12.8 (A, B) The first fixation suture is along the mid-pupillary plane. The needle the passes through the levator aponeurosis, a large purchase should be applied to the levator. The needle also passes through the full thickness and the pretarsal obicularis oculi muscle cuff. (C) Medially, the levator aponeurosis is deep and poorly defined. The fibrofatty tissue is used as the medial fixation point and to the medial muscle cuff.

Complications

Use of perioperative antibiotics, strict sterile surgical technique, and the highly vascularized facial skin are all factors contributing to the infrequency of infection. Hematoma formation is more frequently seen, owing to numerous capillaries in the subdermal plexus. Ectropion is caused by excessive tension on the pretarsal skin by the action of the levator, frequently associated with placement of a high fixation on the levator. Significant ectropion requires early surgical intervention to release the fixation suture and resuturing the fixation suture at a lower level on the levator aponeurosis. Ptosis can be a result from several factors including: infiltration of local anesthesic to the levator muscle, hematoma formation within the levator muscle or aponeurosis, injury to the levator aponeurosis, or developing compensatory ptosis due to asymmetric fixation of the levator. Ptosis due to local anesthesia or hematoma within the levator resolves with time. During double eyelid surgery, disruption of the levator aponeurosis may not be apparent, especially near or over the tarsal margin. Ptosis from injury to the aponeurosis requires identifying the severed ends of the levator, and directly fixating the levator aponeurosis to the tarsus. Ptosis do to asymmetric fixation can be corrected by either placing the fixation suture at a lower position on the nonptotic side, or by placing the fixation suture higher on the levator on the ptotic side. Partial eyelid ptosis can frequently occur medially, obstructing the inner and upper visual fields. To correct this,

medial fixation sutures should be repositioned to a higher level. Suture material may migrate to the surface and cause redness, papules, or pustules. Suture granulomas are generally due to a long suture tail, superficial placement of the knot, thin skin, or a combination thereof. Removal of the suture and a short course of oral antibiotics tend to correct the problem. Suture material may migrate internally causing corneal or conjunctiva irritation.

Some cosmetic complications include asymmetry, shallow fold, release and inferior migration of the supratarsal crease, scarring, multiple folds or dimpling, and hollow eye deformities. Loss of fold or a shallow fold is frequently due to improper fixation techniques. Fixation to the orbital septum or fat compartments to anchor the fixation sutures instead of the levator aponeurosis, leads to loss of fold over time. Multiple folds, dimpling, and deep-set eyes are frequently due to aggressive removal of preaponeurotic fat or excessive obicularis muscle excision.

Cases; (Figure 12.9A,B) (Figure 12.10A,B)

PARK Z-EPICANTHOPLASTY

The medial epicanthal fold runs medially over the medial canthus as an extension of the upper eyelid. It covers the lacrimal lake and attaches to the medial aspect of the lower eyelid. The epicanthal fold is generally present in eyelids of the East Asian population. While it is present in 2–5% of Caucasian eyes, the

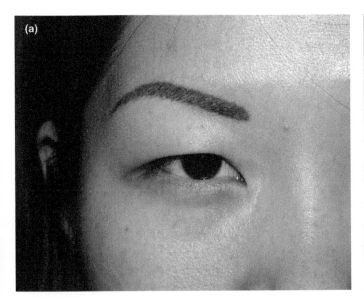

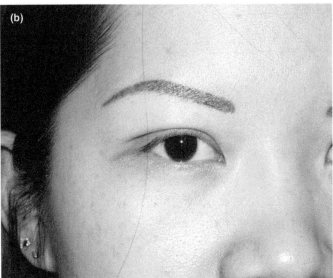

Figure 12.9 (A, B) Patients with OOLA.

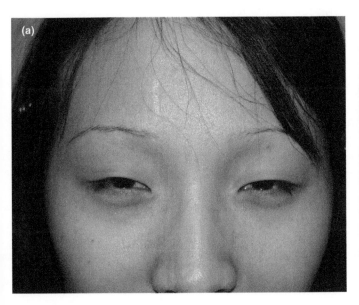

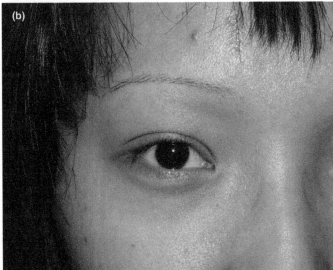

Figure 12.10 (A, B) Patients with OOLA.

incidence of the epicanthal fold ranges from 40–90% in the Asian population.(14, 15) The epicanthal fold has several clinical variations and a classification system has been described. The Asian epicanthal folds are either type II or type III.(16–18) For type II epicanthal folds, the pretarsal skin extends medially to form the epicanthal fold as it partially covers the lacrimal lake before ending at the lacrimal lake's margin (Figure 12.11A). Type III epicanthal folds completely cover the lacrimal lake curving laterally to transition with the lower eyelid (Figure 12.11B).

In the Asian eyelid without a supratarsal fold, the upper eyelid skin and the epicanthal fold region have a similar degree of skin laxity. This degree of skin laxity to the epicanthal folds allows the fold to have a gentle natural curve. Double eyelid surgery does not address the skin laxity to the epicanthal region. As

such, for patients with significant skin laxity to both the pretarsal region and the epicanthal region, performing a double eyelid surgery without addressing the epicanthal will create an unnatural transition from the supratarsal fold to the epicanthal region (Figure 12.12).

Formation of a supratarsal crease with a prominent epicanthal fold creates a narrower and higher appearing palpabral fissure. To create a more natural oval shape to the eye, an epicanthoplasty must be performed to increase the horizontal width of the eye. One of the major drawbacks to this procedure has been the risk of unsightly scars in the medial canthal area.(19) To avoid this potential complication, the senior author designed the Park Z- epicanthoplasty, in which the incisions are limited to the thin upper eyelid skin of the epicanthal fold.(16–18)

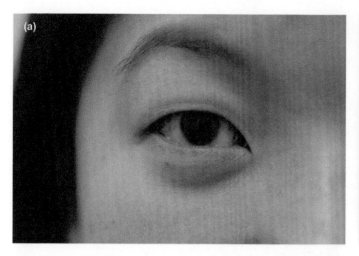

Figure 12.11 (A) Epicanthal fold type II (B) Epicanthal fold type III.

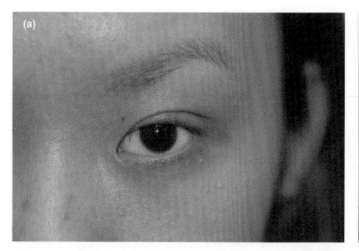

Figure 12.12 A distinct and unnatural appearance noted if a double eyelid fold is created without addressing a significant epicanthal fold.

Marking

Marking is made with the patient in a sitting position. The first marking is done on the surface of the epicanthal fold. Point A is marked as a surface representation of point D (Figure 12.13A). Point D is the medial most point of the lacrimal lake under the epicanthal fold. (Point D is not visible unless the epicanthal fold is stretched with the surgeon's finger (Figure 12.13B). Next, Point B is marked where the epicanthal fold joins the margin of the lacrimal lake in type II or the medial aspect of the lower eyelid in a type III. Point C is marked medial to point A on the eyelid skin. A line is drawn from point A medially toward the nose at a 90-degree angle to the medial curvature of the tarsal margin. Point C is marked on this line, crossed by the medial extension of the line for the double eyelid incision. Point E is marked on the medial aspect of the double eyelid incision line. Point E is a somewhat arbitrary point placed as a curved and upward extension of line AB (Figure 12.14A–C, Figure 12.15A,B). The supratarsal crease line is used for those who already have a double eyelid fold.

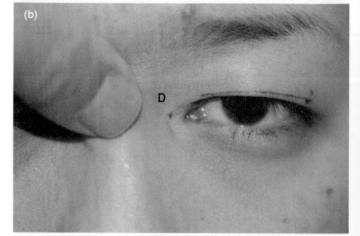

Figure 12.13 (A) Point A is the cutaneous representation of point D. (B) Epicanthal fold retracted. Point D is the most medial position of the lacrimal lake.

Operation

A Z-epicanthoplasty incision is made before the primary incision in a double eyelid operation. This is because the marking is complex and drawn in a small area with erasable ink. The

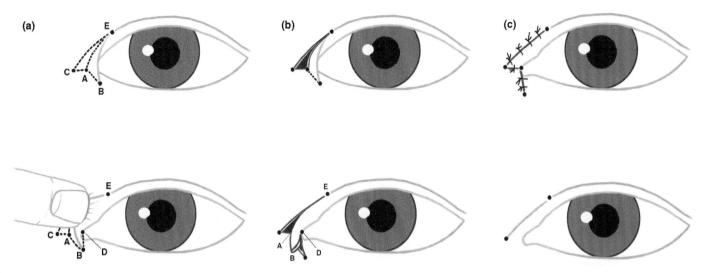

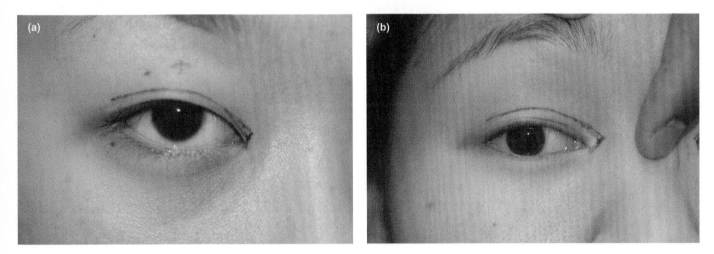

Figure 12.14 (A) Park Z-epicanthoplasty design. Line BD is exposed by retracting the epicanthal fold. (B) The skin paddle of triangle EAC is excised. An incision is made from points A to point B and from point B to point D, creating a flap EABD. (C) The flap is rotated. A suture is passed from point A to point D.

Figure 12.15 (A) Park Z-epicanthoplasty marking. (B) Point D and line BD are shown by pulling the epicanthal fold medially.

incision lines are scored with a blade before the markings are erased by blood. It is crucial to stretch the skin tight so that the incision line follows the marking exactly. Even a minor deviation from the marking could cause a significant scar. Line ECA is excised and discarded. Next, flap EABD is developed. The incision penetrates through the skin and muscle. Incision BD should be made straight by stretching the skin tightly. Point D is exposed by pulling the flap medially. The incision is made by facing the blade toward the surgeon and by beginning from Point D in order to avoid injury to the eyes. The incision is made with small, alternating gentle pushing and rocking motions until the instrument reaches the medial canthal ligament. Next, the muscle under point B is grasped with a pair of fine iris forceps and pulled up gently. At this point the base of the flap EABD rises off the surface of the medial canthal ligament. The surgeon feels a sudden release of the flap when it is completely freed from the ligament. The flap is then rotated to fill triangle ECA. If this flap release has been complete, the flap should fit in place without any fixation sutures (Figure 12.16A,B). Point A should be able to be brought down to point D without tension and line AB aligned with line BD. The flap is sutured with fast-absorbing gut. If a more distinctive crease is desired at the medial aspect of the double eyelid, one 7–0 clear nylon suture may be made between the muscles under the lines EAB and EC. The suture should be placed deep; otherwise suture granuloma develops easily in this area. For the eyelid with an excessively large epicanthal fold, a small portion of the tip of flap EABD may be trimmed. Great care should be made when placing the future from point D to point A, as to avoid injury to the eye. Debulking fat under skin flap CAB with electric cautery may help to level skin thickness with flap ABD.

Complications

Prolonged redness and scar formation are the two most common complications following this procedure. This can be attributed to poor flap design or improper surgical technique. Exact placement of point A and complete detachment of flap EABD are the two most important steps in avoiding a tense closure. If incision

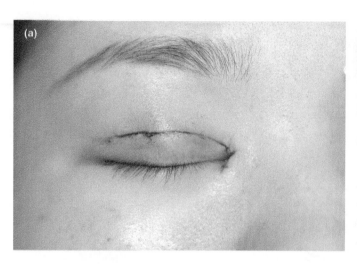
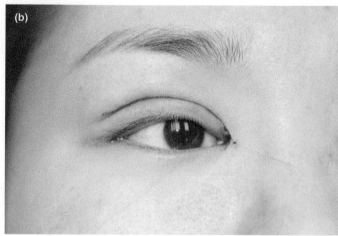

Figure 12.16 (A) The epicanthal fold is held in place quite nicely after being rotated. There is no suture holding the flap in place. (B) View with the eye open.

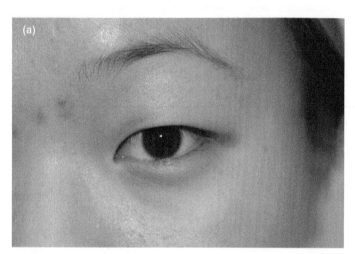
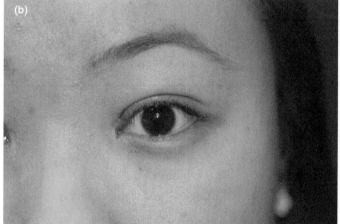

Figure 12.17 (A) Pre and (B) Post Park Z-epicanthoplasty views.

BD is made laterally to extending include the lower eyelid margin, an unsightly scar formation may form resulting in a "sand in the eyes" appearance.

Case; (Figure 12.17A,B)

ASIAN BLEPHAROPLASTY FOR ELDERLY PATIENTS

As skin ages, the double eyelid fold becomes thicker and irregular. Increased eyelid skin redundancy, obstructs a larger portion of the pretarsal skin leading to less pretarsal show. Aging eyelid surgery for both Asians and Caucasians requires excision of redundant skin from the lower portion of the supratarsal eyelid. Because the thickness of the upper eyelid skin differs, the approach to aging eyelid surgery significantly differs. Caucasian upper eyelid skin is generally the same thickness throughout the eyelid. Therefore the remaining skin, which is reapproximated after blepheroplasty surgery, is similar thickness to the removed excess skin preserving the delicate double eyelid fold appearance. In Asian eyelids, the upper eyelid skin and muscle are relatively thin near the supratarsal fold and become thicker closer to the eyebrow.(20) Resection of the delicate skin above the crease leaves the thicker skin to fold

over, which can result in a thickened appearance to double eyelid fold (Figure 12.18A,B). The goal of blepharoplasty for elderly Asian patients is to preserve as much of the thinner skin above the supratarsal crease so as to create a natural appearing supratarsal fold. Brow ptosis is also frequently a concurrent finding in many of these patients, which compounds the dilemma of preserving the thin supratarsal eyelid skin, since brow ptosis necessitates more skin excision. To address this, a concomitant forehead lift can be effective in preserving the thin upper eyelid skin (Figure 12.19A,B; Figure 12.20A,B).

Preoperative care
See that for the OOLA technique.

Marking
Marking is performed with the patient in a seated position and the eyes closed. The eyebrow is lifted with the nondominant thumb until the upper eyelashes begin to rise. A mark is made 7 mm from the ciliary margin at the mid-pupillary line using an extra fine, felt-tipped marker. Next, two additional marks are

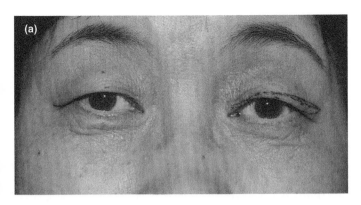
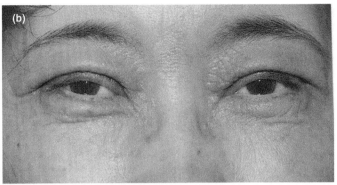

Figure 12.18 Upper lid blepharoplasty in an older Asian patient with significant dermatochalsia. (A) Preoperative, view. (B) One month-post operative view. Use of the thicker upper eyelid skin, results in a full appearance.

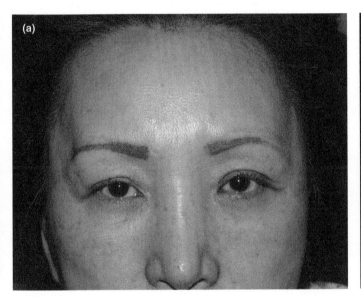
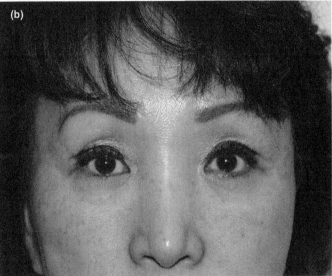

Figure 12.19 Forehead/browlifts can be used concomitantly with aging Asian blepharoplasty to preserve the thinner upper eyelid skin. (A) Preoperative. (B) Postoperative.

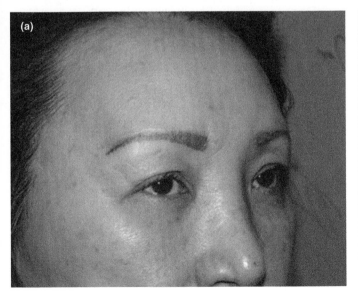
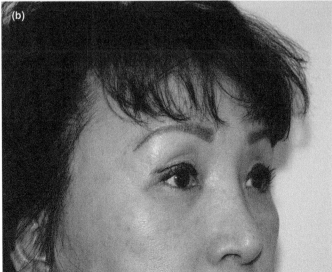

Figure 12.20 Forehead/browlifts can be used concomitantly with aging Asian blepharoplasty to preserve the thinner upper eyelid skin. (A) Preoperative. (B) Postoperative.

made 7 mm above the ciliary margin on the medial and lateral aspect. These three points are connected to make a gently curved line parallel to the ciliary margin. At the lateral end, the line is continued in a gentle upward curve within a rhytid. The patient next is asked to open his or her eyes in a neutral gaze and allow the eyebrow to settle into a neutral position. The three markings (medial, central, and lateral) are made at about 2 mm above the ciliary margin and parallel to the tarsal border. There markings are connected to form an upper incision line. Next the patient is asked to close the eyes, and the eyelid skin is then stretched tight by again lifting the eyebrow upward. The line is extended medially and laterally to join the lower incision marking. Medially the ellipse of the skin island is tapers in and laterally the skin island tapers out. The same amount of eyelid skin is removed bilaterally unless there is asymmetric brow ptosis. The marking of the opposite eyelid may be made with the patient in a supine position in the operating room, as better symmetry may be achieved by comparing the two sides on the operating table. However we recommend marking both eyes in the sitting position if the patient has asymmetric brow ptosis. (The eyebrow symmetry should be documented during the preoperative consultation. If brow asymmetry is present preoperatively, the patient should be made educated on this finding.)

Procedure

After the skin muscle excision is carried out, the standard OOLA procedure is followed. Despite the larger amount of skin excised, the skin edges should still have good apposition following fixation. The skin is closed using in a simple continuous running fashion with 6–0 fast-absorbing gut suture.

ELDERLY ASIAN MALE WITH UPPER EYELID REDUNDANCY

Regardless of the presence of the double eyelid fold, a main concern among elderly Asian males is the correction of droopy upper eyelid skin hanging over the tarsal margin and narrowing of the palpabral fissure. Unless a natural double eyelid is present, the majority of Asian males prefer not to receive a new double eyelid. When the skin excision method described for elderly Asian women is applied to the elderly Asian male patient, unwanted and sometimes unnatural-looking double eyelids are formed. This may happen even in the absence of an OOLA fixation. To avoid this, the lower incision in male patients should be placed lower (about 5 mm from the ciliary margin instead of 7 mm, as generally used in women). The upper incision is also placed lower, about 1 mm above the ciliary margin when the patient's eyes are open and in a primary gaze position. Pretarsal fixation should be conservative. However, adequate amount of skin should be excised laterally to address the increased amount of skin redundancy along the lateral orbital rim region.

REFERENCES

1. Park DH, Choi WS, Yoon SH, Song CH. Anthropometry of Asian eyelids by age. Plast Reconstr Surg 2008; 121(4): 1405–13.
2. Flowers RS. Upper blepharoplasty by eyelid invagination: anchor blepharoplasty. Clin Plast Surg 1993; 20: 193.
3. Zubiri JS. Correction of the oriental eyelid. Clin Plast Surg 1991; 8: 725.
4. Doxanas MT, Anderson RL. Oriental eyelids: an anatomical study. Arch Ophthalmol 1984; 102: 1232–6.
5. Chen WPD. Asian blepharoplasty and the eyelid crease. Philadelpia, PA: Butterworth Heinemann/Elsevier, 2006.
6. Mikamo K. A technique in the double-eyelid operation. J Chugaishinpo 1896; 396: 9.
7. Baek SM, Kim SS, Tokunaga S, Bindiger A. Oriental blepharoplasty: single-stitch, nonincision technique. Plast Reconstr Surg 1989; 83: 236.
8. Boo-Chai K. In: Barron JN, Saad MN. Operative plastic and reconstructive surgery. Edinburgh, Churchill-Livingstone, 1980: 764–8.
9. Mutou T, Mutou H. Intradermal double eyelid operations and its follow-up results. Br J Plast Surg 1972; 25: 285.
10. Chen WP. Asian blepharoplasty – anatomy and technique. J Opthal Plast Reconstr Surg 1987; 3(3): 135–40.
11. Park JI. Orbicularis-Levator fixation in double-eyelid operation. Arch Facial Plast Surg 1999; 1(2): 90–5.
12. Park JI. Orbicularis-Levator Fixation technique. In: Toriumi DW, Park JI. Asian Facial Cosmetic Surgery. Philadelpia, PA: Saunders/Elsevier, 2007: 49–59.
13. Park JI, Park MS. Double eyelid operation: Orbicularis oris-Levator aponeurosis fixation technique. In: Facial Plastic Surgery Clinics of North America. Philadelpia, PA: WB Saunders, 2007: 315–26.
14. Liu D, Hsu WM. Oriental eyelid: anatomic difference and surgical consideration. Ophthal Plast Reconstr Surg 1986; 2: 59–64.
15. Ohmori K. Esthetic surgery in Asian eyelid. In: McCarthy JG. Plastic Surgery. Vol 3. Philadelphia, PA: WB Saunders Co, 1990: 2415–35.
16. Park JI. Z-epicanthoplasty in Asian eyelids. Plast Reconstr Surg 1996; 98: 4, 602–9.
17. Park JI. Park Z-epicanthoplasty. In: Kim DW. Facial Plastic Surgery Clinics of North America. Philadelphia, PA: WB Saunders, 2007: (15):3:343–52.
18. Park JI. Park Z-epicanthoplasty. In: Chen WPD. Asian blepharoplasty and the eyelid crease. Philadelpia, PA: Butterworth Heinemann/Elsevier, 2006: 273–81.
19. Hin LG. Unfavorable results in oriental blepharoplasty. Ann Plast Surg 1985; 14: 523.
20. Hwang K, Kim DJ, Hwang SH. Thickness of Korean upper eyelid skin at different levels. J Craniofac Surg 2006; 17(1): 54–6.

13 Aesthetic eyelid surgery in different ethnic groups
Sterling S Baker and Randal Pham

More than 26% of the US population is nonwhite according to 2006 census.(1) The rate of growth in some minority groups is 18 times faster than the caucasian population. It is estimated that by 2056 more than half of the US population will be nonwhite. In fact, California has already become the first state in the United States with "minority" population surpassing 50%. These demographic changes impact surgical considerations in eyelid surgery as well as in many other areas of aesthetic surgery. Modified surgical techniques for application in darker skin types (Fitzpatrick III through VI) as well as linguistic and cultural competencies are needed to meet the increased aesthetic demands of this diverse population. A complete account of cultural issues involving aesthetic surgery is beyond the scope of this chapter; instead emphasis is placed on defining the doctor-patient relationship through which mutual understandings can be achieved across language and cultural barriers. A large part of this relationship can be established at the first meeting when the surgeon and the patient discuss aesthetic concerns and formulate treatment recommendations. From a philosophical perspective, the population of the United States has historically been diverse. Whether this pluralism is framed in lofty political rhetoric or in the harsh reality of discrimination based on one or more of many variables, economic and social pressures push this country towards homogeneity. Perhaps the collective genius of the founding fathers is embodied in the Constitution which provides for and directs us toward inclusiveness. Recognition of ethnic and cultural heritage remains an active pursuit of many, but even the celebrations that ensue are often inclusive, such as St. Patrick's Day. This process of defining what the population will become genetically and what phenotype will be accepted as the norm is for the foreseeable future a dynamic one. By definition, substantial ethnic diversity will persist. The authors hope that this chapter will provide the surgeon with perspectives that will be useful in understanding the ethnic patient's objectives. While we will be presenting general considerations, we recognize that each patient must be evaluated as an individual.

INTERVIEW THE ETHNIC PATIENT
The interview is the most important part of the entire evaluation process preceding surgery. While it is crucial to know anatomical variations among ethnic patients, the surgeon must also understand the patient's desires and expectations. Unrealistic expectations may be an indication of subtle psychological problems that present as a concern for the patient's appearance.

The patient's ethnic identity and individual desires must be taken into account. The surgeon's goal should be to enhance the patient's appearance within these parameters. The position of the upper eyelid crease in Asians is a widely discussed example of ethnic identity. In those Asians who have an upper eyelid crease, the crease is not as high or prominent as the crease in non-Asians.

The anatomic cause of this variation in Asians is the fusion of the orbital septum with the levator aponeurosis beneath the pretarsal orbicularis oculi muscle between the eyelid margin and the superior border of the tarsus.(2) In contrast, this area of fusion in non-Asians is above the superior margin of the tarsus which lies beneath the preseptal orbicularis oculi muscle. This common anatomic difference causes the Asian patient to identify with people who have low eyelid creases. This appearance may be radically changed by variations in techniques during blepharoplasty surgery. Aggressive upper eyelid skin removal may lead to a high upper eyelid crease and thereby "occidentalize" the patient. The initial interview with the Asian patient should clearly address the desired position of the postoperative lid crease. Some Asian patients will seek surgery to get an upper eyelid crease that looks like a Caucasian while others will choose an upper eyelid crease that retains an Asian appearance.

Another special concern that must be addressed during the interview is whether the patient has had a previous herpetic infection. Many patients for whom English is not a first language may assume that herpetic infections are sexually transmitted diseases. There may be a bias in their culture toward such diseases that may lead them to deny a truthful answer.

African American, Mediterranean and Southeast Asian patients are genetically predisposed to sickle cell anemia, thalassemia, and glucose-6-phosphate dehydrogenase deficiency. Failure to be aware of these hereditary diseases may result in severe complications during and after surgery.(3)

During a discussion of results and complications, patients should be informed of possible dyschromia, scarring, and prolonged erythema that may result from aesthetic eyelid surgery. Many Asian patients are Buddhists who believe in reincarnation, fate and destiny. These patients are taught to accept their appearances and may be embarrassed about having aesthetic surgery. A prolonged postoperative recovery period or a complication may result in isolation that can lead to depression. These postoperative issues should be discussed with the patient and their support system before surgery.

Such an open discussion will help establish a positive doctor-patient relationship.

SKIN VARIATIONS
Histological studies have shown that skin in the malar area of pigmented patients contains large and numerous melanosomes that are spread uniformly throughout the entire epidermis.(4) In contrast, lightly pigmented skin contains melanosomes that are small and sparse and concentrated as clumps in the basal layer of the epidermis. This lightly pigmented skin is prone to develop moderate to extensive solar elastosis with cumulative sun exposure. Darker skin types are less likely to develop this photodamage. Asians and African Americans rarely develop solar elastosis with aging. They

seldom complain about rhytides and treatment is usually not necessary. Lentigenes in the periorbital area, however, are challenges in Asian patients because these blemishes can present earlier in life than the sun damage associated with solar elastosis. Ablative laser resurfacing can be effective therapy but this treatment may expose these patients to postoperative inflammatory hyperpigmentation. (5) Nonablative laser and nonlaser treatments can be attractive alternatives for lentigenes in this population. Hispanic Americans, unlike Asians and African Americans, lack uniformity in skin type in part because their ancestry is mixed. Their skin types can vary from Fitzpatrick I to V. This mixture of skin types requires individual evaluation on a case-by-case basis. Prediction of risk of postinflammatory hyperpigmentation may not be as easy for Hispanic Americans as for Asians.(6)

Keloid and hypertrophic scars cause problems in ethnic groups with darker skin. African Americans are especially affected by these concerns.(7) Eyelid skin is thin and well vascularized, which seems to offer some protection against the development of these unsighted scars as a result of the eyelid incision during blepharoplasty surgery. Some surgeons advocate limiting the lateral extent of the upper lid incision to the orbital rim to avoid potential scarring. We have used many techniques to create blepharoplasty incisions ranging from steel scalpels to electrocautery. Although none of these modalities has created significant scarring, we have always attempted to limit lateral propagation of thermal energy at the wound margin to avoid hypopigmentation as well as scarring. We have found no contraindications to utilizing our preferred technique of CO_2 laser blepharoplasty in pigmented patients.

EYELID ANATOMIC VARIATIONS

Asian eyelid has distinct anatomic variations compared to other racial groups. Millard reported the surgical technique for "revision of the oriental eye" in 1964.(8) Since then numerous reports have been published on the subject of Asian eyelid anatomy. In 1984, Doxanas and colleagues reported the weak or absent insertion of the levator aponeurosis into the preseptal orbicularis and overlying dermis in Asian eyelids.(9) The fuller appearance of the Asian eyelid is due to the low extension of preaponeurotic fat and/or brow fat into the upper eyelid.(2)

In 1998, using high-resolution magnetic resonance images to compare Asian and Caucasian lower eyelids, Carter and colleagues showed two major differences in the lower lid anatomy: (1) there is more anterior projection of orbital fat with respect to the orbital rim in the Asian eyelid as compared to Caucasian eyelid and (2) there is more superior projection of orbital fat to the inferior border of the tarsus with poorly demarcated creases in Asian eyelid.(10) These anatomic differences are responsible for a higher incidence of eyelid malpositions, particularly entropions, in Asians.(11)

UPPER EYELID BLEPHAROPLASTY

The significant difference in Asian eyelid anatomy calls for a different approach to upper eyelid surgery in this population. Surgical planning must take into account the desired height of the upper eyelid, the amount of preseptal and postseptal fat to be removed and the medial and lateral contours defined by skin incision and, at times, orbicularis resection.

Kim et al. reported a high dissatisfaction rate among Koreans who underwent "double eyelid" surgery. The authors claim that their scar revision techniques achieved favorable aesthetic results for 2 years which was the duration of their postoperative followup.(12) McCurdy presented a system for reliable construction of Asian upper eyelids of specific size and shape and a system for staged modification of the epicanthal fold.(13) Lee et al. reported 67 patients undergoing anchor epicanthoplasty, where orbicularis muscle was trimmed and skin attached to deeper tissue in the medial canthal area.(14) Chen et al. outlined a detailed step-by-step approach to Asian upper lid blepharoplasty with special consideration to lid crease formation.(15)

In 2007, Yu et al. compared CO_2 laser blepharoplasty and radiosurgery and found that the CO_2 laser was superior to radiosurgery in terms of less intraoperative bleeding and shorter operative time.(16) Their immediate postoperative evaluation, however, only included 1 hour and 1 week postoperative followups. The erythema and swelling during the first week was not documented. Returning to work early was not evaluated in the older age group in Yu's study. Our experiences with thousands of Asian patients undergoing CO_2 laser blepharoplasty have been that the erythema and swelling during the first 3 days postoperative are crucial in determining when patients could return to their normal activities including presenting for work.

We found no study reporting upper eyelid blepharoplasty in Hispanics or African Americans. From our own series, we have noted satisfactory results with the use of CO_2 laser in the upper eyelid. We have not encountered hypertrophic scars and keloids on the eyelids which we attribute to the vascularity of the eyelid skin and to its thinness, particulary in the subdermis. Further, there are no significant subcutaneous anatomical variations among ethnic groups that predispose to hypertrophic scarring. We emphasize the need to limit the lateral extent of the upper eyelid incision especially in African Americans to avoid adhesive scarring. The removal of portion of orbicularis oculi muscle beyond the orbital rim risks removal of the lateral palpebral artery which can delay revascularization, prolong edema, and retard wound healing. When the periosteum at the rim is exposed, scarring of the skin to the orbital rim can occur. If the thicker skin of the lateral lid and temple are included in the blepharoplasty incision, this portion of the wound must be closed tightly to avoid late retraction of the wound. Our techniques have evolved to include a running locked suture in the extra-orbital portion of the incision.

LOWER EYELID BLEPHAROPLASTY

In 2002, Kang et al. determined the benefit of using the Ultrapulse CO_2 laser in Asian blepharoplasty. The authors noted postinflammatory hyperpigmentation in 10% of their patients that was successfully treated with topical retinoids and hydroquinone cream. (17) Because of the this relatively high prevalence rate of postoperative hyperpigmentation associated with CO_2 laser resurfacing, we prefer to resect excess lower eyelid skin with the CO_2 laser.

In addition to skin resection, orbicularis oculi muscle removal is also useful in addressing orbicularis muscle prominence that is quite common in Asian lower eyelids. To detect muscle prominence, the patient is asked to smile. Orbicularis muscle flexing can be assessed by measuring the amount of lower eyelid bunching, which is characterized by outward projection on lateral view. We recommended

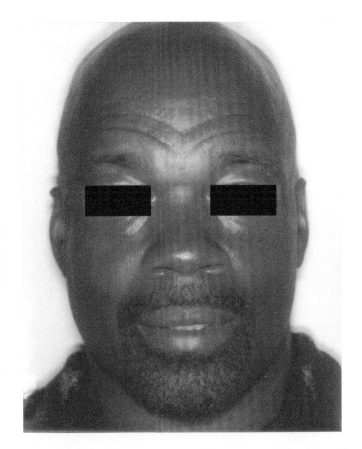

Figure 13.1 Pre-op photograph of 56 year-old African American patient with lower lid fat prolapse.

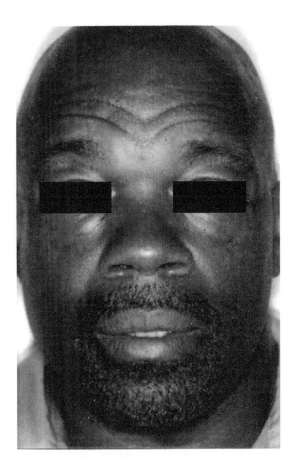

Figure 13.2 Post-op photograph of same patient one day post transconjunctival lower lid blepharoplasty shows improvement of fat prolapse with minimal swelling and ecchymosis.

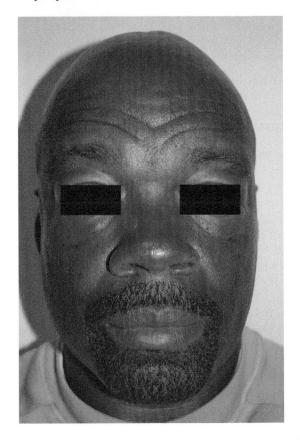

Figure 13.3 Post-op photograph of same patient 3 weeks after surgery shows improvement of fat prolapse.

minimal skin and only superficial orbicularis resections to avoid ectropion formation and extensive scarring, respectively. No more than 30% of orbicularis prominence should be reduced to prevent overcorrection with subsequent orbicularis weakness and contracted scar formation.

In patients with Fitzpatrick skin type VI or above, we prefer transconjunctival blepharoplasty with subsequent use of radiofrequency device such as Thermage to tighten the lower eyelid skin. This approach avoids the possibility of scar formation and pigmentation change in the lower eyelid, which is more difficult to conceal than in the upper eyelid because there is no lid fold (Figures 13.1, 13.2 and 13.3).

PERIORBITAL RHYTIDES
Melanin provides a natural protective mechanism against photodamage. For this reason periorbital rhytides occur much later in life in dark skin patients. Various modes of laser and nonlaser treatments have been studied in Asians and Hispanics. Few studies of rhytide treatment in African Americans have been performed perhaps because rhytides in this population are an infrequent problem.(3)

ABLATIVE LASER RESURFACING

CO_2 Laser Resurfacing
Studies of laser resurfacing in Asians show that postinflammatory hyperpigmentation is a frequent complication when performed in

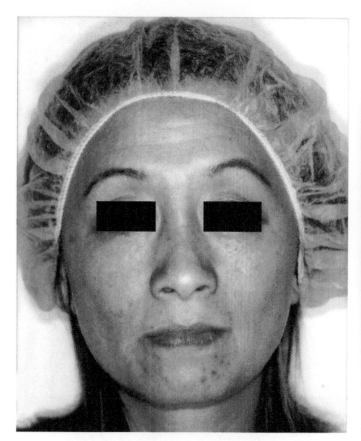

Figure 13.4 Pre-op photograph of 38 year-old Vietnamese female patient with solar lentigenes.

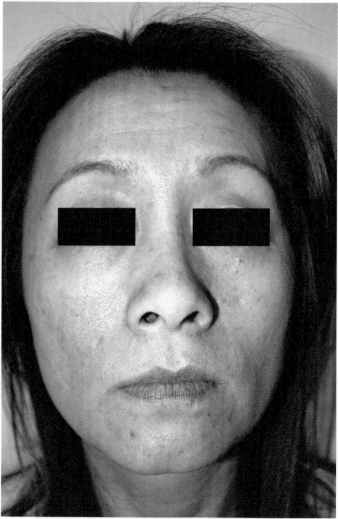

Figure 13.5 Post-op photograph of same patient 4 month post periocular laser resurfacing with Mixto fractionated CO2 laser (Lasering USA).

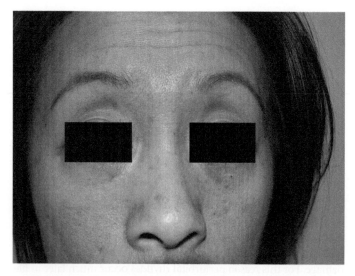

Figure 13.6 Enlarged post-op photograph of same patient 4 months after surgery shows improvement of solar lentigenes with no evidence of postinflammatory hyperpigmentation.

this population. A recent prospective study conducted by one of the authors found that fractionated CO_2 laser resurfacing, when performed with appropriate settings and adequate postoperative care, avoids postinflammatory hyperpigmentation. Six patients, two men and four women, of Vietnamese descent underwent

fractionated CO_2 laser resurfacing with the Mixto laser (Lasering USA, San Ramon, CA) in the periorbital area and were followed over a 6-month period. Preliminary results revealed no postinflammatory hyperpigmentation at 3-month postoperative followup (Figures 13.4, 13.5 and 13.6).

Ruiz-Esparza et al. studied CO_2 laser resurfacing in 36 Hispanics and noted 9 cases of hyperpigmentation. There were also 2 cases of focal hyperpigmention. One of these patients was exposed to the sun in the postoperative period.(6)

Erbium YAG laser resurfacing

Erbium YAG laser resurfacing can be safely performed in Asians with appropriate technique and pre- and postoperative cares. Pham conducted a prospective study involving 15 Asians using the Erbium YAG laser to treat photodamaged skin. Clinical improvement was noted in all patients. Hydroquinone 4% was used in the pre- and postoperative periods to prevent hyperpigmentation. No postinflammatory hypigmentation was noted in this study.(18)

NONABLATIVE LASER RESURFACING

Nd:YAG 1320-Nm Laser Treatment (Cooltouch)

Pham studied nonablative laser resurfacing in Asians using the CoolTouch laser and noted improvement of rhytides could be achieved with no side effect.(19) From this study the combined fractionated 1440 nm and 1320 nm nonablative laser named Affirm was developed by Cynosure (Chelmsford, MA, USA). The author's experience with this laser, however, has not been extensive at the time of this writing.

ND:YAG 1450-NM LASER TREATMENT (FRAXEL)

In 2007, Chan et al. suggested that both density and higher fluence determines the risk of postinflammatory hyperpigmentation.(20) In 2008, Kono et al. treated 30 Asian women with fractionated Nd:YAG 1450-nm and noted patient satisfaction increased significantly with increased fluence but not with increased density. Postinflammatory hyperpigmentation was seen in two patients. Pain, swelling, and erythema were also observed with higher fluences and densities.(21)

RADIOFREQUENCY TREATMENT (THERMAGE)

In 2006, Biesman, Baker et al. treated 63 patients for eyelid skin laxity and dermatochalasis using monopolar radiofrequency and reported modest success in a majority of patients treated. Of these 63 patients, 12 were Hispanics and 3 Asians. Posttreatment erythema was seen in all subjects but resolved within the first day after treatment. Blistering was noted in three patients. No postinflammatory hyperpigmentation was reported.(22) Our experience (SB) since publication of the Biesman study has included a more aggressive protocol with an increase in the number of applications. Our results have continued to show modest improvement in periorbital rhytides with the lower lids being the area most commonly treated.

PERIORBITAL DYSCHROMIA

Lentigenes

Lentigenes are benign actinic damage manifested as small flat uniformly pigmented lesions that can present in the lower lids, malar areas and lateral canthal regions. They occur in young and middle age Asian women and become more abundant with age. These lesions responded well to ablative and nonablative laser resurfacing. One of the authors (RP) noted that focal treatment with CO_2 or Erbium YAG lasers using the smallest spot size available with fluence of 20 J/cm² rarely produced postinflammatory hyperpigmentation.(18) These lesions, however, must be differentiated from malignant tumors such as basal cell carcinoma, squamous cell carcinoma and melanoma. When in doubt an excisional biopsy should be performed.

Melasma

Melasma presents as flat uniformly pigmented macules in the malar areas. Melasma occurs in all ethnic groups but is more prevalent in fair-complexed African American women, as well as Hispanic women and Asian women than in their more darkly pigmented counterparts. Patients who are at high risk of developing melasma are also at high risk of developing postinflammatory hyperpigmentation. In a study of Asian women undergoing Erbium YAG laser treatment for benign pigmented skin lesions one of the authors (RP) noted that medical history played a major role in predicting which patients would develop postinflammatory hyperpigmentation. Postinflammatory hyperpigmentation is the result of an inflammatory process triggered by an injury to the skin. When occurring after laser resurfacing, these lesions respond well to topical hydroquinone and eventually resolve.(18) Melasma, on the other hand, tends to recur when bleaching agent is discontinued.

Eyelid Vascular Lesions

In 2001, Pham reported successful treatments of three Asian patients for eyelid vascular lesions using Nd:YAG 1064-nm laser. One patient was diagnosed with port- wine stains, one with capillary hemangioma and one with a vascularized hypertrophic scar. All patients reported satisfaction with treatments and no adverse effect was noted.(23)

In 2008, Jackson noted that treating black skin for vascular lesions was challenging because melanin competes with hemoglobin for absorption of laser energy. However, port-wine stains, telangiectases, hypertrophic scars, and keloids can be treated with lasers.(4)

Eyeliner Tattoos

Eyeliner tattoos are very popular in Asian women. In 2004, we presented a study noting successful treatment of misplaced or over-applied eyeliner tattoos. In this study six Asian women were treated with the 810-nm diode laser. The treatments were repeated up to four times at 8-week interval. Improvements were noted in all patients treated (Figures 13.7 and 13.8). Loss of lashes, the only side effect, was noted in five lids (20.8%).(24)

Hair Removal Near the Eye

In 2002 one of the authors (RP) reported a prospective study of patients followed with electroretinography (ERG) after laser hair removal in the periorbital region. Pham et al. found no ERG evidence of retinal damage after laser hair removal near the eye when proper eye shield placement was used even when patients subjectively reported seeing "flashing lights" during laser irradiation. In this study all the subjects were Asians with dark choroids capable of intensely absorbing 810 nm infrared laser energy. Large external eye shields were used during the procedure that completely covered the globe and no retinal damage was recorded.(25)

Pham et al. studied the efficacy of the 810-nm laser in removing dark eyelashes in Asian patients and noted 80% reduction of eye lashes with the direct contact technique developed with this laser.(26) Although the technique was developed for trichiasis it could be used for removal of unwanted brow hair and other hair in the periorbital area.

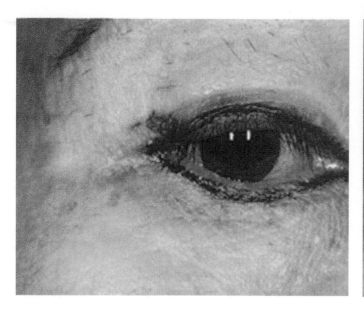

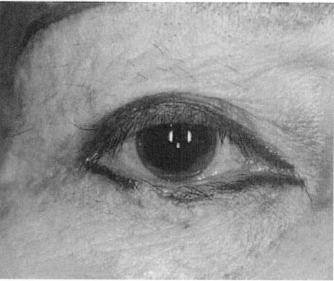

Figure 13.7 Pre-op photograph of 75 year-old Vietnamese female patient with misplaced tattoos.

Figure 13.8 Post-op photograph of same patient two year post-op shows disappearance of misplaced tattoos with scarring and no change in tattoo color.

CONCLUSION

Aesthetic surgery in the periorbital area in ethnic patients can present challenges to both the novice and the experienced surgeon. Emerging data, however, show that aesthetic surgery can be safely performed in different ethnic patients with proven techniques and appropriate pre- and postoperative cares. Further studies are needed to determine the safety and efficacy of new technologies as these modalities become available for treatments of ethnic patients.

REFERENCES

1. Projections of the resident population by race, Hispanic origin, and nativity: Middle series, 2006 to 2010. Washington, DC: Populations Projections Program, Population Division, US census Bureau, 2000.
2. Chen WPD, Khan JA, McCord CD Jr. Eyelid anatomy. In: Chen WPD, Khan JA, McCord CD Jr, eds. Color Atlas of Cosmetic Oculofacial Surgery. Philadelphia (PA): Elsevier, 2004: 5.
3. Jackson BA. Lasers in ethnic skin: a review. J Am Acad Dermatol 2003; 48: S134.
4. Blackmun S. Diverse skin types call for modified aesthetic treatments. Dermatol Times August 1998; 13.
5. Pham RT. Hyperpigmentation in Asians after carbon dioxide laser resurfacing (abstract). J Dermatol Surg 1998; 29: 118.
6. Ruiz-Esparza J, Barba Gomez JM, Gomez de la Torre OL, Huerta Fra Parga Vazquez EG. Ultrapulse laser skin resurfacing in Hispanic patients. A prospective study of 36 individuals. Dermatol Surg 1998; 24: 59.
7. Halder RM, Grimes PE, McLaurin CL, Kress MA, Kenney JA Jr. Incidence of common dermatoses in predominantly black dermatology practice. Cutis 1983; 32: 388.
8. Millard DR. The Oriental eye and its surgical revision. Am J Ophthalmol 1964; 57: 646.
9. Doxanas MT, Anderson RL. Oriental eyelids. An anatomic study. Arch Ophthalmol 1984; 102: 1232.
10. Carter SR, Seiff SR, Grant PE. The Asian lower eyelid: a comparative anatomic study using high-resolution magnetic resonance imaging. Ophthalmic Plast Reconstr Surg 1998; 14(4): 227.
11. Carter SR, Chang J, Aguilar GL, Rathbun JE, Seiff SR. Involutional entropion and ectropion of the Asian lower eyelid. Ophthalmic Plast Reconstr Surg 2000; 16: 45.
12. Kim YW, Park HJ, Kim S. Secondary correction of unsatisfactory blepharoplasty: removing multilaminated septal structures and grafting of preaponeurotic fat. Plast Reconstr Surg 2000; 106(6): 1399.
13. McCurdy JA Jr. Upper blepharoplasty in the Asian patient: the "double eyelid" operation. Facial Plast Surg Clin North Am 2005; 13(1): 47.
14. Lee Y, Lee E, Park WJ. Anchor epicanthoplasty combined with out-fold type double eyelidplasty for Asians: do we have to make an additional scar to correct the Asian epicanthal fold? Plast Reconstr Surg 2000; 105(5): 1872.
15. Chen WPD, Khan JA, McCord CD Jr. Asian blepharoplasty of the upper lid. In: Chen WPD, Khan JA, McCord CD Jr, eds. Color Atlas of Cosmetic Oculofacial Surgery. Philadelphia (PA) 2004: 73.
16. Yu CS, Chan HH, Tse RK. Radiosurgery versus carbon dioxide laser for dermatochalasis correction in Asians. Lasers Surg Med 2007; 39(2): 176.
17. Kang DH, Choi JH, Koo SH, Park SH. Laser blepharoplasty in Asians. Ann Plast Surg 2002; 48(3): 246.
18. Pham RTH. Laser resurfacing in Asians. In: Carniol PJ, ed. Facial Rejuvenation. New York (NY): Wiley-Liss, 2000: 389.
19. Pham RTH. Nonablative laser resurfacing. Facial Plast Surg Clin North Am 2001; 9(2): 303.
20. Chan HHL, Manstein D, Yu CS et al. The prevalence and risk factors of postinflammatory hyperpigmentation after fractional resurfacing in Asians. Lasers Surg Med 2007; 39: 381.
21. Kono T, Chan HH, Groff WF et al. Prospective direct comparison study of fractional resurfacing using different fluences and densities for skin rejuvenation in Asians. Lasers Surg Med 2008; 39(4): 311.
22. Biesman BS, Baker SS, Carruthers J, Silva HL, Holloman EL. Monopolar radiofrequency treatment of human eyelids: a prospective, multicenter, efficacy trial. Lasers Surg Med 2006; 38(10): 890.
23. Pham RTH. Treatment of vascular lesions with combined dynamic precooling, postcooling thermal quenching, and Nd:YAG 1,064-nm laser. Facial Plast Surg 2001; 17(3): 203.
24. Pham RTH. Treatment of eyeliner tattoos using 810 nm diode laser. ASOPRS Fall Scientific Symposium; 2004.
25. Pham RTH, Tzekov RT, Biesman BS, Marmor MF. Retinal evaluation after 810 nm Dioderm laser removal of eyelashes. Derm Surg 2002; 28(9): 836.
26. Pham RTH, Biesman BS, Silkiss RZ. Treatment of trichiasis using 810 nm diode laser: an efficacy study. Ophthalmol Plast Reconstr Surg 2006; 22(6): 445.

14 Ethnic rhinoplasty in patients of African descent

William Lawson and Konstantin Vasyukevich

INTRODUCTION

Aesthetic surgery of the African nose presents a unique set of challenges to the rhinoplasty surgeon. Lack of a unified concept of "facial beauty" for the African face makes it difficult to establish aesthetic objectives and even more difficult to judge the outcome of surgery. The anatomy of the African nose differs sufficiently from its Caucasian counterpart making the use of many surgical techniques developed for Caucasian patients ineffective. Not the least, preservation of ethnic self-identity, desired by most patients, requires the changes to the shape of the nose to conform to a "norm" accepted within the patient's social group.

To establish the aesthetic goals of the surgery both the surgeon and the patient rely on the idealized image of the face that in their minds represents beauty. Assuming that the patient holds the same standard of beauty as the surgeon could results in significant disappointment for both parties, as the desired facial aesthetics may vary widely between the cultures and the countries of origin. The neck rings of Kaya people or the lip plates of Surma women are striking examples of this difference.

Although in our increasingly globalized world certain facial qualities (e.g., facial symmetry) hold nearly universal appeal, important racial and cultural differences still exist.

In Western culture, the quest for the idealized representation of a beautiful face dates back to the classical canons of the Greeks and the neoclassical canons of the Renaissance. The pursuit to define idealized facial proportions, once the domain of artists and scholars, in recent years has been overtaken by ever growing media outlets and fashion magazines in search of the face that appeals to the aesthetic sensibilities of the public.

Needless to say, idealized facial beauty is heavily influenced by the shape and proportions of the western face, which in turn is based on distinctive Caucasian anatomy.

The mass appeal of the fashion and movie industries presenting African models and actresses with nearly western features is largely responsible for an idealization of Western features by many African patients seeking rhinoplasty. However, most ethnic patients would outrightly reject the idea of ethnic transformation to a Western model and wish to retain their overall ethnic look but with improved facial features.

Regardless of one's ethnic origins the images of actors and fashion models that surround us in our daily lives have a profound effect on our perception of beauty. Therein lies the first challenge to ethnic cosmetic surgery as most patients do not want to lose their distinctive ethnic characteristics, but at the same time want their features to be modified to resemble those of the celebrities they admire. Another challenge is the inherent limitations of the surgical techniques as they are applied to the distinctly different anatomical structures of the ethnic face. To overcome these challenges thorough exploration of the patients' expectations and understanding of their esthetic standards is paramount in establishing the appropriate goals for the surgery. Surgeons' understanding of the limitations of the surgical techniques as they apply to the African nose makes accomplishing these goals possible.

WHAT THE PATIENT WANTS?

Cosmetic modification of the African nose is based on a thorough assessment of the nasal components and an understanding of the balance of the nose as it relates to other facial features. Each patient presents a unique set of features to be analyzed and challenges to be overcome. However, despite significant variability in patients' facial features a pattern of changes that the patients desire and which are unique to the African rhinoplasty can be derived.

Stucker reviewed the preoperative records of 100 consecutive African-American patients and 100 Caucasian patients. He found notable differences between the White and Black patients' response to the question "What specifically do you not like about your nose?". The most common complaint by Caucasian patients was hump deformity, followed by tip deformity, nasal obstruction, and a crooked nose. In Black patients the most common complaints were in order of decreased frequency: (a) tip too big and fleshy; (b) base too broad; (c) nostrils round; (d) columella short; (e) dorsum too wide; (f) nose too close to the lip (acute nasolabial angle); (g) depressed dorsum; (h) hump deformity.(1)

Hoefflin provides a detailed description of the nose most commonly requested by patients in his practice.(2)

1. The radix that displays a subtle concavity that is in harmony with the supraorbital ridge.
2. A bridge that is neither too prominent nor too thin but is of uniform and moderate width from the nasion down to the alar groove. The supraorbital ridge should flow and blend in with the bridge.
3. A straight or slightly concave dorsum. Most patients initially want to limit the size of the dorsal graft fearing that their nose will appear too large.
4. A shapely tip with a contoured projection above the dorsal line. Many non-Caucasian patients want more nasal tip projection than one might initially anticipate.
5. Vertical-oblique nostrils that are neither flaring nor pitched. The nasal base should be triangular in shape and should fit within the intercanthal distance dimension.
6. A columella of adequate length that projects slightly below the alar margins.
7. Slightly obtuse nasolabial angle.
8. A maxilla that provides good support to the nasal base.
9. Skin of thin-to-moderate tension that provides good tip definition.

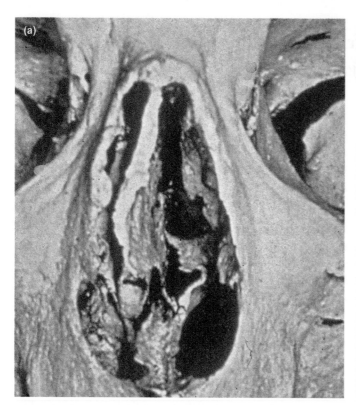
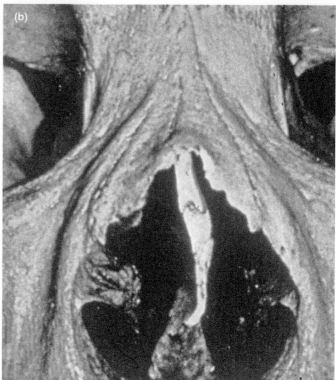

Figure 14.1 Photograph of Caucasian (left) and African (right) skulls illustrating the differences in nasal aperture geometry.

ANTHROPOMETRIC MEASUREMENTS, MORPHOLOGY, AND ANATOMY

Anthropometric Measurements

The scholarly exploration of the anthropometric differences between races has its origins in the late 19th century. The nasal index, popularized by Topinard (1890), attempted to quantitate anthropologic features.(3) The ratio of nasal width to nasal height multiplied by 100 was used to classify a nose into either Leptorrhine(Caucasian): 69.4 to 63; Platyrrhine (Negroid): 108 to 87.9; or Mesorrhine (Mongoloid): 81.4 to 69.3 (4) categories. Although the actual numbers are not intrinsically significant, their use serves as an objective reproducible means of discussing racial differences.

Farkas et al. conducted anthropometric measurements of African male and female faces and compared them to standard Caucasian measurements. He found highly significant differences in almost all the measurements of nasal dimensions between these groups. The African nose was consistently wider and shorter than the Caucasian.(5)

The study of the facial dimensions of 109 males of African-American descent, by J. P. Porter, showed a significantly shorter nasal length, a wider alar width, a shorter nasal tip protrusion, a wider nasal root width, a shorter columella, a more acute nasolabial angle, and a nasal bridge that is less inclined than that of its Caucasian counterpart.(6) In a similar study of 107 African-American females, anthropometric measurements of the noses showed a decreased columella-to-lobule ratio, a wider alar width when compared to the intracanthal distance, a more acute nasolabial angle, and a decreased nasal inclination when compared to the Caucasian standard.(7)

Ofodile and Bokhari compared seven anthropometric measurements of African-American noses to those of the North American adult population reported by Farkas et al.(8) They found the African nose to be wider, with the lateral attachments of the alae placed lateraly to the medial canthus. Contrary to other reports, the length of the African nose approximated that of the Caucasian nose in this patient population.(9)

Nasal Bones and Pyriform Aperture

The study of the width and length of the nasal bones and the pyriform apertures by Ofodile demonstrated remarkable difference in the configuration of the nasal pyramid between the skulls of persons of African descent and their European and Indian counterparts. On average the pyriform apertures in Blacks were wider and more oval-shaped (Figure 14.1), with short nasal bones set at obtuse angle to each other. Caucasian and Indian nasal pyramids were triangular-shaped, narrow, and long.(10)

Lower Lateral Cartilages

Ofodile measured the size of the lower lateral cartilages of 12 African male cadavers and compared them to the Caucasian alar cartilages measurements reported by Zelnik and Gingrass.(11) Contrary to the common belief that the cartilages in African noses are significantly smaller and weaker than in the Caucasian nose, he found only marginal differences in lower lateral cartilage size. When comparing the width of the cartilages in these populations, he found a greater range of the width in the African than in the Caucasian nose (0.9–2.5 cm vs. 1.7–3 cm).(12)

Nasal Morphology

The objective measurements of the nasal dimensions and study of the nasal components substantiate the descriptions of the African nose by experienced rhinoplasty surgeons.

Stucker outlined the following distinctive features of the African nose specified by his patients (1)

1. The tip is too big, fleshy (broad, flat)
2. Base (alae) too broad
3. Nostrils round
4. Collumela short, tip depressed
5. Dorsum too wide
6. Nose too close to lip (nasolabial angle)
7. Depressed dorsum
8. Hump deformity

Hoefflin provides a detailed description of a typical African nose.(2)

1. The radix is usually low, deep, and inferiorly set, with an obtuse nasofrontal angle averaging 130 to 140 degrees. The lack of the radix projection may be further accentuated by a wide intercanthal distance.
2. The bridge is usually wide and flat with short nasal bones. The average bridge width is 2.5 cm. There is often a deficiency in osteocartilagenous support, which is particularly striking in relation to the full tip. Due to the inferiorly set radix the nose is quite short, averaging 5.0 cm from nasion to tip.
3. The dorsum is often flat or depressed, lacking anterior height.
4. The nasal tip is usually thick-skinned, round, and slightly-to-moderately underprojecting, with the apex lying below the dorsal line. The domes are broad, and there is abundant subcutaneous tissue. Because of the fullness, there is minimal definition and a lack of landmarks and sculpting. The average tip height is 2.4 cm. The average tip width is 2.8 cm.
5. The base is wide with thickened alar side walls. The nostrils are usually more horizontal than vertical, causing a flattened appearance. The alar walls usually project beyond the intercanthal line. The nostrils are flaring with a wide interalar distance. The average base width is 3.8 cm.
6. The columella is usually short and recessed with hypoplastic medial crura. There is an alar-columella disproportion resulting in little or no columellar show.
7. The nasolabial junction is usually retructed. The nasal spine is underdeveloped and the maxilla is retrusive. The nasolabial angle is usually less than 90 degrees.
8. The maxilla is usually hypoplastic.
9. The skin is generally thick and bulky, containing vast amounts of fibrofatty tissue and sebaceous glands.

To account for the variability in the nasal morphology among the patients in his study group, Ofodile et al. divided black American noses into three groups: African; Afro-Caucasian; and Afro-Indian.

1. The African nose is usually found in darker pigmented individuals. This nose is short and wide with a concave dorsum and a bulbous tip. The alae are flared and the columella is short resulting in wide and horizontally oriented nostrils.
2. The Afro-Caucasian nose is found more often in light-skinned American blacks. The nose is longer and the dorsum is high, narrow, and often has a hump. The alae are less flared and the columella is longer which results in more vertically oriented narrow nostrils resembling the Caucasian nasal base. The tip is less bulbous.
3. The Afro-Indian nose is usually long and large. The bridge is wide and high with a hump. The alae are flared and the tip is bulbous, but tip projection is greater then in the African nose.(13)

SURGICAL TECHNIQUES

Dorsal Modification

Kamer and Parkes viewed the African nose as an equilateral triangle with the apex removed. They noted that with this configuration of the nasal pyramid, lateral osteotomies with infracturing of the nasal bones failed to increase dorsal projection, or narrowing of the nose. They suggested that placement of a dorsal strut without lateral osteotomies would result in an illusion of narrowing of the nose by closing the apex of the triangle (14) (Figure 14.2a).

Although dorsal augmentation is more common in African rhinoplasty, Stucker noted that about 20% of African patients in his practice required dorsal hump reduction and nearly 50% needed augmentation. For limited dorsal augmention (< 4 mm) he recommended the use of septal cartilage. If more significant augmentation was required (> 5 mm) he had great success using a tightly rolled alloplastic mesh. The mesh was placed over the nasal bones and was tapered for a precise fit in the nasofrontal angle; caudaly it extended to the area just above the tip cartilages (1).

As discussed above, Ofodile divided African noses into three distinct subtypes. A dorsal hump was present is 63% of the Afro-Indian group, 36% of the Afro-Caucasian group, and 18% of the African group. Osteotomies with infracture could be successfully performed in the Afro-Caucasian nose and dorsal augmentation was more commonly required in the African group.(13)

A variety of autogenous and alloplastic materials can be used to augment the dorsum. Septal cartilage provides a convenient source of cartilage for both dorsal augmentation and structural grafting. The most significant drawback to its use is an inadequate amount of material available for high volume augmentation. In the African nose, as noted by Stucker, the septal cartilage is often thinner than in the Caucasian nose (1) which limits its use to subtle augmentation of the dorsal profile and correction of minor irregularities.

The addition of cartilage obtained from the auricular concha can increase the bulk of the dorsal implant and produces minimal donor site morbidity. Layers of the cartilage can be stacked and sutured together to increase the implant thickness. Addition of crushed cartilage or fascia, as advocated by Hoefflin, can increase the bulk and soften the edges of the graft.(2)

Obtaining autogenous bone or cartilage from sources such as the rib or the outer table of calvarial bone can provide additional autogenous material to augment a markedly deficient dorsum. However, it comes at the expense of increased morbidity at the donor site, an unpredictable resorption rate, and possible delayed warping.

To overcome these difficulties, a number of rhinoplasty surgeons have turned to alloplastic implants as their first choice of material for dorsal augmentation. These implants have an unlimited supply, are relatively inexpensive, easy to use, and can be fashioned precisely to fill the defect. As with any implant, concerns of rejection, infection, and extrusion limit their use.

107

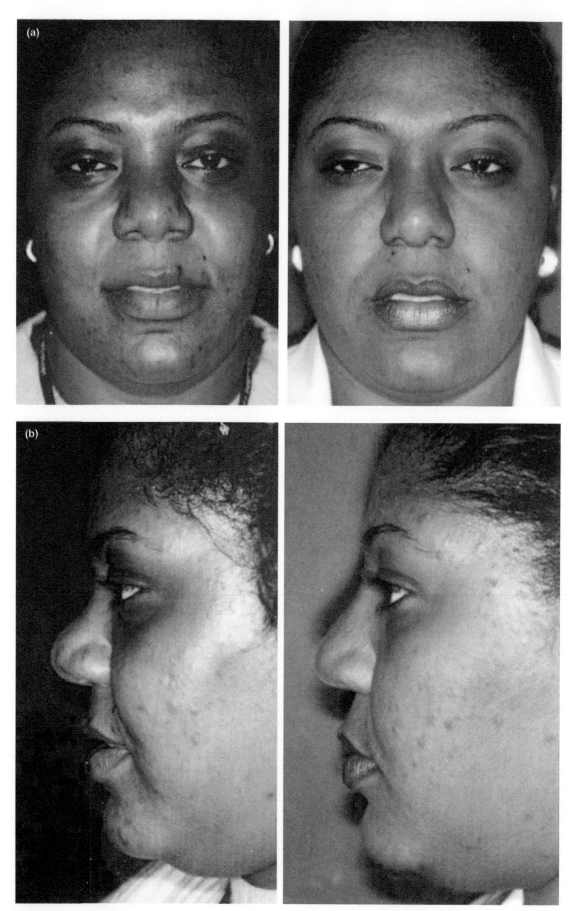

Figure 14.2 Patient underwent Prolene® dorsal graft placement. No osteotomies were performed. (A) Note the appearance of the narrowing of the nose on the frontal view. (B) Augmentation of the dorsum lateral view.

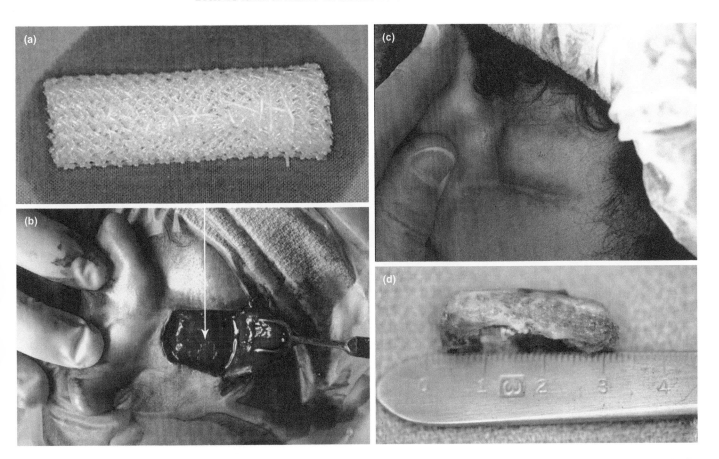

Figure 14.3 Tightly rolled Prolene® mesh (A) can be used primarily, or secondarily, as an autoalloplast (D). The implant is embedded into a postauricular pocket for three weeks (B, C). Following soft tissue ingrowth, the graft looks almost indistinguishable from the surrounding soft tissue (arrow in (B)). Once removed the graft can be easily carved into the desired shape and implanted into a dorsal pocket.

Kamer and Parkes advocated the use of Silastic® for dorsal augmentation. While up to 20% of their patients developed problems with their implants, they believed that timely removal of the implant and re-implantation of the silastic into the same pocket once the acute inflammation subsided provided a way to improve implant retention.(14)

As noted above, Stucker had great success in using tightly rolled Merselene® mesh. In over 400 cases, only 5 implants were lost to infection. No implant that was soaked in an antibiotic solution before placement was lost to infection.(1)

In the authors' experience the majority of patients of African descent desiring a rhinoplasty generally have a platyrrhine configuration and require a significant degree of augmentation. Septal grafts provide insufficient volume and are reserved for the creation of columella struts. Auricular cartilage when employed with mild to moderate defects is divided into segments which are placed transversely along the nasal dorsum.

Patients are generally reluctant to accept the donor site morbidity of calvarial bone and costal cartilage grafts. Consequently, alloplastic implants of Prolene® mesh are inserted primarily in their native form, or secondarily as an autoalloplastic following implantation and fibrous ingrowth in the retroauricular area. This material has been used for 15 years and has been found to have excellent biotolerance and long-term retention (Figure 14.3).

When significant dorsal augmentation is required, osteotomies are not performed as they only produce instability and provide no gain in nasal height. The authors use an endonasal approach in virtually all the cases, inserting the implant through combined intercartilaginous and transfixion incisions, creating a deep and symmetric pocket over the nasal framework which extends from the glabella region to the supratip area. The overlying soft tissue should not be under tension to avoid vascular compromise. Care is taken to bevel and feather the edges to avoid ridges and have a contour confluent with the underlying structures. All implants are soaked in an antibiotic solution before implantation (Figure 14.2a, 2b).

Tip Modification

The various techniques of tip modification that are commonly used in Caucasian rhinoplasty can be applied to the African nose. Increasing tip projection and improving tip definition are the two most commonly sought surgical changes.

Tip projection can be modified by changing its protrusion off the plane of the face, by creating an illusion of increased projection by narrowing the alar base, or by modifying the tip.

Tip modification of the African nose must be approached as creation of the tip-columella complex to create tip protrusion and definition. This entails compensation for the diminished thickness and elasticity of the lower lateral cartilages, lateral displacement of the lateral crura along with the often elongated and horizontal ala and nares, increased interdomal width, and shortened medial crura. These structural deficiencies are enhanced by a short cartilagenous septum and an increased membranous septum failing

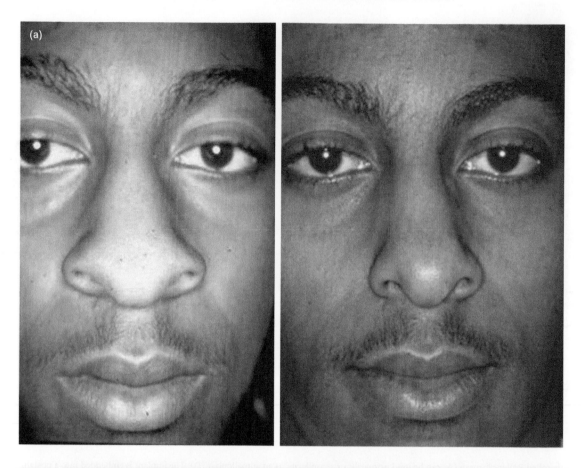

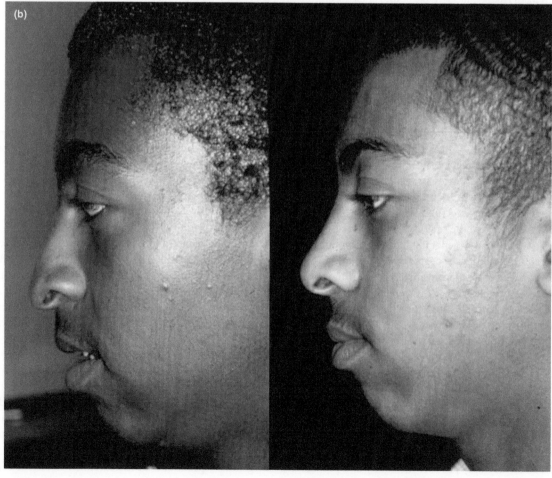

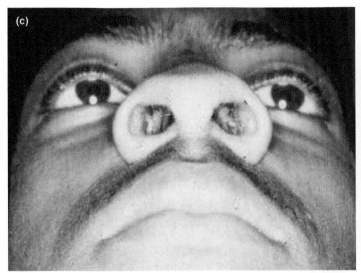

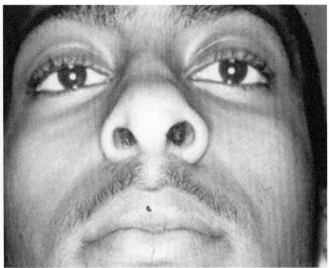

Figure 14.4 Patient underwent dorsal modification with medial, and lateral osteotomies, and a minor hump reduction. The tip was modified with a dome binding suture and a columellar strut. A premaxillary plumping graft was placed at the anterior pyriform aperture. Both alar flare and a wide nasal sill were reduced. (A) Frontal view; (B) Lateral view; and (C) Base view.

to provide caudal septal support to the lower lateral cartilage-columellar complex.

Narrowing of the tip can be achieved either with suture modification of the intact cartilagenous strip, or by cartilage interrupting techniques such as the Goldman tip-plasty, or one of its modifications. Suture modification of the shape of the domes entails placement of an intradomal suture through the junction of the medial and the lateral crura of the lower lateral cartilages. Both domes can also be brought together with one transdomal suture. A suture placed between the domes of the alar cartilages can also increase tip projection especially when a segment of lateral crus is incorporated into the dome resulting in lateral crural steal. In poorly supported tips, a columellar strut can be incorporated into this construct effectively creating a stable structure that resists the gravitational forces on the thick soft tissue envelope (Figure 14.4a,b,c).

Goldman tip-plasty involves complete transection of the alar cartilages just lateral to the domes and suturing the domes together. This releases the spring of the lower lateral cartilages resulting in increased projection of the medial segment. Placement of a columellar strut which is incorporated between the medial crura provides additional tip support projection and narrowing (Figure 14.5). In the senior author's experience this technique provides excellent and long-lasting results in African patients (Figure 14.6a,b,c).

Placement of a columellar strut is the most commonly used technique to increase tip projection. A rigid structure placed between the medial crura can augment the deficiency of the natural spring and length of this paired structure and push the tip off the facial skeleton. In patients with a deficiency or retrusion of the anterior nasal spine the strut can be used in conjunction with the "plumping" graft that is placed at the anterior border of the pyriform aperture and is designed to provide a stable base for the augmented and projected tip. Placement of the precrural "shield" graft is another way of increasing tip projection and improving tip definition. This can be designed as an

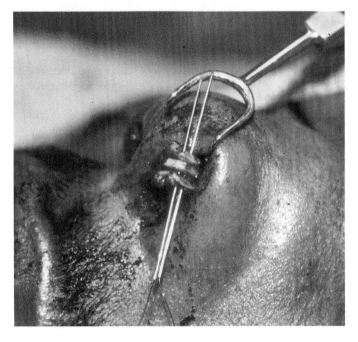

Figure 14.5 Goldman tip-plasty. Lower lateral cartilages transected and the columellar strut is placed between the medial crurae. The lower lateral cartilages–strut complex is secured with a permanent suture.

extended graft serving also as a columellar strut.(15) In patients with bimaxillary protrusion it might be impossible to eliminate an acute nasolabial angle and a combined columellar strut and a pyriform rim graft are necessary to achieve tip projection, columella "show" and a more harmonious profile.

The structural grafts used to improve tip support and projection require material of sufficient rigidity which can be fashioned into the desired shape. As in dorsal grafting, the nasal septum is the most convenient source of cartilage. However when multiple grafts are required the surgeon may "run out" of cartilage and seek other sources of usable material within the same operative

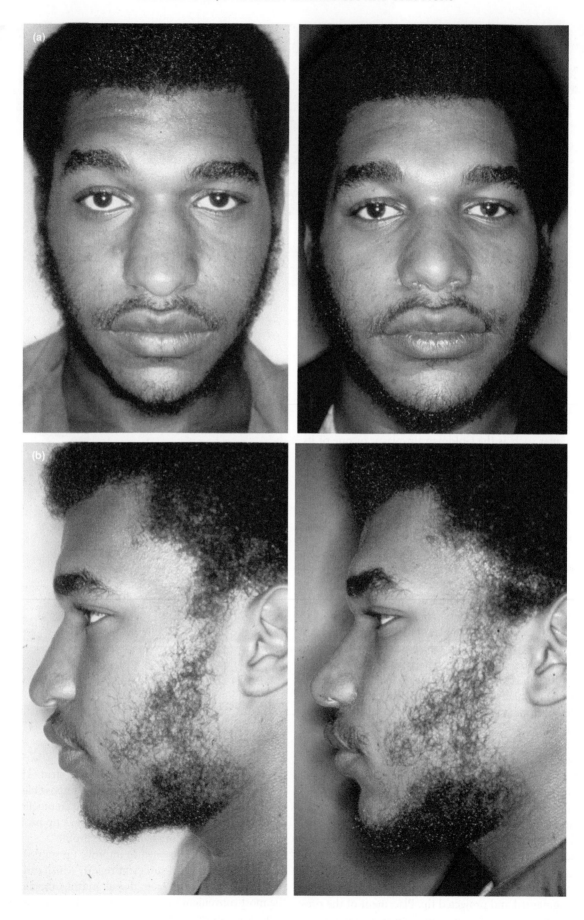

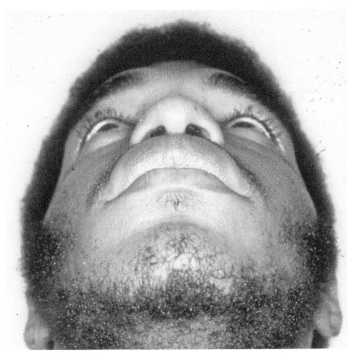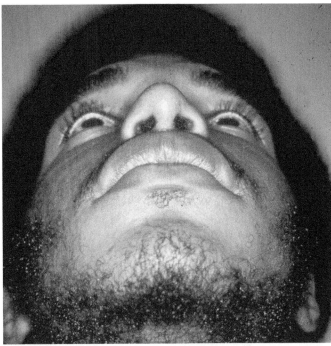

Figure 14.6 Patient underwent dorsal modification with medial and lateral osteotomies. The tip narrowing and projection were achieved with a Goldman tip-plasty with a columella strut. The alar base was modified by reducing an excessively wide nasal sill. (A) Frontal view; (B) Lateral view; and (C) Base view.

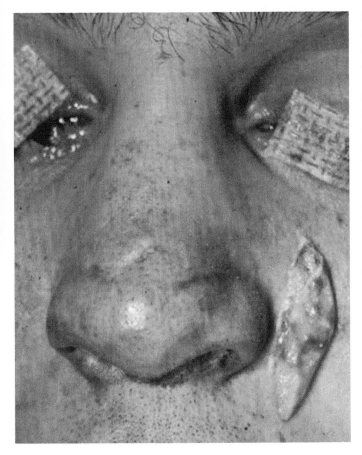

Figure 14.7 The bone of the inferior turbinate can be harvested and fashioned into a columellar strut in patients with a limited amount of septal cartilage.

field. In the senior author's experience, the bone of the inferior turbinate may provide such a source of grafting material for the columellar strut. When placed into the pocket between the medial crura it provides excellent support to the tip (16) (Figure 14.7).

Improving the definition of the nasal tip in the African patient can be a daunting task due to the thick sebaceous skin that covers the cartilaginous framework of the tip. Conservative thinning of this fibrofatty tissue overlying the domes in conjunction with dome narrowing can result in improvement of tip definition in these patients.

Alar modification

The reduction of the nasal base can be broadly subdivided into two types: the reduction of excessive alar flaring (Figure 14.8) and reduction of the excessively wide nasal sill (Figure 14.6c). A combined resection of both the sill and the alae can also be performed with excessively wide and flared alae (Figure 14.5c). Aside from the actual reduction of the width of the nose, alar resection creates an illusion of improved nasal tip projection. However, it should be noted that with alar resection (Weir excision) the actual nasal projection is reduced (Figure 14.8). Analysis of the nostril shape aid in preoperative planning and helps to select proper procedure for each patient. Farkas et al. devised a system of classifying nostril types based on their inclination.(8) Types VI (horizontally oriented) and VII (inverted axis) nostrils were the most common subtypes in Black patients, together accounting for little over 70% of all African nostril types (Figure 14.5c and 14.6c). This shape of the nostril requires reduction of the excessively wide nasal sill often coupled with reduction of the alar flare

113

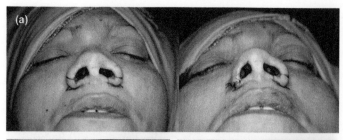

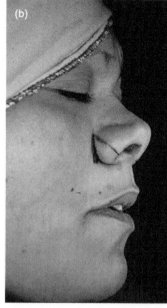
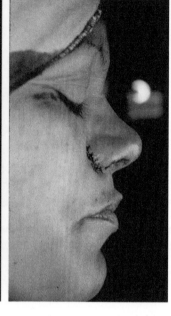

Figure 14.8 (A) The Weir excision reduces alar flare. (B) It can also result in decreased tip projection.

to reduce the very wide nasal base and produce more attractive vertically oriented nostrils.

CONCLUSION

Rhinoplasty in the African nose should not be a global transformation of the nasal shape but rather a selective correction of specific features to achieve harmonious nasal form that is in balance with the ethnic face. In authors' opinion attempts to reshape the African nose to fit Caucasian esthetic standards not just fraught with difficulty due to anatomic dissimilarities but often lead to facial disharmony and, as a result, an unhappy patient and a frustrated surgeon.

REFERENCES

1. Stucker FJ. Ethnic Considerations in African American Patient in: Matory M.D., Considerations in Facial Aesthetic Surgery. Lippincott Williams & Wilkins; 1998; 197–211.
2. Hoefflin SM. Ethnic Rhinoplasty Springer-Verlag; 1 edition (January 15, 1998).
3. Topinard P. Anthropology. Chapman and Hall, London 1890: 256.
4. Hodge FV, Swanton JR. American anthropologist. Lancaster, PA., 1910: 360.
5. Farkas LG, Katic MJ, Forrest CR. Comparison of craniofacial measurements of young adult African-American and North American white males and females. Ann Plast Surg 2007; 59(6): 692–8.
6. Porter JP. The average African American male face: an anthropometric analysis. Arch Facial Plast Surg 2004; 6(2): 78–81.
7. Porter JP, Olson KL. Analysis of the African American female nose. Plast Reconstr Surg 2003; 111(2): 620–6.
8. Farkas LG, Hreczko TA, Deutsch CK. Objective assessment of standard nostril types–a morphometric study. Ann Plast Surg 1983; 11(5): 381–9.
9. Ofodile FA, Bokhari F. The African-American nose: Part II. Ann Plast Surg 1995; 34(2): 123–9.
10. Ofodile FA. Nasal bones and pyriform apertures in blacks. Ann Plast Surg 1994; 32(1): 21–6.
11. Zelnik J, Gingrass RP. Anatomy of the alar cartilage. Plast Reconstr Surg 1979; 64(5): 650–3.
12. Ofodile FA, James EA. Anatomy of alar cartilages in blacks. Plast Reconstr Surg 1997; 100(3): 699–703.
13. Ofodile FA, Bokhari FJ, Ellis C. The black American nose. Ann Plast Surg 1993; 31(3): 209–18.
14. Kamer FM, Parkes ML. The conservative management of the Negro nose. Laryngoscope 1975; 85(3): 551–8.
15. Pastorek NJ, Bustillo A, Murphy MR, Becker DG. The extended columellar strut-tip graft. Arch Facial Plast Surg 2005; 7(3): 176–84.
16. Jones ME, Westreich RW, Lawson W. Augmentation of nasal tip projection using the inferior turbinate: review of technique and evaluation of long-term success. Arch Facial Plast Surg 2008; 10(1): 34–7.

15 Rhinoplasty in patients of hispanic descent
Konstantin Vasyukevich and William Lawson

"Nothing is rarer than a real perfect nose, and that a perfect nose is one which unites harmony of form, correctness of proportion and proper affinity with other features".(1)

The concept of the perfect nose finds its origin in the early Egyptian and Greco-Roman civilizations. During the artistic explosion of the Renaissance, artists and aesthetists, such as Botticelli and Leonardo da Vinci, planted the seeds for today's concepts of perfect human form with its idealized features. Modern perceptions of facial beauty and the "aesthetic ideal" are based heavily on their work.

The nose, as the most prominent feature, received a great deal of attention from the scholars of the human face. The late Eighteen Century physiognomist and poet Johann Kaspar Lavater believed the nose to be the "foundation of the brain". He passionately states that for a thousand beautiful eyes there is one great nose and that such nose "… is worth more than of a kingdom."(2) Perhaps more than any other feature of the face the shape of the nose in western culture became a hallmark of nobility and was often viewed as symbol of social status.

Advances in surgical techniques and preoperative care at the turn of the century made it possible to alter one's facial features by mean of an operation.

The pioneers of rhinoplasty in America such as John O. Roe and Robert F. Weir described endonasal techniques for dorsal augmentation and modification of an unsightly nasal tip.(3, 4)

Rhinoplasty quickly became a way not just to improve ones appearance but also to alleviate the social stigmata associated with a deformed nose. The "saddle" nose was a recognized sequela of tertiary syphilis. The shape of the nose could also reveal an unfavorable ethnic descent. It is likely that the history of so called "ethnic rhinoplasty" originated in early 20th century America. Surgical modification of the shape of the nose with the goal of approaching the Anglo-Saxon "norm" perhaps could advance one's social standing or improve prospects of gainful employment.(5)

The present day Latino population has evolved genetically and ethnically from the South and Central American Indians. They are believed to have descended from Indian tribes that migrated over the Bering Straits. These tribes rarely intermingled until about the 15th and 16th centuries when the Spanish Conquistadors invaded their territory. The mixing of Indians and Europeans created a new ethnic group collectively referred to as *mestizo* or "mixed", from the Latin word "mixticus". In the late 17th and early 18th century further ethnic variations were introduced by the African slave trade. This was most evident in the Caribbean, especially in Puerto Rico. The term *mestizo* now came to represent the mixture of three races: Indian, Caucasian, and Negro. In the late 18th century the expansion of Dutch, British, French and other European settlers into Central and South America created an ethnic subgroup with distinct nasal and facial characteristics.

The growing economic prosperity of Hispanic immigrants in the United States and their developing interest in cosmetic facial surgery creates a need to address the aesthetic concerns of this population. Understanding the facial anthropometric and morphologic variability in the Hispanic face and nose can greatly enhance the surgeon's ability to meet patients' expectations. Understanding inherent limitations of such intervention can also prevent disappointment and frustration by both both the surgeon and the patient (Table 15.1).

There is a relative paucity of reports on Hispanic rhinoplasty in the Anglo-American literature. Two early reports by Ortiz-Monasterio (1977) and Alberto E. Sanchez (1980) provide a wonderful outline of the key features of a typical Hispanic nose.(6, 7) Ortiz-Monasterio in his work "Rhinoplasty of the Mestizo Nose" stresses the concept of evaluating the nose in the context of the whole face. The typical *Mestizaje* face is described as being broad and convex with prominent malar eminences. Prognathic dental arches are common. This creates the appearance of a sharp nasolabial angle, underrotated nasal tip, and accentuates the appearance of a receded chin. The nasal base is wide and the domes of the lower lateral cartilages are broad with short medial crura. The nasal skin is moderately thick with the subcutaneous fat tissue covering the prominences of the osteocutaneous framework resulting in the overall impression of thickness. Alberto E. Sanchez summarized the key anatomic features of the "Chata" nose of the Caribbean as follows:

1. The tip is very wide, flat, poorly supported, and somewhat fatty.
2. The alaes are wide based, flaring, overhanging, and thick.
3. The dorsum is wide, depressed and in some cases, even saddled.
4. The columella is wide and hidden.
5. The nostrils are round or transversely elliptical.
6. The skin cover is thick.

Even though these descriptions are remarkably similar, significant differences are apparent. Milgrim and Lawson studied variations in nasal appearance in a geographically diverse

Table 15.1 Limitations to Hispanic rhinoplasty.

Desired	Constraint
Narrow nose	Broad pyriform aperture
Higher Dorsum	Bimaxillary protrusion
Defined tip	Diminished nasal vault
Projected, defined tip	Short septum/columella
	Thick skin

Hispanic population. Based on the anthropometric measurements the patients were divided into three distinct subtypes: Caribbean, Central American, and North American.(8) In a study of "Hispanic Rhinoplasty in the United States with emphasis on the Mexican American Nose "Rollin Daniel reviewed the photographs of 25 consecutive rhinoplasty patients and devised three distinct morphologic subtypes.(9) Type I (Castilian) has a profile with a normal radix, high bridge, and normal tip projection. Type II (Mexican-American) has a low radix height, a nearly normal bridge, and a dependant tip Type III (Metizo) was distinguished by broad base, thick skin and a wide tip.

The use of the nasal index popularized by Topinard, in 1890, attempted to quantitate anthropologic features.(10) The ratio of nasal width to nasal height multiplied by 100 was used to classify a nose into either Leptorrhine(Caucasian): 69.4 to 63; Platyrrhine (Negroid): 108 to 87.9; or Mesorrhine (Mongoloid): 81.4 to 69.3.(11) Although the actual numbers are not intrinsically significant, their use serves as an objective reproducible means of discussing racial differences.

Anthropometric analysis supports classification of the Latino nose as mesorrhine.(8) It is wider than the Caucasian nose, but narrower than African-American nose. While this classification scheme permits generalization for the collective Latino population, it does not account for intra-ethnic variability. By separating the subjects into subgroups based on the geographic area, it becomes apparent that the Latino nose ranges from subplatyrrhine to paraleptorrhine type. The total nasal length (nasion to subnasal point) of Caribbean Latinos approximated that seen in African Americans, reflecting the increased interracial mixing between Caribbean Latinos and black Africans. In contradistinction, the low rate of interracial mixing with blacks in Central and South America produced nasal measurements that approached the Caucasian norms, especially in the South American group. Comparatively, the Central American nose, though more closely related to the Caucasian than the African-American nose, structurally maintains a position midway between Caribbean and South American nasal features.

The differences in nasal characteristics between these subgroups are summarized in Table 15.2 and 15.3. The typical Caribbean nose is wide, with a flat nasal dorsum, wide base and short septum. The tip is bulbous and often overrotated (Figure 15.1). The Central American nose has less dorsal flatness, the nasal root and alar base are narrower, the tip is often poorly supported and underrotated (Figure 15.2). The South American nose approaches the Caucasian norms in most measurements. The nasal root is narrow and a dorsal hump is often present (Figure 15.3).(8)

NASAL AESTHETICS

Applying the observations on facial proportions set forth by da Vinci, Michelangelo and others, Broadbent and Mathews (12), in 1957, introduced aesthetic nasal concepts that are part of modern nasal surgery. Their ideas led to the theory of nasal alignment as it relates to the eyes, ears, and chin. They proposed that the nose should be (1) half as long as the distance between the chin and glabella; (2) have its widest portion (lateral alar edges) in line with the medial canthus of the eye; and (3) lie at the level of the earlobe. These observations formed the basis of the subsequent concepts of aesthetic beauty.

Gonzales-Uloa (13) also studied the "formulas of beauty" espoused by the Renaissance artists and expanded on the Broadbent

Table 15.2 Ethnic characteristic: geographical differences.

	Caribbean	Central American	South American	Caucasian
Dorsal hump	48%	64%	68%	60%
Bulbous tip	95%	34%	53%	55%
Thick skin	78%	32%	39%	47%
Poor tip support	54%	68%	58%	22%
Bimaxillary protrusion	27%	0%	7%	0%

Table 15.3 Clinical and morphological differences between Latinos, Caucasians, and African Americans.

Nasal Feature	Caribbean	Central American	South American	African American (17)	Caucasian (18)
Nose length	Short	Mid-sized	Mid-sized/long	Short	Long
Narrow	Wide, no hump	Wide, possible hump	Hump	Wide/low	Narrow
Tip	Bulbous, poor support, very poor projection	Bulbous to thin, moderate support, moderate projection	Bulbous to thin, good support, good projection	Bulbous, poor support, poor projection	Thin, good support, good projection
Columella	Short, obtuse columella-labial angle	Moderate to long, normal range of columella-labial angle	Moderate, length, normal to acute columella-labial angle	Short, acute columella-labial angle	Long, normal range to obtuse columella-labial angle
Ala	Fatty, hooded, slightly flared	Thin to fatty, not hooded, slightly flared	Thin not hooded, slightly flared	Fatty, hooded, flared	Thin, not hooded, not flared
Skin	Thick, oily	Thick not oily	Thin, oily	Thick, oily	Thin, not oily
Septum	Short, poor height, septal angle does not add to tip projection	Moderate length, good height with hump, septal angle adds slightly to tip projection	Moderate length, good height with hump, septal angle adds to tip projection	Short, septal angle does not add to tip projection	Longer, septal angle contributes to tip projection
Face	Round, bimaxillary protrusion	Round to oval	Oval	Round to oval, bimaxillary protrusion	Oval

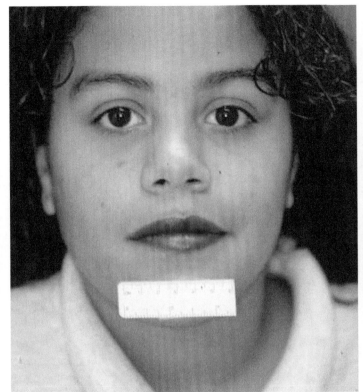
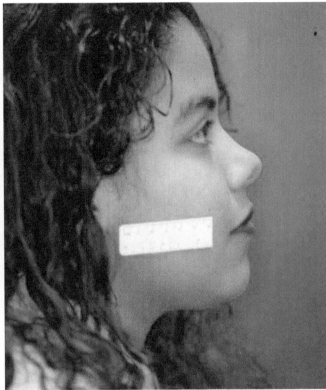
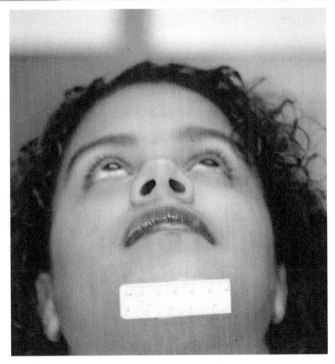

Figure 15.1 The Caribbean nose is wide with a flat dorsum and short septum. The tip is bulbous and often overrotated.

and Mathews perceptions; he published his findings, in 1962, under the term "quantitative principle". By taking two perpendicular intersecting lines, as seen on the lateral view of the face, he was able to combine nasal, forehead, lip, and chin features into one cohesive concept. The two lines used were the Frankfort line, from the tragus to the infraorbital rim, and the vertical line dropped perpendicular to the Frankfort line from the nasion. Gonzales-Uloa believed that certain facial features should approximate this line, namely the alar crease of the nose, the nasion to the vermilion border of the upper and lower lips, and the pogonion. He termed the modification of facial disharmonies by this principle: profileplasty.

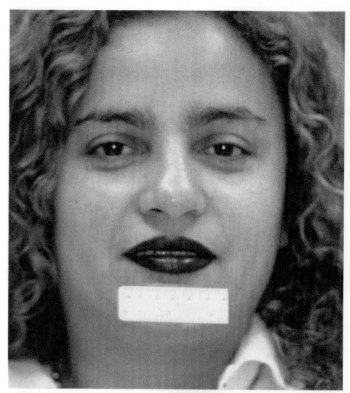
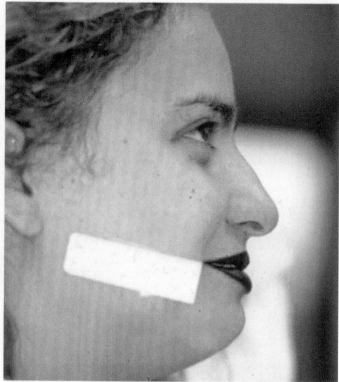
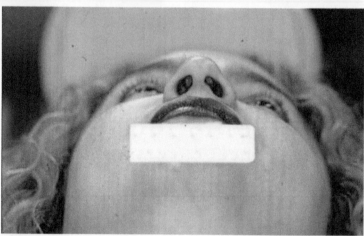

Figure 15.2 The Central American nose has less dorsal flatness, the nasal root and alar base are narrower, the tip is often poorly supported and underrotated.

Modern nasal aesthetics integrates the balance between the nasal length, tip protrusion, nasal angles, and total size of the nose. In 1988, Crumley and associate (14) envisioned the aesthetic nose as a 3:4:5 triangle, with vertices at the nasion, the alar crease and the tip-defining point. This triangle gives information regarding the optimal size and length of the nose, the optimal tip protrusion, and the optimal nasal angle needed to create a cosmetically pleasing surgical result for any given nose.

These attempts at creating the aesthetically pleasing nose have been derived from Anglo-European models. They reflect the distinctive characteristics of the underlying nasal anatomy of a Caucasian nose, such as long and narrow bony pyramid, well-developed lower lateral cartilages, and a defined tip. The question is whether these concepts can be applied to nonwhites and still obtain satisfying results. The answer is a qualified no. All these concepts are applicable only if one removes outside influences on facial form, i.e., ethnic variability. Once racial variations in facial and nasal morphologic characteristics are introduced, the concept of the ideal nose becomes meaningless. However, given the universal appeal of the Western mass media in a culturally globalized world, approximation of Caucasoid nasal proportions is desired by many patients. Although there are anatomical constraints that hinder the achievement of this goal, surgical modification can be accomplished that is not ethnically disharmonious.

Anthropometrically, structural differences exist in the Latino face that influence nasal alignment. In a study of Milgrim and Lawson, Latino nasal indexes were intermediate between African-American and Caucasian values. Caribbean indexes approach or

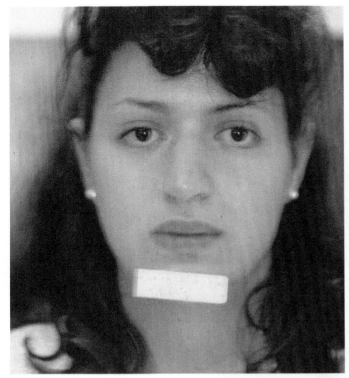

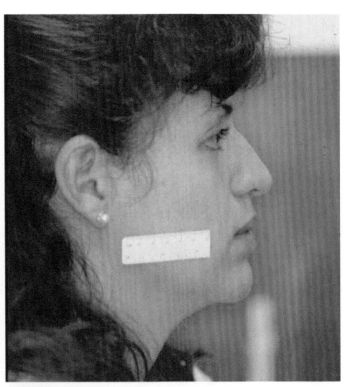

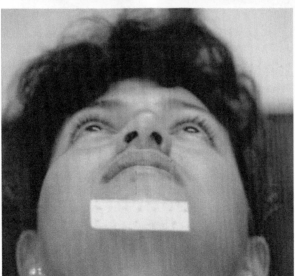

Figure 15.3 *The South American nose approaches the Caucasian norms in most measurements. The nasal root is narrow and a dorsal hump is often present.*

sometimes were even lower than African-American values. South American indexes reflect Caucasian values, and Central American indexes fell somewhere in between. In approximately one forth of Caribbean Latino faces, bimaxillary protrusion is present, which acts to push the nose off the face. Herein lies the discrepancy between the hypothesized aesthetic ideal and the ethnically derived nose. This protrusion of the nose off the face serves to (1) increase the nasolabial angle, (2) lower the bottom of the ala, which in turn reduces the columella-ala angle (3) raises the position of the supratip point. Table 15.3 details the clinical and morphological differences between Latinos, Caucasians and African Americans.

SURGICAL TECHNIQUES

Thorough discussion of the goals and aesthetic objectives of the patient should precede surgical planning. Despite significant Western influence, strong individual or cultural preferences influence the patients' desire for a change in the shape of their nose. Patients' goals should be measured against what is possible given their nasal anatomy and facial structure. Successful rhinoplasty is a compromise between what is desired and what is possible.

Approximation of the Western ideal with the preservation of ethnic identity is commonly sought by our patients. That often

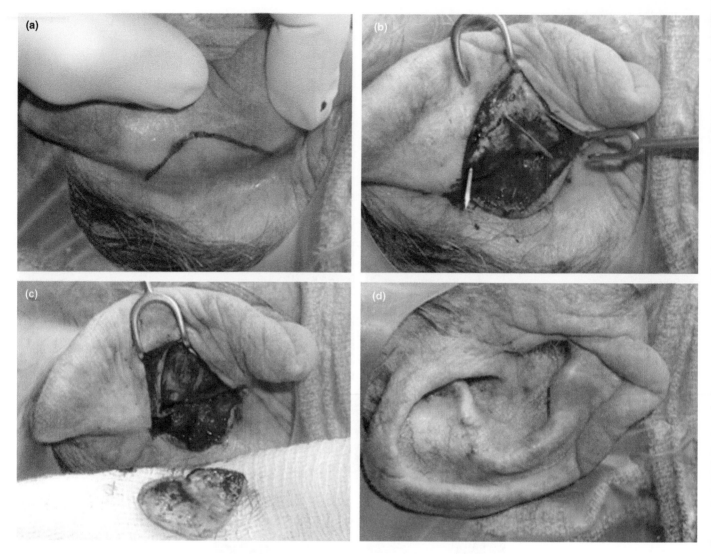

Figure 15.4 Ear cartilage harvest. (A) Incision outline. (B) The needles are inserted "through-and-through" to mark the outline of the conchal bowl. (C) The conchal cartilage excised. (D) The conchal bowl contour is unchanged.

includes augmentation of the dorsum, achieving better tip projection and definition, and narrowing of the nasal base. However, given the wide variability in nasal morphology among ethnic subgroups no single "recipe" for Hispanic rhinoplasty can be devised. Instead, analysis of the individual nasal subunits should be undertaken in each case.

We have chosen to address surgical correction of Latin noses by subdividing them into three geographically defined subgroups. Although a wide range of phenotypical variability exist within each geographic region (9), each subgroup represents a predominant phenotypical and morphological set of features.

CARIBBEAN NOSE (SUBPLATYRRHINE)

Nasal Dorsum

The dorsum is typically flat with short nasal bones and a wide pyriform aperture. Narrowing and increasing the height of the dorsum is commonly requested by the patient. In our experience osteotomies alone do not accomplish either, with dorsal

augmentation often necessary. In addition to increasing dorsal height, dorsal augmentation also downwardly displaces an over-rotated tip. A variety of materials can be used for augmentation of the entire dorsum, or the radix. Septal cartilage is the most accessible material for nasal augmentation. It is located within the same surgical field and can be easily harvested with little risk of donor site morbidity. It can be shaped to augment the specific area of the dorsum. Warping, resorption, displacement, or overgrowth are well-recognized potential sequela of this graft. In patients who are septal cartilage depleted or when the amount of augmentation exceeds the available supply, auricular cartilage can be successfully used. The resulting conchal cartilage deficiency and the scar are negligible and well accepted by most patients. (Figure 15.4) When more material is needed, cartilage harvested from the patient's rib can be used at a price of increased donor site morbidity and potentially increased warping (Figure 15.5a,b). Calvarial bone grafts can also be used.

A variety of alloplastic materials have been used over the years with variable success. Silastic, GorTex®, Medpore®, Merseline® or

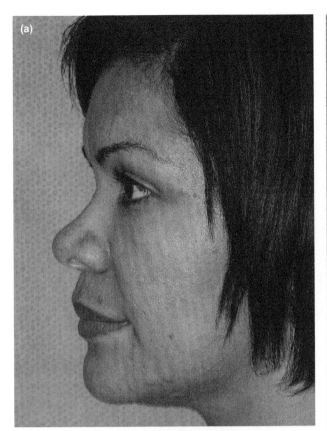
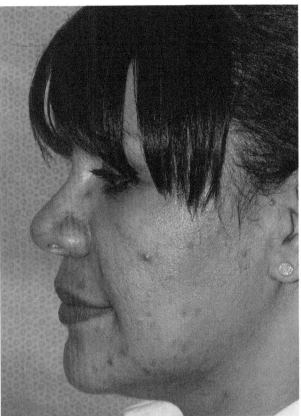

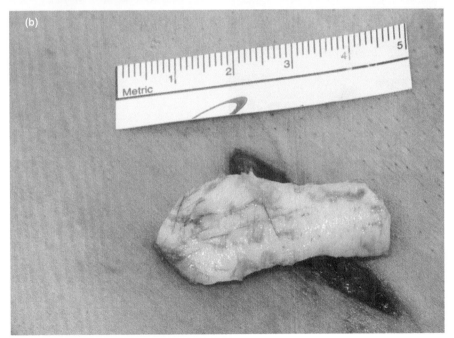

Figure 15.5 (A) Nasal dorsum augmentation: rib graft. Before and after. (B) Rib graft harvest.

Proline® mesh and others were successfully used in dorsal augmentation (Figure 15.6). However, concerns over infection and extrusion have dampened the enthusiasm for alloplastic implants. When faced with the cartilage depleted patient in need of augmentation, proline mesh is our material of choice.

Midvault

Resection of the cartilaginous dorsum or the upper lateral cartilages is usually unnecessary in this type of nose. Maintaining the attachment of the upper lateral cartilages to the nasal septum also serves to support and stabilize dorsal onlay grafts.

121

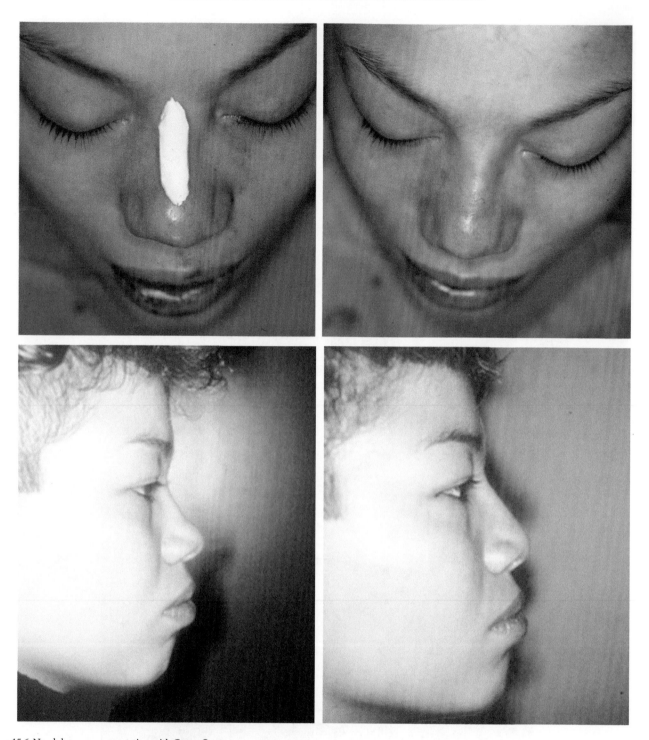

Figure 15.6 Nasal dorsum augmentation with Gortex®.

Nasal tip

In The Caribbean nose, the lobule is broad and the tip is under-projected and poorly supported. Tip modification is mandatory in almost every case if an aesthetically pleasing result is desired. Improving definition and projection of the tip without over-rotating the lobule is the surgical goal. The thick skin of the lobule and structurally soft lower lateral cartilages limit the degree of modification. Surgical objectives can be met with cartilage interrupting techniques such as Goldman's tip-plasty, or its modifications (Figure 15.7).(15, 16) In the senior author's experience excellent

longevity of tip projection can be achieved with this technique. Alternatively, suture modification of the domes is an excellent way to improve the definition and shape of the nasal tip. The shape of the domes can be altered by the strategic placement of an intradomal suture through the junction to the medial and the lateral crura of the lower lateral cartilages. Both domes can also be brought together with one trans-domal suture. (Figure 15.8). A variety of grafts can be used to project, augment and shape the tip. A columella strut is almost universally required in the Caribbean nose given the structural weakness of the medial crura of the

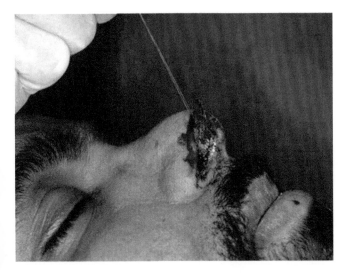

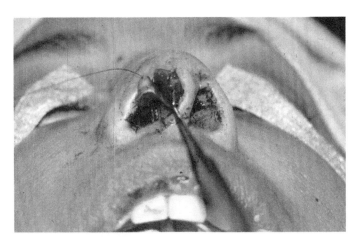

Figure 15.7 Goldman's tip plasty: intraoperative view. The lower lateral cartilage strip is transected at the domes and sutured together.

Figure 15.8 Suture modification of the lower lateral cartilages. A single permanent horizontal mattress suture is placed through the cartilage immediately adjacent to the domes.

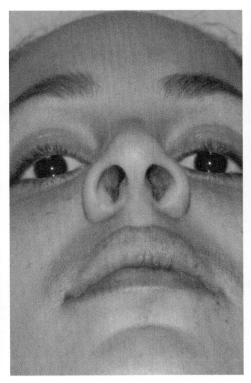

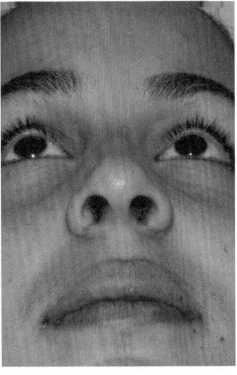

Figure 15.9 Alar flare reduction: before and after.

lower lateral cartilages. The strut is usually fashioned form septal cartilage and is placed between the medial crura. It serves to support and project the nasal tip. In a cartilage depleted patient, bone harvested form the inferior turbinate can be used as an alternative to septal cartilage. Increasing columella show can be achieved if a wider strip is used. A shield graft can also be used to improve the projection and definition of the tip and to lengthen the nose.

Nasal base

The widened nasal base is often present in the Caribbean nose. The perception of a wide base is exacerbated by the relatively short and flat dorsum. The wide nasal base can be the result of an excessively wide nasal sill or increased ala flaring (Figure 15.9, 15.10).

Reduction of the nasal sill or resection of the alar segment narrows the nasal base producing a more harmonious appearance (Figure 15.10). About 25% percent of the patients in the Caribbean subgroup had significant bimaxillary protrusion.(8) The placement of a premaxillary graft is often necessary to provide a stable base for increased tip projection and columella show. Both autologous and alloplastic materials can be used. The graft is placed just inferior to the nasal spine through an extended transfixion, or hemi-transfiction incisions.

Chin

Chin implant can be placed to improve receded chin appearance, and balance the nose and the lower part of the face (Figure 15.11).

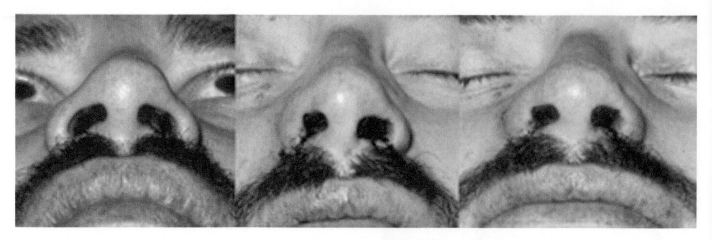

Figure 15.10 Nasal sill reduction: preoperative base view; intraoperative view after reduction of the right side; intraoperative view after bilateral reduction.

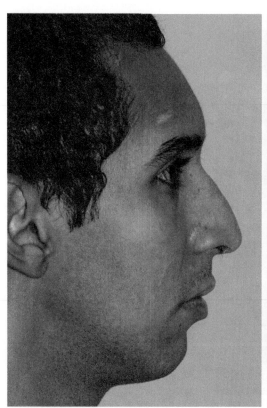

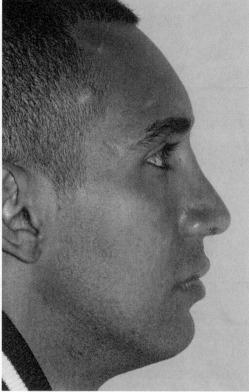

Figure 15.11 Dorsal hump reduction and a chin implant: before and after.

CENTRAL AMERICAN NOSE (MESORRHINE)

Nasal dorsum

The dorsum is higher than in the Caribbean nose and a small dorsal hump or a pseudohump is often present. The nasal bones are often wide but are longer than in the paraplatyrrhine Caribbean nose and the desired narrowing can be accomplished by osteotomies and bone infracture Conservative dorsal hump reduction can be undertaken if a straight dorsum is desired. A dorsal hump can be reduced with an osteotomy, rasping, or the combination of both (Figure 15.12).

A deep nasofrontal angle and a dependent tip are common in the Central American nose and can result in the pseudohump appearance (Figure 15.13). This is corrected by augmentation of the nasofrontal angle and by improving tip projection.

Midvault

The cartilaginous hump is reduced and the dorsal part of the upper lateral cartilages is trimmed if necessary. Midvault narrowing can be accomplished by separating of the upper lateral cartilages from the septum.

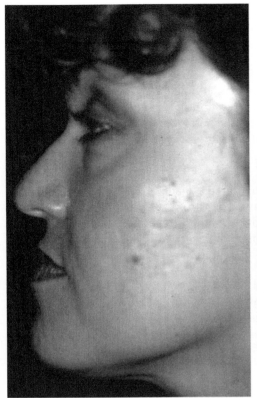
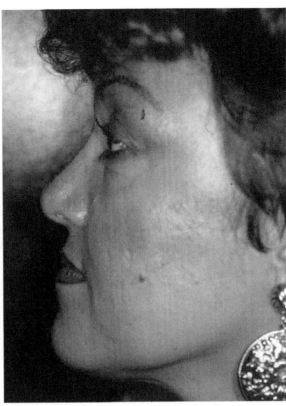

Figure 15.12 Central American nose: before and after.

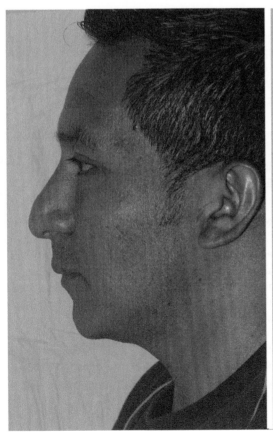
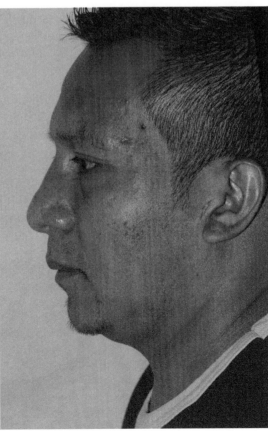

Figure 15.13 "Pseudo hump" appearance was addressed with naso-frontal angle augmentation, minimal dorsal hump reduction, and projection of poorly supported tip. Before and after.

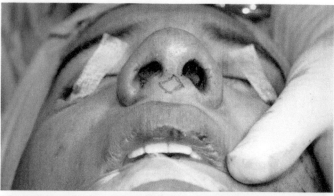

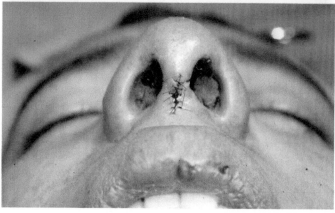

Figure 15.14 External reduction of the wide columella: intraoperative view.

Nasal tip

The nasal tip is often in a dependent position producing the appearance of supratip fullness and an acute nasolabial angle. The dependency of the tip is related to the deficiency of the caudal septum which requires augmentation. Lower lateral cartilages unsupported by the caudal septum often bend or flare under the weight of the tip (Figure 15.14). Therefore a columella strut is an essential component to achieve tip projection. As previously discussed, tip-plasty can be accomplished by cartilage strip interrupting techniques (Goldman's) or by suture modification. The lateral crura often have increased width and require cephalic trim.

Nasal Base

Excessive columella width or medial crural flare can be addressed by an external columella reduction or an endonasal columella modification. External reduction is performed by excising a rhomboid segment of the base of the columella. The resultant scar is vertically oriented and is well accepted by patients. Endonasal medial crural flare reduction is accomplished through a full or hemi-transfixion incision. An absorbable or permanent mattress suture is placed approximating the feet of the medial crura and then fixing both crura to the caudal septum.

SOUTH AMERICAN NOSE (PARALEPTORRHINE)

South America is a geographically large area having diverse immigration patterns and racial admixtures. Countries along its northern section and the Andean range often show a predominant influence of the indigenous Indian population. The noses resemble those of Central America and are modified similarly. The lower part of the continent (Argentina, Chile) had a greater influx of Europeans and noses show paraleptorrhine features the correction of which will be discussed in this section.

Nasal Dorsum

The nasal dorsum in the South American nose approaches Caucasian proportions. A narrow bony vault with long nasal bones and significant dorsal hump is typically present. Reduction of the hump is commonly requested by the patients and can be accomplished with dorsal and lateral osteotomies and nasal bone infracture (Figure 15.15). In patients with a significant dorsal hump and a shallow nasion area, deepening of the nasofrontal angle is often required to prevent the so-called "Greek nose" appearance. In our experience this is best accomplished with the removal of the bone in the naso-frontal area with a narrow rongeur.

Midvault

Cartillagenous hump reduction is accomplished with conservative reduction of the protruding dorsal septum and upper lateral cartilages.

Nasal tip

The tip in the South American nose is well supported by a relatively long caudal septum and strong medial crura of the lower lateral cartilages. The domes are often well defined and the tip is narrower than in the previous groups. Tip modification can be accomplished through previously described tip-plasty techniques.

Nasal Base

The nasal base is typically narrow, with oblique nares and no alar flare. Base reduction is uncommonly necessary and can be performed by reduction of the nasal sill.

CONCLUSION

The aesthetic surgery of the ethnic nose necessitate thorough analysis of the facial and nasal morphological characteristics in each individual case. The difference in facial structure, nasal anatomy, and skin characteristics between Caucasian and Hispanic patients would destine most attempts at ethnic transformation to fail. Therefore, the improvement of the nasal shape within the framework of the individual ethnicity should be a realistic surgical goal. Although no single approach to a Hispanic nose could be devised, we found that dividing patients into categories based on the ethnic origin helped to determine the most optimal surgical intervention to accomplish our goals.

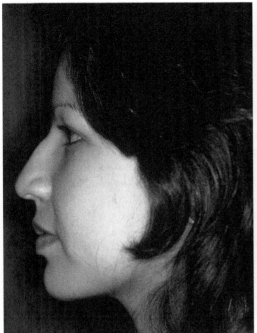 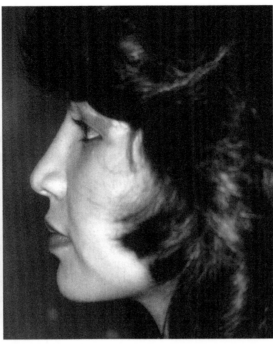

Figure 15.15 South American nosee. Dorsal hump reduction with medial, lateral osteotomies and infracture: before and after.

REFERENCES

1. Linn C, Stevans CM. Encyclopedia of superstitions, folklore, and the occult sciences of the world. J.H. Yewdale & Sons Publishers, 1908: 1701.

2. John Caspar Lavater (translated by Thomas Holcroft). Essays on physiognomy: designed to promote the knowledge and love of mankind. William Tegg and Co. London, 1850: 390–1.

3. Roe JO. The deformity termed 'pug nose' and its correction by a simple operation. By John Orlando Roe, 1887. Arch Otolaryngology Head Neck Surgery 1989; 115(2): 156–7.

4. Weir RF. On restoring sunken noses without scarring the face. 1892. Aesthetic Plast Surg 1988; 12(4): 203–6.

5. Haiken E. Venuss envy. The Johns Hopkins University Press, Baltimore and London, 1997: 181–5.

6. Ortiz-Monasterio F, Olmedo A. Rhinoplasty on the mestizo nose. Clin Plast Surg 1977; 4(1): 89–102.

7. Sanchez AE. Rhinoplasty in the "Chata" Nose of the Caribbean. Aesthetic Plast Surg 1980; 4: 169–77.

8. Milgrim LM, Lawson W, Cohen AF. Anthropometric analysis of the female Latino nose. Revised aesthetic concepts and their surgical implications. Archives of Otolaryngology Head Neck Surgery 1996; 122(10): 1079–86.

9. Daniel RK. Hispanic rhinoplasty in the United States, with emphasis on the Mexican American nose. Plast Reconstr Surg 2003; 112(1): 244–56.

10. Topinard P. Anthropology. Chapman and Hall, London, 1890: 256.

11. Hodge FV, Swanton JR. American anthropologist. Lancaster, PA, 1910: 360.

12. Broadbent TR, Mathews VL. Artistic relationships in surface anatomy of the face: application to reconstructive surgery. Plast Reconstr Surg (1946). 1957; 20(1): 1–17.

13. Gonzales-Ulloa M. Quantitative principles in cosmetic surgery of the face (profileplasty). Plast Reconstr Surg Transplant Bull 1962; 29: 186–98.

14. Crumley RL, Lanser M. Quantitative analysis of nasal tip projection. Laryngoscope 1988; 98(2): 202–8.

15. Goldman IB. Surgical tips on the nasal tip. Eye Ear Nose Throat Mon 1954; 33: 583–91.

16. Chang CW, Simons RL. Hockey-stick vertical dome division technique for overprojected and broad nasal tips. Arch Facial Plast Surg 2008; 10(2): 88–92.

17. Ofodile FA, Bokhari FJ, Ellis C. The black American nose. Ann Plast Surg 1993; 31(3): 209–18.

18. Farkas LG. Anthropometry of the head and face. New York, NY: Raven Press, 1994.

16 Management of the twisted nose

Stephen A Goldstein and Paul J Carniol

Management of the twisted nose can be a challenging endeavor for experienced rhinoplasty surgeons. To be effective, the surgeon must first understand the etiology of the deformity, which varies from patient to patient. Once established, treatment of the external nasal deviation can be better guided to achieve the desired result. External nasal deviations arise from two broad categories: traumatic and developmental.(1) Traumatic deformity is quite common as the position of the nose off of the facial plane makes it susceptible to injury. Adult injuries tend to involve the upper half of the nose while pediatric injuries result in displacement of the lower half. Since facial asymmetry is prevalent in more than 90% of the population, it must be identified and discussed before undertaking repair.(Figure 16.1) These types of asymmetry may be inherited or due to abnormal growth patterns in the midface after childhood injury.

When planning the correction of an external nasal deviation, an accurate diagnosis of the anatomical causes for the deviation is essential to a successful outcome. It has been stated that "90% of nasal surgery is accurate diagnosis and 10% execution."(23) Goals for the correction of an external nasal deviation must be carefully outlined with the patient. It is important to communicate that the nose will be "straighter," but may not be perfectly midline. Second, in the preoperative evaluation, it is important for the patient to understand the differences between functional and aesthetic nasal surgery. Conversely, it is important for the surgeon to understand the patient's goals.

ANATOMY

Comprehension for normal anatomy and the relationships of the bony cartilaginous skeleton in the nose is crucial for accurate diagnosis.(2, 3) The paired nasal bones fuse to the frontal bone at the radix and attach laterally along the ascending maxillary process of the skull. This relationship becomes important when discussing osteotomies.

The lower two-thirds of the external nasal skeleton is cartilaginous, composed of the paired upper and lower lateral cartilages. The quadrangular cartilage of the septum should divide these structures in the midline. The nasal septum is also the architectural wall that supports the nasal dorsum and tip. The septum is composed of a quadrangular cartilage with two bony contributions. The anterior septal angle sits below the nasal tip, while a properly positioned posterior septal angle rests in the midline, attached to the anterior nasal spine.

The nasal spine may also be slightly paramedian in patients with mild midfacial asymmetries. Disruption of the vomerian groove from an incomplete cleft defect may also play a role in septal displacement and growth patterns. The septal bones include the vomer inferiorly and the perpendicular plate of the ethmoid, which inserts onto the skull base. Care must be taken when manipulating the perpendicular plate to prevent traumatic injuries at the skull base. This may lead to disturbances of olfaction and possibly a CSF leak.(5, 7, 24, 25) It is important to identify and record the patient's olfactory status preoperatively. When disturbed it often

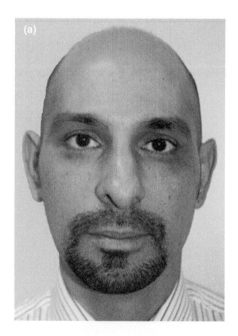
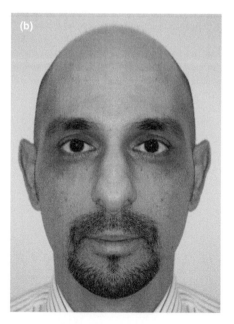
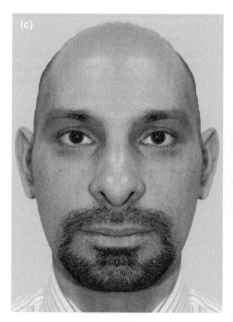

Figure 16.1 (A) Asymmetries of the mid face and nasal subunits provide a sense of imbalance and are easily seen on frontal view. (B) and (C) Split face analysis of the right and left mirror images further demonstrate how varied one side of the nose and face is from the other.

returns with in several weeks or months but may be permanently impaired. Maintaining integrity at the junction of the bony cartilaginous dorsum is crucial for dorsal support.(5)

The dorsal septum provides one of the primary support mechanisms for the tip as it provides projection off the maxillary crest. At minimum, dorsal support is best maintained with an intact cartilaginous L strut. Stability from blunt force is strongest when at least a 15-mm cartilaginous segment remains attached at the dorsal perpendicular plate, with preservation of overlying mucoperichondrium.(4)

The septum also controls the vectors which create the dorsal line. The upper lateral cartilages (ULCs) attach to the dorsal septum and have fibrous connections under the nasal bones. At their caudal aspect they are typically with in 1–3 mm of the anterior septal angle. The upper lateral cartilages connect and interdigitate with the cephalic margin of lower lateral cartilages forming "the scroll." This attachment is also one of the three major tip supporting mechanisms. In a well-balanced nose, the tip should rise 1 to 2 mm above the dorsum on lateral view, creating an aesthetically pleasing supratip break.

PRE OP EVALUATION

Aside from acute nasal injuries, a good history may identify potential mechanisms for previous injury. Prior nasal fractures often occur from participation in sports, although a large percentage of patients do not recall suffering a specific traumatic event. A preoperative CT scan of the sinuses may identify any anatomical variants or abnormalities which can contribute to the deformity. A concha bullosa of the middle turbinate can cause displacement at the mid-septum, contributing to the twisted nose. (Figure 16.2) Birth trauma and previous surgery can also cause an asymmetric or crooked nose. Underlying facial asymmetries often result in discrepancies between the size and length of the nasal subunits as seen in Figure 16.1. The nasal septum may be offset from the midline if there is significant facial asymmetry.

Identifying the anatomic cause of the twisted nose depends on an accurate examination both visually and with palpation. A systematic approach of evaluating the external and internal nose allows precise surgical planning. The external appearance of the nose is not a good indicator of internal septal position, and septal position should be viewed both with a nasal speculum and a nasal endoscope.

During the initial consultation, discussion of the patient's desires regarding both function and position of their nose balanced by the overall aesthetics are reviewed. The twisted nose undoubtedly has a deviated septum with possibilities of nasal valve impingement. Acute nasal trauma often results in contusion of the soft tissues with or with out fractures. A convexity at the rhinion may be present as edema alone or in combination with the fracture, adding the illusion of a more significant curve. Given this is process one should allow resolution of edema before proceeding with the procedure for a more accurate outcome.

Septal injuries can range along a spectrum from simple deviation to subluxation off the maxillary crest all the way to more significant comminuted fracture. When moderately displaced the dorsal septum may twist while loss of dorsal support in the tip or midvault regions of the nose is often seen. When the dorsal cartilage is

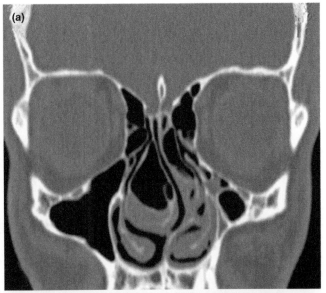

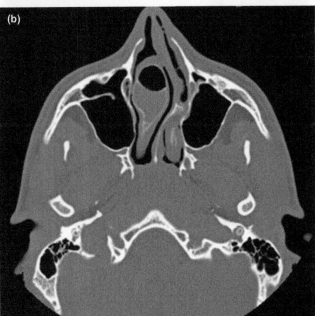

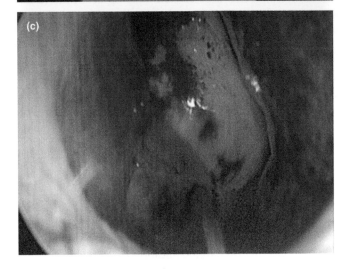

Figure 16.2 (A–C) The large right concha bullosa is visualized by CT scan and endoscopically. The degree of septal displacement can easily explain the developmental malposition of the patient's nose.

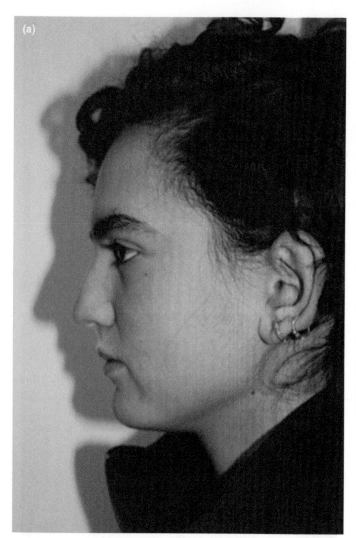

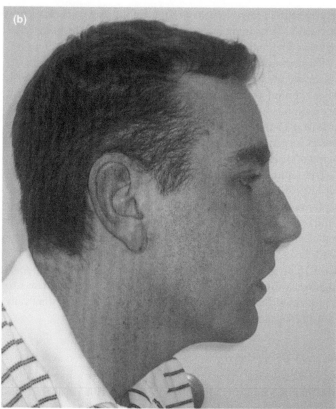

Figure 16.3 (A) The dorsal and tip projection are lowered from subluxation of the cartilaginous septum causing a pseudo hump at the rhinion, compared to an overprojected nose on lateral view. (B) The frontal view seen in Figure 16.10 shows the crooked nasal pyramid and asymmetric tip.

decreased in height or projection, the nasal bones appear as a dorsal convexity. It is important to differentiate this type of "bump" from the overprojected dorsum, which is due to hypertrophy of the quadrangular cartilage and nasal bones.(Figure 16.3) Patients with an overprojected nose or even nasal tip deformity (a bulbous or wide tip) can be corrected at the time of surgery, but this is not a necessity for straightening the nose internally. Tip procedures help give a more balanced appearance, but it is important to discuss the difference preoperatively with the patient. When a dorsal convexity is present in a twisted nose the best result is usually achieved if the convexity is resected or rasped. Ethnic traits or "the family" nose may be of great psychological importance to patients. Discussion preoperatively or even computer imaging is educational for the patient and surgeon before surgery.

Often in traumatic injury, septal displacement along the maxillary crest may result in deformities affecting both the septum and the nasal tip. This may be identified preoperatively on base view as a caudal septal deflection. Flattening in the supra tip region from a minor saddle deformity, may also occur if tip projection is lost with subluxation. A swinging door type procedure, first introduced by Safian and its modifications are reliable techniques for repositioning the lower third of the nose.(3, 9, 17, 20) If the quadrangular cartilage is tilted or buckled along the dorsum, internal nasal valve collapse is also likely to be found.

"As the septum goes, so does the nose," Cottle describes the overall role of its shape and location. Preoperatively, it is helpful to recognize whether the septum is "C" or "S" shaped. The difficulty with the curved septum is its ability to twist and rotate around both the horizontal and vertical axis. The surgeon must recognize which axis has the majority of torsion so it can be released and stabilized to minimize postoperative failure.(Figure 16.4) When curvature at the bony cartilaginous junction is present it has a certain potential energy stabilizing the injured anterior quadrangular cartilage too the fixed and rigid bony septum, placing the septum under tension. When separated the curvature most often releases but unfortunately, further destabilization can result. Structural grafting for added support is vital for stabilizing the septum in its new position.(16)

The areas of septal curvature may benefit from many techniques including simple scoring partial resection to submucosal resection. Maintaining contralateral perichondrial flap attachment was first advocated by Metzenbaum for caudal deflection repair.(20) Lawson has described the benefit of leaving the flap intact when making complete vertical incisions to straighten the septum.(26) Most often bilateral flap elevation is required to access the deformities. As the deformity of the nose and septum increase in complexity, an open approach to the dorsal septum is very helpful for increased visibility and manipulation.

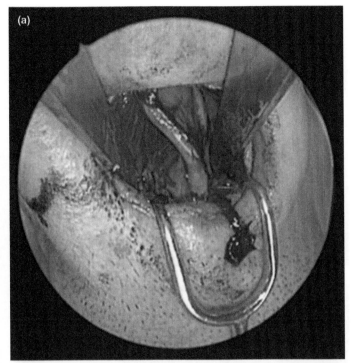

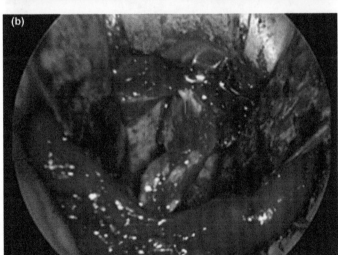

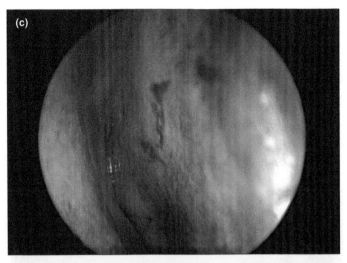

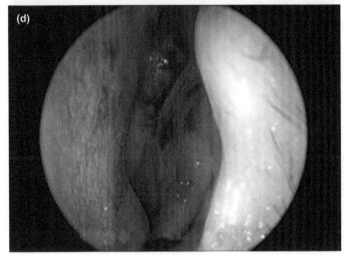

Figure 16.4 The septum can be curved and rotated in either the x and y axis or both. (A) demonstrates a vertical S shape septal deformity. Injuries' causing C shape deformities along the horizontal axis is seen in (B) while a vertical C displacement is noted in (C–D).

Many techniques exist to reshape and stabilize septal cartilage. They include cutting, cross-hatching on the concave side, incomplete fracture of the cartilage, grafting, and splinting.(1, 9–12, 21, 22) Any physical alteration of the cartilage can weaken its inherent structural support and lead to further instability.(5) These changes can be counteracted by the placement of autogenous cartilage grafts or posterior septal bone for reinforcement.(Figure 16.5) Another method for stabilization of the septum is to provide external septal fixation once the intraoperative reconstruction is complete. This may be achieved through the use of external fixation devices such as nasal splints, nasal packs, or taping methods. In addition, quilting sutures are most commonly employed to further stabilize the repositioned septum. The surgeon who relies on the splints and sutures to provide the long-term stabilization will often be disappointed. Release and correction of the underlying injury is the key to success.

Schwab has stated that due to the unpredictability of septal cartilage, none of these techniques will always achieve the desired results.(5) The unpredictability, in part, comes from "the memory effect" of cartilage. This is not well understood, but accounts for the warping of the cartilage back to the preoperative state after septoplasty. This represents one of the reasons why recurrent deformities and deviations can occur. Unfortunately, this is a circumstance that is not always under the control of the surgeon.(7) Given this problem with septorhinoplasty, it should be explained in as part of the informed consent.

To account for septal unpredictability, many surgeons have compensated clinically by overcorrecting the septum. This complication of septoplasty particularly affects younger patients, as they are at a higher risk. The overall incidence of septal overcorrection is 2%, while the incidence for patients under the age of 20 is 7.3%.(8) It is theorized that the need for overcorrection in younger patients is related to the growing quadrangular cartilage. According to Lee et al., the central quadrangular cartilage has a high level of metabolic activity, cell replication, and proliferative capacity, all of which decline with age. The anterior free end of the

131

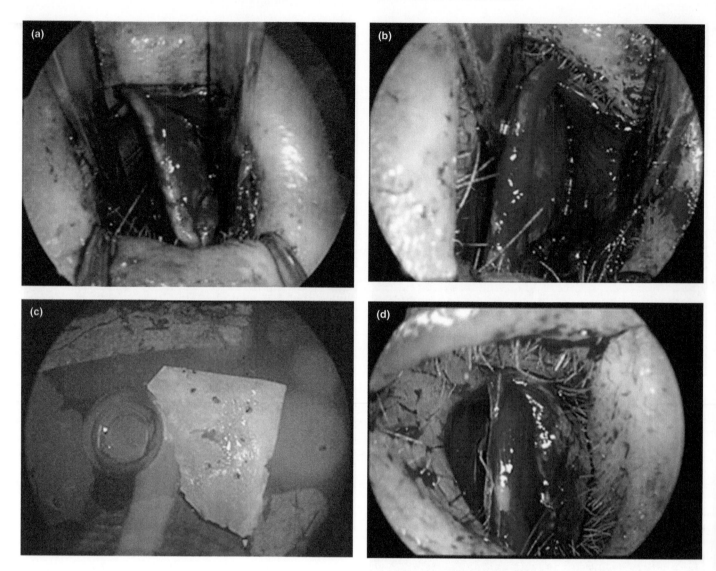

Figure 16.5 (A) This caudal septal deflection is due to a fracture seen inferiorly. (B) The scar tissue was released and figure of eight sutures placed for support. (C) This was followed by additional structural grafting with an ethmoid bone graft. (D) Note the graft adds 2 mm of tip projection which was lost after the fracture.

cartilage, however, retains high levels of these aspects throughout the aging process.(8) When overcorrection does occur, it usually will present with symptoms of nasal obstruction on the side opposite of the initial deviation. This may occur at least 1 month after surgery. To avoid midfacial growth disturbance, surgeons often advocate waiting until the age of 16 or 17 is achieved. Our recommendations are to discern if the patient has also obtained >90% of adult stature relative to their family. We prefer avoid overcorrection and just correct the septum as needed.

When the nasal bones are shifted to one side, a discrepancy in the slope of the sidewall is seen. The depressed side is concave while the contralateral side is elevated and possible convex. The upper lateral cartilages may be partially avulsed in such an injury causing a subtle convexity. This is seen just lateral to the rhinion and caudal to the nasal bones. This must be differentiated from an elevated nasal bone.(Figure 16.6) Correction of the ULC deformity involves the release and repositioning back into its anatomical position. In refractory cases an onlay graft can be used to camouflage the defect. In the lower portion of the nose, the lower lateral cartilages (LLC) possess innate asymmetry

which may accentuate the twisted appearance of a nose. This is further compounded when the septum is fractured or significantly displaced. The tip is pushed off the midline with an additional torsion or rotation around the anterior septal angle. If injury is localized to the anterior septal angle widening and flattening of the supratip will occur.(1) Fractures in the infra-domal medial crura will also create flattening in the supratip and additional tip ptosis . Suture repair of the medial crura and placement of a columellar strut graft provide the necessary tip support.(Figure 16.7)

Septal fractures most commonly occur at the bony cartilaginous junction but may occur along the length of the nose. It is the natural internal "crumple" zone of the nose serving as a protective role for the brain in facial injury. As the force increases more complex facial fractures may occur. A fracture at the bony-cartilaginous junction or anterior quadrangular cartilage often displaces the caudal septum, twisting the lower 2/3 of the nose. A swinging door with a figure of eight suture to the nasal spine, Wright stitch, may be necessary to stabilize the nose in the midline. It is often necessary to add tip support in these cases. If a

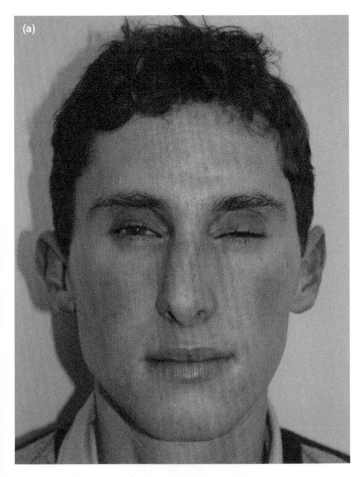
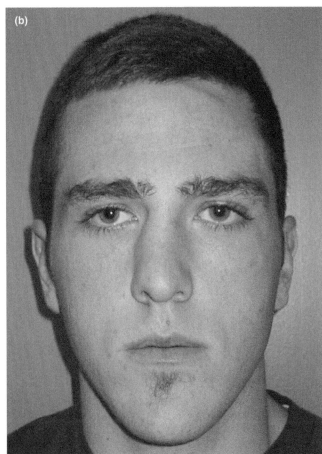

Figure 16.6 A crooked nose involving the upper 2/3 of the nose may cause an avulsion of the upper lateral cartilage requiring repair (A) Osteotomies alone will not release the fibrosis. If the cartilage is not avulsed, only the nasal bones need to be repositioned (B).

high septal deflection has occurred, obstruction of the nasal valves is also common and is repaired with a spreader or cross bar graft.(12) Anterior septal fractures are fixed with a combination of suture and structural grafting techniques. Figure of eight suture is also best applied when stabilizing end to end cartilage fragments.(Figure 16.8)

TIMING OF REPAIR
After a traumatic nasal injury, many patients report displeasure over the appearance of their nose or complain of new nasal obstruction. When a patient presents acutely with a fracture, a closed nasal reduction is the treatment of choice within 2 to 3 weeks. Closed reductions may be performed under local anesthetic in an office setting unless significant septal injury is noted or the patient is anxious. If significant septal injury is diagnosed, a septoplasty with the closed reduction is performed in the OR under IV sedation or general anesthesia. Since edema may camouflage dorsal irregularities ample time should lapse to allow for adequate resolution of nasal edema. This allows accurate repositioning of the nasal framework. If there is a significant septal injury or the injury is old, than a combined septoplasty with possible open approach techniques will provide the best outcome, minimizing the need for revision surgery.(14)

If the patient has missed their window of opportunity for acute fracture reduction, then the patient should delay a potentially more extensive reconstructive procedure until the initial healing process is completed usually in 2–3 months. If the secondary procedure is performed too early there can be increased associated risks. These can be small irregularities not seen from the edema or even uncontrolled osteotomies going through a partially healed nasal fracture line.

THE REPAIR
Many papers have been written describing algorithms for correction of the crooked nose. A varied sequence of surgical steps and multiple options attest to the complexity of these cases.(1, 2, 13, 15) The risks for weakening the support, further impairing breathing are also well described.(12) A systematic repair of the twisted nose begins after identifying the areas of displacement and twisting. Release of these injuries and any scar tissue holding the nose in its current position hopefully allow the nose to return back to a more normal position.

The mucoperichondrium overlying the septum provides significant structural integrity. In a crushed septal fracture injury, extra careful elevation of the flap is required. The cleavage plane is frequently disrupted with scarring of the mucoperichondrium into the fracture line. These scars are cut sharply with a knife while at the same time avoiding perforation the flap or cutting into the cartilage causing further instability. The cartilage provides a certain "spring" or support to the nose. There is a "memory" effect with

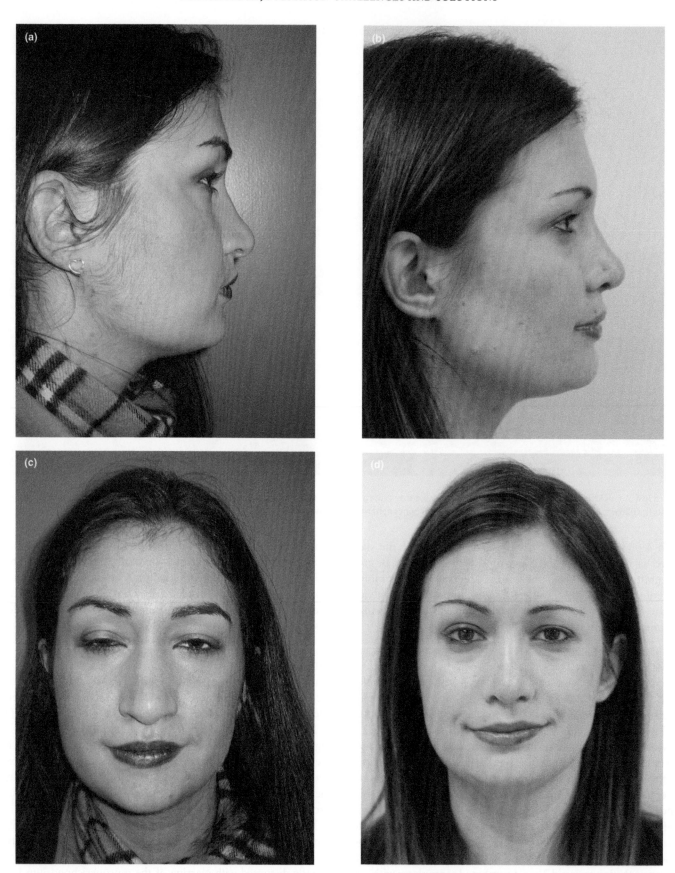

Figure 16.7 This patient present with loss of nasal projection and caudal septal support. At the time of surgery she was found to have injuries of the infradomal portion of the lower lateral crura along with a subluxation of the caudal septum. Projection was restored with suture repair of the domal fractures and a columellar strut graft. Pre- and postop views are shown.

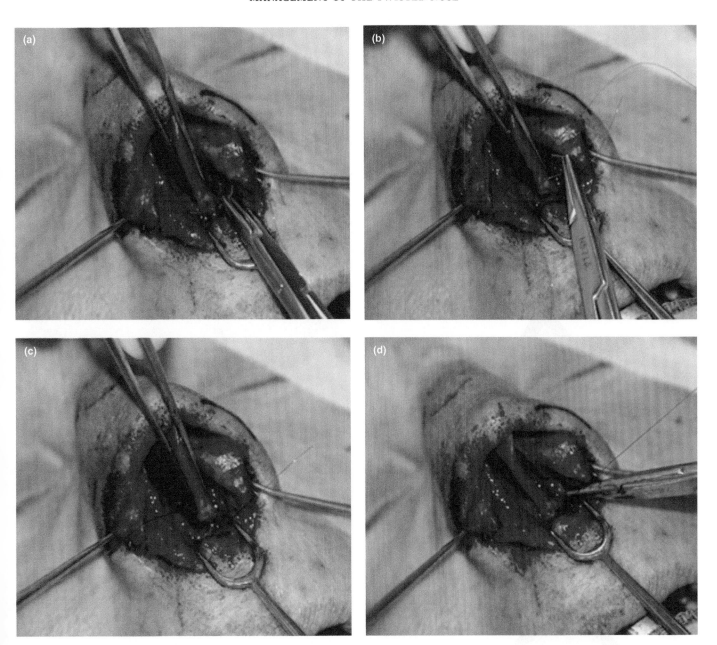

Figure 16.8 When the posterior septal angle is displaced from the maxillary crest a Wright suture (figure of 8) can be utilized to re-secure it to the midline. The double hook retracts the soft tissue and maintains orientation. (A) The sequence starts with the first throw through the periosteum of the nasal spine. (B) The second throw comes back from the same direction. The surgeon should be ~3 mm from the edges of the posterior septal angle to avoid splitting the cartilage with the needle or when tying down the stitch. A third pass of the needle through periosteum crossing the first throw at a midline point will fixate the posterior septal angle. Please note the anterior septal is not in the mid line secondary to a fracture which needs repair. To obtain a straight dorsum, it is more important to ensure the anterior septal angle is closest to midline.

in scarred or fractured cartilage that often limits the long-term results and is the bane of the surgeon regardless of technique. Once the septal flap is freed it is necessary to identify the points of bony and cartilaginous displacement. Sequential release of the displaced segments controls and resets the tensegrity or innate energy (spring) in this dynamic system.(1, 16) The least amount of cartilage resected to open the nasal passage while releasing the twist is removed. This maintains stability and can minimize the cicatricial contracture after careful closure of the mucoperichondrial flaps.(1, 2, 9, 17)

Twisting of the septum occurs from disruption of its normal structural attachment points to the skull and nasal bones due fractures of the cartilage and bones. Evaluation of the septum after topical mucosal decongestion with local injection aids in accurate diagnosis. Definitive sites of injury are identified setting the stage for surgical sequence. Addressing septal position first is the most critical for building a long-term foundation. Release of septal attachments will allow surrounding structures the ability to hopefully reposition back in a straighter position. A prolonged waiting period from injury allows increased scar contracture making this more difficult to control.

The procedure is most often begun with a hemi-transfixion incision when access to both sides of the nose and caudal septum is needed. After raising septal flaps the surgeon must decide whether an endonasal or open approach will better allow access to correct the underlying deformities. There are four points of

(a)

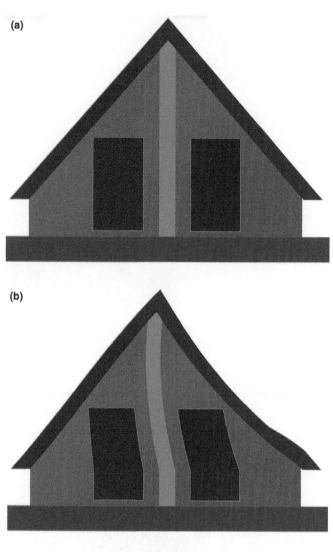

(b)

(c)

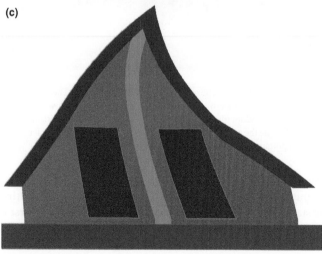

(d)

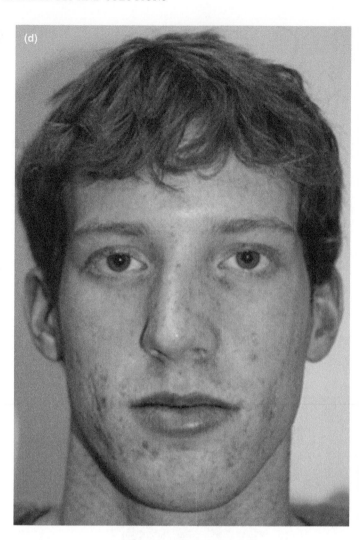

Figure 16.9 An A frame model is shown as an analogy for the nasal pyramid; (A) Normal position, (B) mild displacement and (C) severe depression of the left. A patient with a moderate shift in the nasal pyramid is shown in (D). As the depression increases, an intermediate osteotomy before lateral osteotomies is beneficial for repositioning of the nasal side walls. Medial osteotomies are also recommended with more severe injuries.

septal attachment to the skull: the maxillary crest, skull base, nasal bones and the upper lateral cartilages. Sequential release of septal attachments only necessary for mobilization is performed. This limits surgical injuries and maintains intact structures. Septal fracture lines are then either resected or scored followed by cartilage or bone strut stabilization.

Once septal flaps have been elevated, septal dissection along the maxillary crest for displacement off the midline is performed first when needed. This can be seen before elevating the flaps and may be avoided if no injury is present. If a dorsal resection is required some author's have advocated doing this step first given the increased support.(1) Injuries at the bony cartilaginous junction require additional

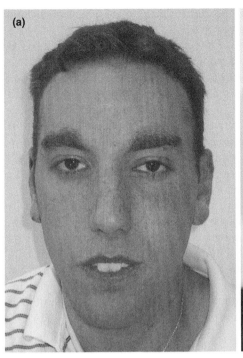 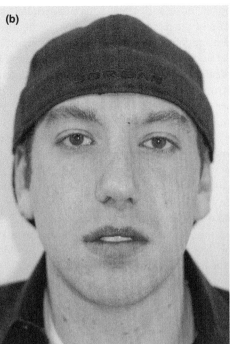 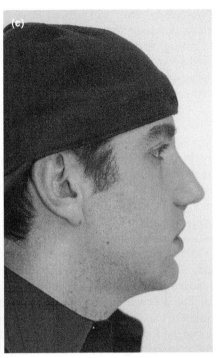

Figure 16.10 This patient had a crooked, overprojected nose but did not wish to have any tip work performed with his surgery. The frontal view reveals persistent asymmetries in both the midvault and tip area despite the straighter dorsum. The postoperative lateral view (C) can be compared with the preop view in Figure 16.3B.

separation of this joint. Release of the bony cartilaginous junction is completed with a Cottle elevator allowing movement toward the midline. When the bony septum is injured, then a controlled incision through the perpendicular plate of the ethmoid bone is made first. This minimizes injury to the cribiform plate thus preserving olfaction and minimizing CSF leaks.(5, 7, 24, 25) The vomer can then be gently back fractured or resected if a spur is present. Resecting part of the cartilage along this line is often necessary to both prevent recurvature and scarring.(18) The surgeon must preserve the dorsal septal attachments. If a significant angulation is observed, total septal reconstruction may be advocated.(19)

If only the lower two third of the nose is displaced from subluxation of the septum off the crest, an endonasal approach may avoid unnecessary exposure of the tip structures especially if tip techniques are not being utilized.(1, 20) If significant injuries or revision surgery are encountered the nose is often best corrected with the open technique. Which technique to utilize, open versus endonasal rhinoplasty, is still a source of debate. In these cases reconstitution of nasal tip support with structural grafting to either the septum or overlying cartilaginous framework is more quickly completed. The endonasal approach may still used for simpler injuries even when graft placement is needed. In the case of caudal deflections a swinging door technique, avoiding injury to the posterior septal angle is completed. The less experienced surgeon needs to recognize that caudal septum is curved and not a perfect rectangle. This often places the posterior septal angle further into the nose than expected. A keel of cartilage is left along the maxillary crest for additional support when possible. If over-resected loss of tip projection occurs causing a pseudo hump.

With significant twisting in the middle third of the nose, the upper lateral cartilages (ULC) are often divided from their septal attachments. This allows the ULC to regain their normal length

if they were avulsed, twisted or scarred. The twisted midvault will have a convex and a concave side. Patients often complain of obstruction bilaterally but typically worse on the concave side as it is being pulled across the midline narrowing the internal valve. Release of the cartilage if avulsed or twisted creates a space for the placement of spreader or septal crossbar graft which will support and help realign the midvault.(6, 12)

Once the septum is fully released, it is secured in the midline to the anterior nasal spine with a figure of eight stitch (Wright suture). Careful attention to asymmetries of the nasal spine should be identified when defining the midline. If a significant fracture has occurred along the caudal septum, a supporting graft is required first to support the caudal septum minimizing re-curvature. Either ethmoid bone or a strong cartilaginous graft can be employed. This provides appropriate tip projection. Rotation can also be adjusted as deemed necessary.(Figure 16.5)

Fractures of the caudal quadrangular cartilage often cause displacement of the anterior septal angle. This often results loss of nasal tip projection and with flattening of the supratip. Appropriate tip projection can be accomplished either with an extended spreader graft when the caudal strut is intact. Otherwise a vertically placed batten graft is needed at the caudal septum.(21) This should extend across the fracture line, re-establishing the caudal septum. Either cartilage or bone grafts may be utilized for creating structural integrity. Alloplastic implants are avoided when possible. Accurate placement of these grafts is important for controlling nasal tip rotation and projection. If counter rotation is needed the extended spreader graft or a caudal septal extension graft is used. A sheen type shield graft is also an option when increased nasal length is needed.

The accurate repositioning of the nasal pyramid is intimately tied to the position of the nasal septum as previously discussed.

Osteotomies alone will seldom fix a crooked nose and often proves fruitless. When evaluating the position of the nasal bones an analogy that patients easily comprehend is the A frame model for the roof of a house. The slope of the nasal side wall varies with the projection of the nasal dorsum. When dealing with an injury to the nasal pyramid, both sides are shifted from the midline with one side concave (in fractured) and the other slightly convex (out fractured). The convex side has a steeper slope and often rises 1–2 mm higher.(Figure 16.9)

The combination and sequence of osteotomies depends both on the degree and location of nasal bone fractures, size and shape. Osteotomies are typically one of the last maneuvers in a standard rhinoplasty. This recommendation is made to minimize edema before splinting. Edema can mask potential dorsal irregularities which require fine rasping.

In a slightly crooked nasal pyramid, only lateral osteotomies may be required to shift the bones back to the midline. If there is a more significant deformity of the nasal bones separation in the midline is beneficial first. The surgeon should first evaluate the height of the nasal pyramid on lateral view. If the patient wants a dorsal reduction, the hump may be rasped or resected. This often creates an open roof deformity, avoiding the medial osteotomies. When the dorsal projection is appropriate on the lateral view or the patient prefers a slight convexity, medial osteotomies followed by lateral osteotomies are used to move the nasal bones back to its appropriate position without rasping.

Medial osteotomies are performed before closing the septum to maintain visualization along the twisted dorsal septum. In severe curvatures it is helpful to also perform the lateral osteotomies at this point to ensure straightening of the dorsal septum. When a persistent concavity is noted, an additional spreader graft is placed to straighten and support the dorsal line. Dorsal onlay grafts can also be utilized to camouflage any dorsal or midvault irregularities at the end of the case. Although they provide a straight appearance functional valve collapse may persist if this is the only technique used.

As the depressed side wall becomes significantly concave, an intermediate osteotomy is required and performed before the lateral osteotomy. This allows the nasal bone to be broken into two segments providing a better contour. (26, Park) It is important to bring the lateral osteotomy into the ascending process of the maxilla to ensure good mobilization. Some authors recommend percutaneous osteotomies to maintain periostial connection to the bone. In cases where dorsal resection is not performed, either a limited medial oblique or a transverse percutaneous osteotomy at the nasion to minimize greenstick is performed last. These maneuvers help when the root of the nose is significantly injured.

In cases of facial asymmetry, the smaller or possibly underdeveloped side of the face tends to have a shorter nasal bone. The nasal pyramid will lean or be "crooked" in that direction. Using the A frame model, the overprojected nose will look more like a steeple than an A frame. When these patients have fractures to their noses, one side elevates and appears steeper, like a Swiss ski chalet while the other is concave and depressed. Dorsal resection in these noses often aids in repositioning of the nose back toward the midline while providing a more appropriate dorsal height. (11) Patient preferences should be noted preoperatively as the overprojection can provide a sense of ethnicity and should be maintained. Batten grafts are included to assist in alar/ side wall support in the subtype of noses.

Ethnic variations of the nose affect all nasal subunits. As already mentioned it is important to discuss the patient's goals and possible outcomes before any procedure. The final position of the dorsum is paramount when straightening the crooked nose. Once the cartilaginous portion of the nose has been repositioned, attention is turned to the nasal bones and dorsum. If the patient has an overprojected dorsum, some resection will provide the most ideal result. If maintaining an ethnic appearance is important then a conservative approach aimed at leaving ethnic characteristics is employed.

Tip asymmetries and alar base disparities also contribute to the final product. When these problems are not addressed the illusion of crooked nose, despite a straight dorsum will remain.(Figure 16.10) Patients with a more platyrrhine nose often require augmentation-type rhinoplasty with additional tip support. When performing lateral osteotomies on a platyrrhine nose, a low-to-low sequence, is recommended given the shorter length of their bones in relation to the piriform aperture.

CONCLUSION

At the completion of the procedure, a secondary survey of the nose is completed to ensure everything is in place. The nose is taped and splinted for the first postoperative week. Thin Silastic splints can be sewn to the septum lending additional support in the first week of healing but can also be a source for scarring. They help minimize formation of synechial bands when tears in the mucoperichondrium have occurred during flap elevation. They too are removed at 1 week.

The careful follow up of patients over months to years is important. This is beneficial for identifying early or late recurvature of a nose. When subunits of the nose have persistent edema, injections with triamcinolone can be judiciously given. Conversely, small depressions can be filled once edema has settled complimenting the nasal contours.

Acknowledgements: I thank Dr Jacob Steiger (Del Ray Beach, Florida) for his help in editing this manuscript.

REFERENCES

1. Converse JM. Corrective surgery of the nasal deviations. Arch Otolaryngol 1950; 52: 671–708.
2. Maliniac J. Role of the septum in rhinoplasty. Arch Otolaryngol 1948; 48: 189.
3. Cottle M, Loring R, Fischer G, Gaynon I. The "Maxilla-Premaxilla" approach to extensive nasal septum surgery. Arch Otolaryngol 1958; 68: 301–432.
4. Mau T, Mau S, Kim D. Cadaveric and engineering analysis of the septal L-strut. Laryngoscope 2007; 117(11): 1902–6.
5. Schwab JA, Pirsig W. Complications of septal surgery. Facial Plast Surg 1997; 13(1): 3–14.
6. Sheen JH. Spreader graft: a method of reconstructing the roof of the middle nasal vault following rhinoplasty. Plast Reconstr Surg 1984; 73: 230–7.
7. Rettinger G, Kirsche H. Complications in septoplasty. Facial Plastic Surgery 2006; 22(4): 289–97.
8. Lee BJ. Chung YS. Jang YJ. Overcorrected septum as a complication of septoplasty. Am J Rhinol 2004; 18(6): 393–6.
9. Goldman I. New techniques in surgery of the deviated nose. Arch Otolaryngol 1956; 64: 183–89.
10. Lawson W, Reind AJ. Correcting functional problems. Facial Plast Surg Clin North Am 1994; 2: 501.

11. Constantian MB. An algorithm for correcting the asymmetrical nose. Plast Recon Surg 1989; 83(5): 801–11.

12. Boccieri A, Pascali M. Septal crossbar graft for the correction of the crooked nose. Plast Reconstr Surg 2003; 111(2): 629–38.

13. Jang YJ, Wang JH, Lee BJ. Classification of the deviated nose and its treatment. Arch Otolaryngol 2008; 134(3): 311.

14. Reilly MJ, Davison SP. Open vs. closed approach to the nasal pyramid for fracture reduction. Arch Facial Plast Surg 2007; 9(2): 82–6.

15. Higuera S, Lee EI, Cole P, Hollier L, Stal S. Nasal trauma and the deviated nose. Plast Reconstr Surg 2007; 120(7): 645–755.

16. Beaty MM, Dyer WK 2nd, Shawl MW. The quantification of surgical changes in nasal tip support. [Evaluation Studies. Journal Article] Arch Facial Plast Surg 2002; 4(2): 82–91.

17. Fomon S, Syracuse V, Bolotow N, Pullen M. Plastic repair of the deflected nasal septum. Arch Otolaryngol 1946; 44: 141.

18. Eisbach E. Cartilaginous septum in the reconstruction of the nose. Arch Otolaryngol 1946; 44: 207–11.

19. Rees T. Surgical correction of the severely deviated nose by extramucosal excision of the osseocartilaginous septum and replacement as a free graft. Plast Recon Surg 1986; 78(3): 320–30.

20. Metzenbaum M. Replacement of the lower end of the dislocated septal cartilage vs submucous resection of the dislocated end of the septal cartilages. Arch Otolaryngol 1929; 9: 282–96.

21. Byrd SH, Salomon J, Flood J. Correction of the crooked nose. Plast Reconstr Surg 1998; 102(6): 2148–57.

22. Kim D, Toriumi D. Management of the posttraumatic nasal deformities: the crooked and saddle nose. Facial Plast Surg Clin N Am 2004; 12(1): 111–32.

23. Eugene Tardy. Lecture: American Academy of Otolaryngology Fall Meeting, San Antonio, Texas, 1998.

24. Gulsen S, Yilmaz C, Aydin E, Kocbiyik A, Altinors N. Meningoencephalocele formation after nasal septoplasty and management of this complication. Turk Neurosurg 2008; 18(3): 281–5.

25. Onerci TM, Ayhan K, Ogretmenoglu O. Two consecutive cases of cerebrospinal fluid rhinorrhea after septoplasty operation. Am J Otolaryngol 2004; 25(5): 354–6.

26. Ammar SM, Westreich RW, Lawson W. Fan septoplasty for correction of the internally and externally deviated nose. Arch Facial Plast Surg 2006; (8)3: 213–16.

17 Lasers, light sources, radiofrequency devices and new technologies for skin of color

Vic A Narurkar

INTRODUCTION

The past decade has witnessed significant advances in the safety and efficacy of lasers, light sources and radiofrequency devices for the treatment of darker skin. It is now evident that the term "skin of color" is becoming more inclusive and a better term is "global skin" to characterize the ever growing population of all skin types. Moreover, the traditional Fitzpatrick skin type classification is also becoming obsolete, as there are so many variations in these traditional skin types and how they respond to devices. Newer classification systems, such as the Roberts classification system, are slowly gaining acceptance as we realize the diaspora of global skin. We are getting closer to truly "color blind" devices with the advent of sophisticated cooling mechanisms, selection of color blind chromophores, and the advent of new technologies such as fractional photothermolysis, photopneumatic therapy, radiofrequency, and cryolipolysis.

REDEFINITION OF SKIN OF COLOR AS GLOBAL SKIN AND NEWER SKIN CLASSIFICATION SYSTEMS

Traditional skin of color classification has been identified as Fitzpatrick skin types IV, V, VI with types IV reflecting darker Mediterranean skin, type V reflecting Asian skin and type VI reflecting African skin. It is clearly evident that this skin typing system is obsolete, as there are so many variations within these traditional skin types. Moreover, skin types which may appear to be lighter on visual inspection may elicit clinical responses similar to darker skin tones, because of complex ethnic backgrounds. This is particularly evident with lasers and light sources and incidence of hypopigmentation and hyperpigmentation. A newer skin classification system was introduced in 2008 entitled the Roberts skin classification system, which employs a variety of factors in determi ning skin response to therapeutic treatments and injury. (1) While the Fitzpatrick classification system relies primarily on phototyping, the Roberts system is a four part serial system that comprehensively identifies a patient's skin type characteristics and provides information to predict the skin's likely response to injury and inflammation, which makes it a perfect system for predicting safety and efficacy of devices. The four elements are phototype, hyperpigmentation, photoaging, and scarring and the four part serial profile is constructed based on a combination of quantitative and qualitative assessments leading to the patient's skin type classification. This includes a review of ancestry, clinical history, visual examination, test site reactions, and physical examination of the patient's skin.

CLASSIFICATION OF DEVICES

The basic premise for modern day laser and light based therapies is predicated on the theory of selective photothermolysis (SP) (2),

whereby in theory any target in the skin can be selectively destroyed if an optimal thermal relaxation time of the target is matched with the optimal biological chromophore (water, oxyhemoglobin, and melanin). It is now evident that while there are more complex mechanisms, especially when competing chromophores are present, such as in hair reduction where melanin is present in the epidermis and the hair follicles. The concept of thermokinetic selectivity (3) is critical in such instances, where larger targets with the same biological chromophore retain heat longer and thereby require longer pulse durations to be destroyed. The parameters in device based therapies are (a) absorption of the biological chromophore, determined by the wavelength; (b) thermal relaxation time of the target, determined by the pulse duration; (c) speed of the energy delivery, determined by frequency (d) energy required to destroy the target, determined by fluence, and (e) protection of unwanted thermal damage, determined by the type of cooling. In darker skin, typically devices require longer pulse durations, lower fluencies, and optimal cooling to prevent complications. Despite the advent of longer pulse duration devices with sophisticated cooling, bulk heating is still possible. Thus, some newer technologies have been introduced to further refine selective photothermolysis. These include selective fractional photothermolysis, photopneumatic therapy, and the use of optical clearing agents. Selective fractional photothermolysis treats a segment of skin and leaves the rest of the skin intact, allowing for reduction in bulk heating.(4) Photopneumatic therapy employs vacuum treatment at the time of light delivery, making photons more energy efficient. (5) Optical clearing agents reduce the amount of energy necessary to destroy the desired target.(6)

HAIR REDUCTION

The most popular laser and light source treatment performed worldwide is laser and light based hair reduction. The mechanism for hair reduction by devices is predicated on thermokinetic selectivity and selective photothermolysis. The biological chromophore is melanin in the hair follicle, which needs to be selectively destroyed with sparing of epidermal melanin. Several devices can be used with safety and efficacy for hair reduction in darker skin (Table 17.1) Melanin absorption shows an exponential drop as one travels down the electromagnetic spectrum from visible light to near infra-red light. The optimal chromophores for hair reduction in darker skin employ longer wavelengths such as the 1,064 nm wavelength. However, in addition to the wavelength, pulse duration and epidermal cooling are equally important. Longer pulse durations, if employed with shorter wavelengths can make these wavelengths safer in darker skin (Figure 17.1). Cooling of the skin is critical, as unwanted thermal injury to the skin can produce blistering and pigmentary changes. Types of cooling include continuous contact cooling, dynamic

Table 17.1 Devices of hair reduction in darker skin.

Device	Mechanism for greater safety in darker skin
Extended pulse 800nm lasers	Pulse durations of 100 to 400 milliseconds
Long Pulse 1064nm lasers	1064nm wavelength with lowest co-incidental absorption of melanin and extended pulse durations
Pulsed light with dichroic filters	Greater selectivity of filters and contact cooling
Photopneumatic therapy and suction based lasers	Pneumatic pressure allowing for more effective delivery of fluence at lower energies

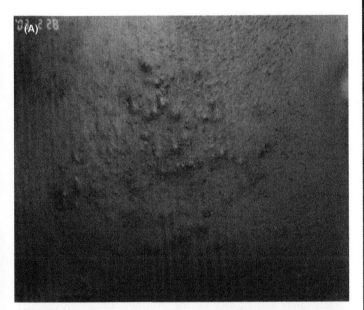

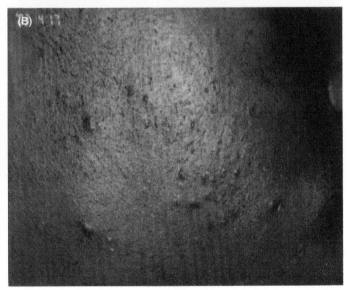

Figure 17.1 Pre and Post 5 treatments 400msec 800nm diode laser hair reduction/ PFB skin type VI.

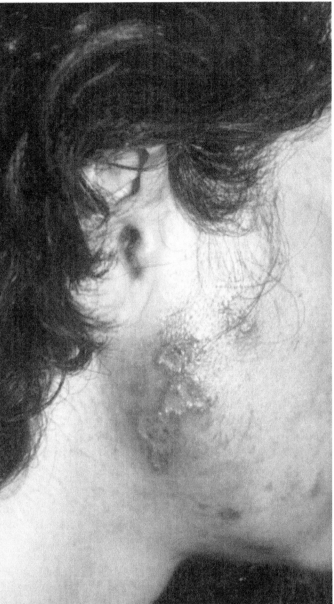

Figure 17.2 Full thickness scars from long pulsed 1064nm laser.

cooling with cryogen spray and cold air cooling. If cooling is suboptimal or does not function, even the safest wavelengths such as the 1,064 nm laser can produce side effects leading to scars and pigmentary changes (Figure 17.2). Darker skin typically requires lower fluencies for hair reduction than lighter skin and therefore requires more treatments. However, one unusual side effect which can occur at suboptimal fluencies

is the phenomenon of paradoxical hair regrowth.(7) This has been particularly reported in Mediterranean, South Asian, and Middle Eastern patients. The mechanism may be a stimulatory effect of low energy on the hair follicle. Pulsed light devices can be used safely in darker skin with the advent of contact cooling, photon recycling, and better filters. While lasers employ, a single wavelength of light, pulsed light employs a broad band of light. Traditional pulsed light systems were not safe for hair reduction in darker skin due to poor filters, higher spikes in energy, and inadequate cooling. Newer generation pulsed light systems have overcome these limitations by the use of more selective filters optimal for the mid to far infra-red region, longer pulse durations with a smooth pulse of delivery and optimal contact cooling to prevent burns and blisters.(8) Photon energy can also be made to be more efficient with pulsed light or lasers using pneumatic energy. Photopneumatic therapy is based on the theory that when vacuum is applied at the time of light

141

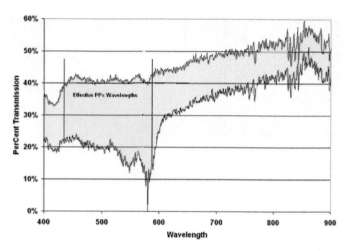

Figure 17.3 Effects of photopneumatic therapy on increasing safety and efficacy of lower wavelength photons.

Table 17.2 Devices for pigmented lesions in darker skin

Device	Mechanism for darker skin
Q switched 755nm lasers	Longer wavelength for less co-incidental melanin absorption
Long pulsed 755nm lasers and 800nm lasers	Extended pulse durations and less co-incidental melanin absorption
Pulsed light sources with dichroic filters and contact cooling	Greater selectivity of filters and contact cooling for epidermal protection
Photopneumatic therapy	Lower fluence and evaporative cooling
Nonablative fractional lasers (1440,1540 and 1550nm)	Color blind chromophore and microthermal injury

Table 17.3 Devices for vascular lesions in darker skin.

Device	Mechanism for safety in darker skin
Long pulsed 532nm lasers	Extended pulse durations and contact cooling for epidermal protection
Long pulse 755nm and 800nm lasers	Moderate affinity for hemoglobin and lower coincidental melanin absorption
Long pulse 1064nm lasers	Off peak hemoglobin absorption and lowest coincidental absorption of melanin
Pulsed light with dichroic filters and contact cooling	Greater selectivity of filters and contact cooling for epidermal protection

based treatment, targets are closer to the skin surface and thereby require less energy (Figure 17.3). Moreover, when lower wavelength photons are used in combination with vacuum, they behave as longer wavelength photons but require less energy. Finally, photon delivery can be made more efficient with the use of a topical agent coined an optical clearing agent (OCA). These OCAS are under development and should be compatible with any device.(9) Optical clearing reduces the optical scattering of biological tissues, thereby making energy delivery safer and more effective at reduced energies of laser and light.

PIGMENTED LESIONS
The treatment of benign pigmented lesions is of great demand in all skin types, but particularly challenging in darker skin because of significant melanin overlap. Several devices (Table 17.2) can be used with safety and efficacy in darker skin. Q-switched devices employ an optomechanical shutter, enabling the delivery of nanosecond pulse durations. Unlike hair reduction, where longer pulse durations are necessary for target destruction, pigmented lesions require shorter pulse durations. With lasers, Q-switched devices at appropriate wavelengths can be safe and effective in darker skin. The 755 nm (alexandrite) wavelength is the safest in conjunction with Q-switching. Pulsed light devices can also be used with safety and efficacy in darker skin. However, it is critical to use longer pulse durations than with lighter skin and to use contact cooling.

VASCULAR LESIONS
Darker skin tones typically do not manifest severe vascular lesions such as essential facial telangiectasias. However, vascular malformations such as port wine stains, angiomas and venous ectasias can be bothersome in all skin types. Traditional vascular devices employ lower wavelengths and can be risky in darker skin types because of too much melanin overlap. Longer wavelength lasers such as the 755 nm, 800 nm, and 1,064 nm (Table 17.3) lasers at longer pulse durations and lower fluencies, can be used with safety and efficacy but will require more treatments than lower wavelength devices due to reduced absorption of vascular

targets. Pulsed light sources, as with pigmented lesions, used to be very risky in darker skin tones. The advent of photon recycling, optimal dichroic filters and contact cooling has allowed for the greater safety and efficacy for the treatment of benign vascular lesions in all skin types.

SKIN RESURFACING
Skin resurfacing can be divided into ablative, nonablative, and fractional modes. Ablative fractional resurfacing was introduced in the 1990s and employed 2,940 nm and 10,600 nm wavelengths (10) with shorter pulse durations to prevent complications. As these devices became used widely, hypopigmentation and depigmentation were reported in all skin types and therefore were not appropriate for resurfacing in darker skin types.(11) Non ablative resurfacing was introduced in the mid 1990s and produced disappointing results for resurfacing and was better suited for the treatment of vascular and pigmented lesions. Fractional photothermolysis was introduced in the 2000s and is rapidly gaining acceptance of the preferred mode of skin resurfacing, regardless of skin types.

Fractional photothermolysis can be further divided into nonablative fractional and micro-ablative fractional. In the author's opinion, non ablative fractional resurfacing is safe and effective in darker skin types, while the jury is still out regarding the safety of microablative resurfacing in dark skin. Non ablative fractional resurfacing employs the following criteria- (a) a non ablative mode of injury, where the stratum corneum is left intact (b) creation of microthermal zones producing microscopic epidermal necrotic debris (MENDS), and (c) a true resurfacing with extrusion of epidermal and dermal contents.(12) The reepithelialization should occur within 24 hours and the density of treated versus untreated skin can be adjusted. Modes of

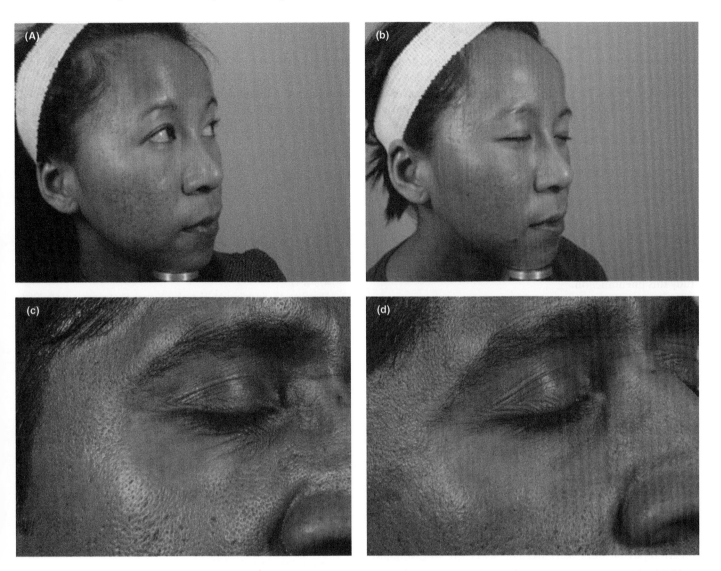

Figure 17.4 (A, B) Pre and post 3 treatments with 1550nm fractional laser for acne scars skin type V. (C, D) Pre and post 3 treatments 1550nm fractional laser resurfacing

fractional delivery can be performed in a scanned random pattern or in a stamped pattern. The wavelengths include 1,440 nm, 1,540 nm and 1,550 nm, all having excellent affinity for water and poor affinity for melanin. In darker skin, fluencies can be kept at equivalent levels to those of lighter skin, but energy densities need to be adjusted to prevent the risks of hyperpigmentation. To this date, no reports of hypopigmentation have been reported and incidence of PIH is reduced with lower treatment densities. Indications for non ablative fractional resurfacing in darker skin include non facial and facial skin resurfacing, treatment of distensible and non distensible acne scars (Figure 17.4), surgical and traumatic scars, striae and therapy resistant melasma. Segmental and isolated areas can be treated without leaving permanent lines of demarcation. A series of three to five treatments is usually necessary. Recently, microablative fractional resurfacing using 2,940 nm and 10,600 nm was introduced with the advantage being the need for one or two treatments. At this juncture, the safety and efficacy of microablative fractional resurfacing in darker skin has not yet been firmly established.

SKIN TIGHTENING

Skin tightening by devices remains a controversial topic, regardless of skin color. Unipolar radiofrequency, bipolar radiofrequency, laser and light sources have been utilized for this indication. In theory, skin tightening devices are truly color blind, as there is no interference with the melanin chromophore, but carried risks independent of skin typing due to bulk heating. The safety of skin tightening devices has increased with protocols such as those employing lower fluencies and multiple passes to avoid bulk heating and subcutaneous atrophy. Monopolar capacitive radiofrequency is the most widely studied and longest utilized device for skin tightening, where selective heating of the dermis and subcutaneous tissue occur with radiofrequency with protection of the epidermis with cooling to preserve epidermal integrity. Initially this device utilized high fluencies which produced significant pain and some adverse effects such as subcutaneous atrophy and unpredictable outcomes. Newer protocols have been developed using low energy delivery with multiple passes and show more consistent and predictable outcomes as well as safety in all skin types.(13) The device is also gaining popularity for non facial indications such as body contouring of the abdomen, arms and buttocks. Single treatments have shown greater efficacy with these new protocols. Combined bipolar radiofrequency and optical energy with lasers and light sources (electro-optical synergy) has also been used for skin tightening but requires a series of treatments. Alternative modalities for skin tightening have employed broad band light sources in the 1,100 to 1,800 nm both in non fractional and fractional modes, for more superficial tightening. Most recently, combination therapies using fractional lasers and unipolar radiofrequency are being developed with the premise of dual modalities having a synergistic effect in collagen remodeling, with fractional resurfacing producing more superficial injury and radiofrequency producing deeper injuries for greater skin tightening. Long term studies are underway to study this phenomenon.

CONCLUSIONS

Devices for darker skin types are undergoing a renaissance, with the advent of newer lasers, light sources and radiofrequency devices. The term "global skin" better describes skin of color, as it is becoming increasingly evident that traditional skin types based purely on phototyping are inadequate. The Roberts skin classification employs multiple parameters to identify features in various skin types to determine the course of treatment, post-procedure sequalae and optimization of outcomes. This system is ideal for device based medicine, as it establishes a scale in response to injury to the skin based on phototype, photoaging, pigmentation response and scar response. The basis of devices is predicated on the theory of selective photothermolysis. It is now evident that this is highly simplistic for modern device therapy, especially in darker skin. Extension of the theory of selective photothermolysis includes thermokinetic selectivity to distinguish competing chromophores, fractional photothermolysis to reduce bulk heating, photopneumatic therapy and optical clearing to maximize photon efficiency and radiofrequency to promote skin tightening. The development of optimal cooling devices has also extended the safety and efficacy for devices in darker skin, by preventing unwanted epidermal injury. In the future, new directions include the development of devices which may be able to detect melanin and erythema content of the skin to further refine optimal setting s for all devices for safety and efficacy.

REFERENCES

1. Roberts WE. The Roberts skin classification system. J Drugs Dermatol 2008; 7(5): 452–6.
2. Anderson RR, Parrish JA. The optics of human skin. J Invest Dermatol 1981; 77(1): 13–9.
3. Goldberg DJ. Laser and light based hair removal: an update. Exper Rev Med Devices 2007; 4(2): 253–60.
4. Narurkar VA. Nonablative fractional resurfacing. Dermatol Clin 2009; 27(4): 473–8, vi.
5. Shamban AT, Enokibiri M, Narurkar V et al. Photopneumatic technology for the treatment of acne vulgaris. J Drugs Dermatol 2008; 7(2): 139–45.
6. Khan MH, Choi B, Chess S, et al. Optical clearing of in vivo human skin and implications for light based diagnostic imaging and therapeutics. Lasers Surg Med 2004 34(2): 83–5.
7. Lolis MS, Marmur ES. Paradoxical effects of hair removal systems: a review. J Cosmet Dermatol 2006; 5(4): 274–6.
8. Ancona D, Stover R, Trelles MA. A multicentre trial of the epilation efficacy of a new large spot consistent spectrum IPL device. J Cosmet Ther 2007; 9(3): 139–42.
9. Khan MH, Chess S, Choi B, et al. Can topically applied optical clearing agents increase the epidermal damage threshold and enhance therapeutic efficacy. Lasers Surg Med 2004; 35(2): 93–5.
10. Tierney EP, Kouba DJ, Hanke CW. Review of fractional photothermolysis: treatment indications and efficacy. Dermatol Surg 2009; 35(10): 1445–61.
11. Biesman BS. Fractional ablative skin resurfacing complications. Lasers Surg Med 2009; 41(3): 177–8.
12. Narurkar VA. Nonablative fractional resurfacing for total body rejuvenation. J Drugs Dermatol 2008; 7(4): 352–5.
13. Hodgkinson DJ. Clinical applications of radiofrequency: non surgical skin tightening (Thermage) Clin Plast Surg 2009; 36(2): 261–8; viii

18 Cosmetic procedures in skin of color

Heather Woolery-Lloyd and Mohamed L Elsaie

INTRODUCTION

Patients with skin of color are increasingly seeking procedures to address the cosmetic concerns unique to this patient population. Improved technology, scientific advances, and reduced costs have also contributed to the rising demand. Patients with skin of color who seek cosmetic procedures have various motivations and goals. They want to reduce the signs of aging, achieve an even skin tone, and create balance in various parts of the face and body. For the clinician, cosmetic procedures in skin of color can be a challenge due to the increased risk of hyperpigmentation and scarring in this patient population. This chapter will review the recent advances and trends in cosmetic procedures for skin of color.

LASERS IN ETHNIC SKIN

The use of lasers in patients with darker skin types has been quite challenging. The main obstacle with cutaneous laser surgery in darker skinned patients is epidermal melanin absorption of laser energy. The absorption spectrum of melanin ranges from 320 to 1200 nm with the greatest absorption observed in the lower end of this spectrum. The main objective in treating patients with skin of color is to avoid epidermal melanin absorption of laser energy and resultant thermal injury. Laser surgery in darker skinned patients must be approached carefully to avoid this unwanted side effect of postinflammatory pigment alteration. In this section, we will review the advances in lasers for ethnic skin with special emphasis on the treatment of acne scars, photorejuvenation, skin tightening, and hair removal.

Acne scars

Ablative devices

CO_2 laser has been used for the treatment of acne scars in skin of color. The laser's usefulness has been limited due to the risk associated with hyperpigmentation and scarring. For that reason other modalities have been investigated for optimum acne scar treatment in ethnic skin.(1)

Fractional devices

Nonablative fractional resurfacing is used for photorejuvenation in all skin types and is especially useful for the treatment of acneiform scarring in ethnic skin.(2) Nonablative fractional resurfacing is performed with a midinfrared laser, which creates microscopic columns of thermal injury. These zones of thermal injury, called microthermal zones (MTZs), have a diameter that is energy dependent and ranges from 100 to 160 µm. At the energies commonly used for facial rejuvenation (8–12 mJ/MTZ), the depth of penetration ranges from 300 to 700 µm.(3) Relative epidermal and follicular structure sparing account for rapid recovery

without prolonged downtime. Melanin is not at risk of selective, targeted destruction; therefore, fractional resurfacing has been used successfully in patients with skin of color.

There are several fractional devices available; however, the most extensively studied is the 1,550-nm erbium-doped fiber laser (Fraxel, Reliant Technologies Inc., San Diego, CA). One study specifically examined Fraxel in skin of color. This study included Japanese patients with acne scars. One treatment consisted of four passes of the device to attain a final microscopic treatment zone of thermal injury with a density of 1000–1500/cm². The fluence was 6 mJ per microscopic treatment zone. The treatment was repeated up to three times at 2–3-week intervals. Clinical improvement was achieved in all the patients. Rare adverse events included mild transient erythema. No patients showed scarring or hyperpigmentation as a result of treatment.(4)

Another study evaluated the 1,550-nm erbium-doped fiber laser (Fraxel, Reliant Technologies Inc., San Diego, CA) for acne scars in 27 Korean patients with skin types IV and V. Patient self-assessments demonstrated excellent improvement in 30%, significant improvement in 59%, and moderate improvement in 11% of patients. In this study no patients developed hyperpigmentation.(5)

Although the safe and effective use of nonablative fractional resurfacing in Asian patients is well documented, there are few published studies in skin types VI or African-American patients. In one retrospective review of 961 treatments in patients of all skin types, the rate of hyperpigmentation was 11.6% in skin type IV ($n = 8$) and 33% in skin type V ($n = 3$). The ethnicities of these patients were not specified.(6)

Nonablative fractional resurfacing offers Asian patients with skin of color an excellent option to treat acne scars and photoaging. In both Asian and non-Asian patients with skin of color, conservative settings (low densities) are necessary to minimize the risk of hyperpigmentation.(7)

Nonablative Devices

One study comparing the 1320 nm Nd:YAG and the 1450 nm diode laser in the treatment of atrophic scars included skin types I–V. In this study both devices offered clinical improvement without significant side effects.(8)

A short pulsed nonablative Nd:YAG (Laser Genesis, Cutera, Inc., Brisbane, CA) has been studied in skin types I-V for the treatment of acne scars. Settings were 14 J/cm², 0.3 ms, 7 Hz with a 5-mm spot size. Each side of the face was treated with a total 2,000 pulses. Nine patients were treated every 2 weeks for a series of eight treatments. Three blinded physician observers used photographs to rate scar severity. Using a grid on the pictures, observers counted scars at baseline and after the final treatment. Overall there was a 29% improvement in the scar severity score. Eight of nine patients reported improvement in their acne scars ranging from 10 to 50% improvement. This nonablative Nd:YAG laser offers another safe and

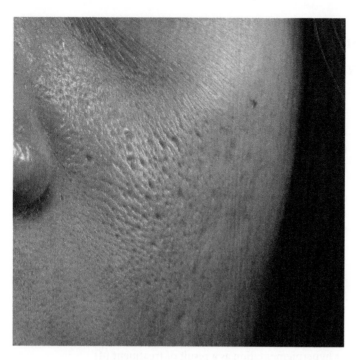

Figure 18.1 Acne scars: patient before treatment.

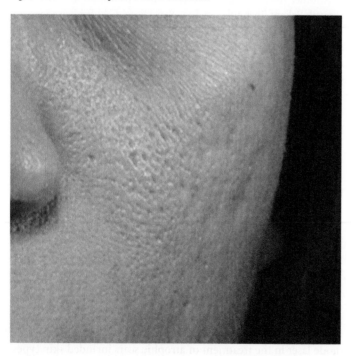

Figure 18.2 Acne scars: patient after treatment with nonablative NdYAG.

well-tolerated option to treat acne scars in patients with skin of color (Figures 18.1 and 18.2).(9) It is important to note that a series of 8 or more treatments are required to achieve improvement. This device has an excellent safety profile in all patients including skin type VI and is most effective in shallow acne scars. Deep ice pick acne scars remain a challenge with all laser modalities in skin of color.

Photorejuvenation

In general, all races are susceptible to photoaging. However, it is clear that in patients with Fitzpatrick's skin phototypes IV to VI

photoaging is delayed and less severe. This is due to the photoprotective role of melanin. Published studies on photoaging in blacks have been limited to African Americans. In African Americans, photoaging is more prominent in lighter-complexioned individuals. In addition photoaging may not be apparent until the late fifth or sixth decade of life. Clinically, the features of photoaging in African Americans can include fine wrinkling, mottled pigmentation, and dermatosis papulosa nigra. In Asian and Hispanic patients, photoaging is also manifested by solar lentigos and prominent pigmentary changes.(10)

Fractional devices

Kono et al. have described the use of the Fraxel in 35 type III and IV Asian skin patients for photorejuvenation. It was noted that increased density was more likely to produce swelling, redness, and hyperpigmentation when compared to increased energy. In this study, the authors concluded that patient satisfaction is significantly higher when their skin is treated with high fluences, but not when treated with high densities. Overall they concluded that fractional photorejuvenation can be safe and effective in darker ethnic skin types.(7)

Light emitting diode (LED)

LEDs offer another advancement in visible spectrum, monochromatic light therapy for photoaged skin. Typically, LEDs in devices are arrayed in panels. Each LED emits visible light in a ± 10 to 20 nm band around the dominant emitted wavelength. Energy output is <25 W, representing a fluence of about 0.1 J/cm².(11) The mechanism of this device is thought to act by targeting stimulation of fibroblast mitochondrial metabolic activity. In addition concomitant upregulation of procollagen and downregulation of matrix metalloproteinase I has been demonstrated.(12) Although there are no studies on LED in ethnic skin, based on the mechanism of action, these devices should be and are generally considered safe in skin of color.

Laser-Assisted Hair Reduction

Alexandrite

The Alexandrite laser has been studied in Fitzpatrick skin types IV to VI. In one study, a long-pulsed 755 nm laser with a 40 ms pulse width was used to treat 150 patients with skin types IV to VI. A test site with a fluence of 16 J/cm² was first performed and energy fluence was selected according to response. The authors reported an overall complication rate of 2.7%; however, only two patients with skin type VI were included in the study and both developed blistering.(13) A smaller study of the Alexandrite (755 nm, 3 ms pulse width) included 4 women with Fitzpatrick skin type VI. In this study, lower fluences were used (8–14 J/cm²) and no side effects were noted.(14) Although treatment of skin types IV to VI is possible with the Alexandrite, the associated risk is still great in these patients.

Diode

The Diode laser has been studied with greater success in the treatment of darker skinned patients. The 800 nm diode laser

146

was studied with pulse widths of 30 ms and 100 ms. Adrian et al. reported that although both settings could be used safely, longer pulse widths (100 ms) allowed higher fluences to be utilized with less complications.(15) Another study utilized the 810 nm Diode laser to treat eight patients with skin types V and VI. These patients were treated with low fluence of 10 mJ/cm^2 and a pulse width of 30 ms. Transient blistering and pigment alterations were noted in some patients despite the lower fluence utilized.(16) Overall, the diode laser offers increased safety over the Alexandrite laser in African-American patients; however, complications remain an issue.

Nd:YAG

The long pulsed Nd:YAG is the safest laser for hair removal in darker skin types. Two factors contribute to the safety of the long pulsed Nd:YAG in darker skin types. First, the wavelength of the Nd:YAG (1064 nm) is at the end of the absorption spectrum of melanin. This wavelength is sufficient to achieve significant thermal injury in dark coarse hairs while sparing epidermal pigment. Second, the adjustable pulse width of long pulsed Nd:YAG lasers allows the laser energy to be delivered over an longer period of time allowing for the heat to dissipate and sufficient epidermal cooling to occur.

The long-pulsed Nd:YAG is the treatment of choice for hirsutism and psuedofollicultis barbae in African Americans with Fitzpatrick Skin Types V and VI. Due the typically coarse dark hair in this patient population, the long pulsed Nd:YAG is safe and highly effective at achieving permanent hair reduction after a series of treatments (Figures 18.3 and 18.4).(17, 18)

Challenges with the long pulsed Nd:YAG in daker skin types arise in those patients with dark skin but fine hair. This is typically seen in patients of Southeast Asian descent. In these patients, permanent hair reduction is more challenging because the fluence and pulse width that are necessary to achieve permanent reduction of fine hair are risky in darker skin types. In these patients, it is important to educate the patient on the limitations of laser-assisted hair reduction. Patients must have realistic expectations and understand that lasers can offer an excellent hair management program but may not offer permanent long term removal of fine hairs. Many patients who fall into this category still prefer laser due to the elimination of irritation and dyschromia frequently seen with shaving, waxing or threading.

Skin Tightening

Many patients with skin of color seek treatment of skin laxity. In contrast to photoaging, increasing skin laxity with advanced age is equally common in all skin types. Older patients seek treatment for the jowls and nasolabial folds which are a prominent sign of aging in this patient population. Younger patients seek treatment of the abdomen postpregnancy. Many patients with skin of color seek nonsurgical interventions due the significant risk of scarring in this patient population.

The concept behind noninvasive skin tightening devices is to spare epidermal injury with the desired injury occurring only at the site of maximal energy absorption in the dermis. This injury is speculated to create new collagen and elastic fibers and may contribute to immediate tightening due to denaturation and contraction of existing collagen fibers.(19, 20) A number of devices

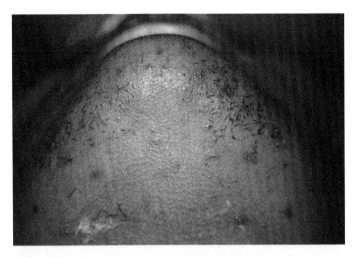

Figure 18.3 Laser hair removal: patient before treatment.

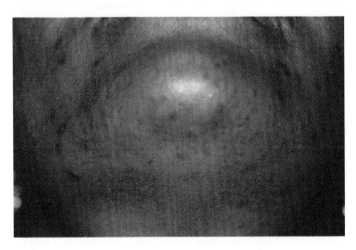

Figure 18.4 Laser hair removal: patient after four treatments with NdYAG.

were created for this purpose; however appropriate patient selection is crucial to achieve significant success with skin tightening. The ideal patient has mild to moderate skin laxity and lack of underlying redundant fatty tissue.

Radiofrequency (RF)

RF is electromagnetic radiation in the frequency range of 3 kHz to 300 GHz. These devices induce dermal heating, denature collagen and induce collagen remodelling.(19) Wound healing mechanisms promote wound contraction, which ultimately clinically enhances the appearance of mild to moderate skin laxity. One device (Thermacool, Thermage Inc, Hayward, CA, USA) has reported efficacy in the treatment of laxity involving the lower face and neck.(21) Because RF energy is not dependent on a specific chromophore interaction, epidermal melanin is not targeted and treatment of all skin types is possible.

Kushikata et al. reported the use of RF in a series of 85 Asian patients of skin types III and IV. Blisters occurred in one patient, a burn occurred in one patient, and hyperpigmentation occurred in 2 of the 85 patients. The skin types of these patients were not specified; however, in all of these cases the complications were transient and healed without permanent sequelae. Objective physician evaluation found relatively good improvement at 3 months post-treatment, and even better improvement at the 6-month evaluation. The authors concluded that RF treatment was effective for skin tightening in Asian facial skin. RF offers safe and effective treatment of skin laxity in ethnic skin.(22)

Infrared Tightening

Titan, (Cutera, Inc., Brisbane, California) uses infrared light to volumetrically heat the dermis. It is designed to thermally induce collagen contraction, with subsequent collagen remodeling and neocollagen synthesis. The epidermis is protected via pre-, parallel, and posttreatment cooling. With this device, improvements in skin laxity and facial and neck contours have been achieved. Response rates are variable and can be influenced by patient selection.(23) Chua et al. investigated the use of infrared light on 21 patients of Fitzpatrick skin types IV and V. At 6-month follow-up, 86% of patients had improvement as measured by the physician assessment. They concluded that Titan was effective to achieve mild to moderate gradual clinical improvement of facial and neck skin laxity.(24) The procedure is associated with minimal downtime and is safe for use in darker skin, including skin types V and VI.

Infrared tightening can be used in all skin types with excellent safety. The settings range from 32–40 J and are determined by patient tolerance and not the skin type. Liberal use of gel appears to improve patient tolerability. In all skin types, multiple sessions (3–5) are needed for best results.

In summary, laser and light therapy can be challenging in skin of color. In this patient population it is important to choose devices that have been studied and have demonstrated safety in skin of color. The lasers discussed in this chapter offer treatment options that have been shown to be safe and effective. Despite this, any laser in skin of color can cause significant complications if the appropriate settings are not utilized. When treating darker skinned patients the use of conservative settings to achieve the desired results is prudent. Following these guidelines, the clinician is most likely to achieve a favorable result with the least unwanted side effects.

Chemical Peels in Ethnic Skin

The use of chemical peeling in ethnic skin dates back to ancient Egypt and Africa. Cleopatra, the famous Egyptian queen was very well known for bathing in sour milk to smoothen and tone her skin (later on scientifically related to the alpha hydroxy-acid properties of sour milk).(25) Chemical peels are an especially popular cosmetic procedure in ethnic skin due to its beneficial effects on hyperpigmentation and acne. Familiarity with the peeling in ethnic skin is essential to ensure its safety and efficacy.

Chemical peels are commonly performed in darker racial-ethnic groups. Serial superficial glycolic acid, salicylic acid, Jessner's solution, and TCA peels (when appropriate) offer substantial benefits for postinflammatory hyperpigmentation, melasma, acne, pseudo-folliculitis barbae, oily skin, and texturally rough skin. Superficial peels are considered safe and effective for darker skinned patients. However, given the labile nature of melanocytes of darker complexioned individuals, medium-depth and deep peels are more likely to induce substantial complications and side effects.

Alpha-hydroxy Acid

Alpha hydroxyl acids are a group of naturally occurring acids including lactic acid (present in sour milk), malic acid (present in apples), citric acid (present in oranges), tartaric acid (present in grapes), and glycolic acid (present in sugarcane). Of these, glycolic acid is the most readily available and utilized commercial peeling agent.

Glycolic Acid

Glycolic acid, an alpha-hydroxy acid has become the most widely used organic carboxylic acid for skin peeling. Glycolic acid formulations include buffered, partially neutralized and esterified products. Chemical peeling can be accomplished with concentrations ranging between 20 and 70% of glycolic acid. Both the concentration and the pH of glycolic acid peels determine the extent of injury. The extent of tissue necrosis of the glycolic acid peel is directly proportional to the concentration of the free acid in the solution. Lower pH products contain more free acid and are more likely to cause crusting and necrosis. It has been shown that a pH under 2.0 favors an increase in tissue destruction and necrosis.(26) In patients with skin of color, lower pH peels are not desirable due to the risk of postinflammatory hyperpigmentation following deeper injury and tissue necrosis.

Glycolic acid peels must be timed and neutralized. Unless neutralized with bicarbonate or water, the effect of glycolic acid will continue keratolysis and desquamation which can lead to complications.(27) Burns et al., treated 19 black patients for PIH with glycolic acid peels. The control group was treated with a topical formulation of 10% glycolic acid and 2% hydroquinone while the active group received the glycolic acid/hydroquinone topical formulation in addition to six serial glycolic acid peels. Greater satisfaction with no observed side effects was obtained on the side with the glycolic acid peels.(28)

Glycolic acid peels are well tolerated in darker skin types. Side effects are minimized when the concentrations of equal to or <30% are used. Glycolic acid peels of >30% or peels with a low pH should be used with caution in patients with skin of color as the risk of postinflammatory pigment alteration increases dramatically.

Lactic acid

Lactic acid is an alpha-hydroxy acid that has similar activities to glycolic acid, but surprisingly it has not been used as much as glycolic acid in peeling treatments.(29) One study used lactic acid to evaluate the efficacy of lactic acid chemical peels and Jessner's solution in melasma in skin type IV. In part of the study, lactic acid was applied to one half of the face in patients with melasma while Jessner's solution was applied to the other half for comparison. The investigators reported that lactic acid peels were equally safe, effective, and tolerable as the Jessner's solution.(30)

Jessner's solution

Jessner's solution was formulated by Dr. Max Jessner in a combination of 14% resorcinol, 14% salicylic, and 14% lactic acid. Jessner's solution has been used extensively since the 1940's.(31) Jessner's solution offers a superficial peel; however this formula

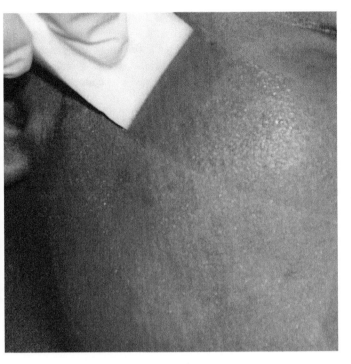

Figure 18.5 Salicylic acid peel.

can be used as a medium depth peel in combination with other agents.

Jessner's peels are safe and effective in skin of color. In these patients, Jessner's peels are particularly useful in patients with acne and/or hyperpigmentation. In patients with skin of color, it best to start with one to two coats and to increase the number of coats at successive treatments. Typically a series of three to five peels are necessary to achieve the desired results.(32)

Salicylic acid

Salicylic acid is a member of the beta-hydroxy acid family and is a commonly used chemical peel. Salicylic is a naturally occurring substance that is derived from the willow tree. In smaller concentrations salicylic acts as a keratolytic and comedolytic agent. Salicylic acid is one of the oldest documented chemical peels and was used by Unna, the German dermatologist in the 19th century. Being a flexible peeling agent, salicylic acid can be formulated in many different vehicles.(33) Salicylic acid solutions are most frequently used as peeling agents to treat acne and melasma in dark skin (Figure 18.5).(34)

As a keratolytic and comedolytic agent, salicylic acid exhibits an affinity to pilosebaceous units and thus is the peel of choice in patients with acne and hyperpigmentation. A total of 20–30% salicylic peel solution is typically applied to the skin with a sponge applicator. The resultant "frost" is actually the salicylic acid powder once the solution has dried. A true frost can occur with a salicylic acid peel and represents denatured protein at the level of the dermis. The true frost is more often observed when patients utilize a retinoid before the chemical peel. In ethnic skin, perifollicular frosting is acceptable and is commonly observed in patients with acne. More extensive frosting of the skin should be avoided as this can result in deeper peeling and possible postinflammatory pigmentation. For all

patients new to chemical peels, retinoids should be held for 7–10 days before the peel. Further recommendations on retinoid use for follow up treatments should be guided by patient response. For example, in sensitive skin patients who are more likely to frost, patients should continue to be advised to avoid retinoids seven to ten days before each peel. In patients with more resistant skin, avoiding a retinoid 2–3 days before the peel is sufficient. A series of three to six treatments at 3–4 week intervals offers the best results. Clinicians should start at a 20% peel and titrate up to 30% as tolerated.

Trichloroacetic acid (TCA)

Roberts, first described TCA in 1926.(35) TCA is an inorganic crystalline compound that is frequently used for chemical peeling. In darker skin, lower concentrations of 10–15% can be utilized. TCA precipitates epidermal proteins and causes necrosis of cells. An end point of TCA is the white frost created after applying the solution; however it is very important to realize that this effect is not desired in darker skin tones as it is associated with postpeel hyperpigmentation and scarring. TCA peels are useful in skin types I-III, but should used with caution in skin types IV-VI.(36) Grimes et al., utilizes a combination of salicylic acid 20% and 30% and a low strength TCA. This combination peeling produces more efficacy rather than using TCA alone and minimizes the side effects of scarring and/or dyschromias. TCA peels should be used with much caution in skin of color and reserved for patients who have failed conventional therapies.(36)

MICRODERMABRASION

Microdermabrasion is increasing in popularity among the ethnic skin population due to the simplicity and safety of the technique. Microdermabrasion improves the absorption of topicals by mechanically removing the stratum corneum layers. In one study, the flux and skin deposition of vitamin C across microdermabrasion-treated skin was approximately 20-fold higher than that across intact skin.(37) There are a variety of microdermabrasion devices available including aluminum oxide-based, salt-based, and crystal-less systems.

Benefits of multiple, regular microdermabrasion treatments in improving dyschromia, facial scarring and facial photodamage have been reported.(38, 39) One study evaluated the efficacy versus safety of microdermabrasion in skin types II–IV. 88% of the patients were of the skin type IV. Abrasion of the whole face was done with a vacuum pressure setting of 30 mmHg, four passes and a vacuum pressure of 15 mmHg and 2 passes over the periorbital skin. Colorimetry values as well as the investigator and patients ratings for safety and efficacy were analyzed and demonstrated a significant improvement in texture and photoaging. Minimal side effects were reported, and the authors concluded that microdermabrasion is as a safe efficient modality in different skin types including skin type IV.(40)

Microdermabrasion is especially useful in patients with sensitive skin. In sensitive skin patients who also have acne, melasma or postinflammatory hyperpigmentation chemical peels are often not well tolerated. In these patients, microdermabrasion offers a less aggressive and better tolerated adjunct to topical therapies.

Although, microdermabrasion is generally considered a safe treatment in skin of color, aggressive treatments at high pressures can lead to streaking in darkly pigmented patients. As with any device in skin of color, very aggressive settings should be avoided in this patient population.

BOTULINUM TOXIN IN ETHNIC SKIN

Botulinum toxin injection was the most commonly performed cosmetic procedure in 2007 representing 23.7% of all cosmetic and noncosmetic procedures. Patients with skin of color represented almost 21% of all patients who performed that procedure with an increasing trend.(41)

In Asian patents, Botulinum toxin type A (BTX-A) has been used for localized recontouring of the upper and lower face. Some Asian patients desire a more open, Eurasian eyelid. This can be achieved with the injection of 1 to 2 units of BTX-A into the mid lower lid to open the eye slightly. However, there is a significant risk of ectropion and this should only be performed by an experienced physician.(42) Another technique that can be utilized in patients that seek a wider eye is the lateral brow lift.

A prominent mandibular angle and jaw fullness is a common concern in Asian women who seek aesthetic treatments. Masseter hypertrophy is a cause of jaw fullness in this patient population. Intramuscular masseter injections with BTX-A can improve contours of the lower facial profile by reducing the bulkiness of masseteric muscles. Results last up to 6 months and cause only mild reduction in bite force that do not interfere with activities of daily living.(43)

BTX-A is also an effective treatment for dynamic wrinkles in African-American and Hispanic patients. African-American patients are less likely to seek treatment for the crows feet as these rhytides are more dependent on photoaging. The most commonly treated sites in African-American patients include the forehead and glabellar areas. In phase III BTX-A clinical trials of the glabella, 21 out of the 405 patients in the trial were African American. Analysis compared the overall efficacy of those 21 subjects to the remaining Caucasian subjects and showed no statistically significant differences in the efficacy or safety responses.(44)

BTX injections represent an effective procedure for the treatment of dynamic wrinkles, independent of sex, age, or race.

SOFT TISSUE AUGMENTATION IN SKIN OF COLOR

Soft tissue augmentation restores volume loss in the face. Volume is primarily restored in areas of fat loss and atrophy.(45) Ethnic patients, particularly African Americans, have a tendency toward midface aging with sagging of the malar fat pads toward the nasolabial folds, upper lid laxity, and jowl formation.(46) With aging, fat atrophy causes hills and valleys to develop on the face producing demarcations between the cosmetic units.

Skin laxity, a sign of aging observed equally in all skin types makes soft-tissue tissue augmentation a popular procedure in all skin types. Based on the skin type, some soft tissue fillers will achieve better results than others. Collagen has an opaque white color which can be seen when injected superficially in skin of color. Hyaluoronic acid, and poly-L-lactic acid are transparent and are better choices for this reason in patients with skin of color. Calcium hydroxyl-appetite is another excellent choice for ethnic skin patients with deep rhytides.

Hyaluronic acid (HA) represents the most frequently used soft tissue augmentation filler and ranks second overall in surgical and nonsurgical cosmetic performed procedures.(41) Due to the susceptibility for scar formation and hyperpigmentation even after minor trauma, some have suggested that injected HA may be more risky in dark skinned individuals. Studies suggest, however, that this is not the case. In a study of 60 patients injected with nonanimal, stabilized hyaluronic acid (Restylane ®), 40 patients were of skin types I–III and 20 were of skin types IV-VI. Of skin types I–III, 2 of the 40 patients had transient adverse events and no patients had permanent adverse events. Of the twenty patients with skin types IV–VI no transient or permanent adverse events were observed. The authors concluded that HA is safe and efficient for darker skin types.(47)

All of the fillers discussed offer a safe and effective treatment options for soft tissue augmentation in skin of color. Consequently, physicians can focus on the individual needs of the patient when choosing a filler in patients with skin of color.

CONCLUSION

The best approach to cosmetic procedures in skin of color involves thorough knowledge of the appropriate devices and modalities to treat various cosmetic concerns. To fully master any cosmetic procedure or laser therapy, knowledge of these treatments in skin of color is essential. Although safe and effective cosmetic treatments in ethnic skin can pose real challenges, it is essential that clinicians feel competent in this group of individuals. Both locally and globally there will continue to be increased demand for cosmetic procedures in skin of color.

REFERENCES

1. Kim JW, Lee JO. Skin resurfacing with laser in Asians. Aesthetic Plast Surg 1997; 21(2): 115–7.
2. Manstein D, Herron GS, Sink RK et al. Fractional photothermolysis: a new concept for cutaneous remodeling using microscopic patterns of thermal injury. Lasers Surg Med 2004; 34: 426–38.
3. Fisher GH, Geronemus RG. Short-term side effects of fractional photothermolysis. Dermatol Surg 2005; 31: 1245–9.
4. Hasegawa T, Matsuka T, Mizuo Y et al. Clinical trial of laser device called fractional photothermolysis system for acne scars. J Dermatol 2006; 33(9): 623–27.
5. Lee HS, Lee JH, Ahn GY et al. Fractional photothermolysis for the treatment of acne scars: a report of 27 Korean patients. J Dermatolog Treat 2008; 19(1): 45–9.
6. Graber EM, Tanzi EL, Alster TS. Side effects and complications of fractional laser photothermolysis: experience with 961 treatments. Dermatol Surg 2008; 34(3): 301–5.
7. Kono T, Chan HH, Groff WF et al. Prospective direct comparison study of fractional resurfacing using different fluences and densities for skin rejuvenation in Asians. Lasers Surg Med 2007; 39(4): 311–4.
8. Tanzi EL, Alster TS. Comparison of a 1450 nm diode laser and a 1320 nm NdYAG laser in the treatment of atrophic facial scars: a prospective clinical and histological study. Dermat Surg 2004; 30: 152–7.
9. Lipper GM, Perez M. Nonablative acne scar reduction after a series of treatments with a short-pulsed 1,064-nm neodymium:YAG laser. Dermat Surg 2006; 32(8): 998–1006.
10. Kligman AM. Solar elastosis in relation to pigmentation. In: Fitzpatrick TB, Pathak MA, eds. Sunlight and man. Tokyo: University of Tokyo Press, 1974: 157–63.
11. Gentlewave approval FDA Gentlewave FDA approval, 2005. Cosmetic surgery-news. Available at: http://www.cosmeticsurgery-news.com/article2357.html.

12. Weiss RA, Weiss MA, Geronemus RG, McDaniel DH. A novel non-thermal non-ablative full panel led photomodulation device for reversal of photoaging: digital microscopic and clinical results in various types. J Drugs Dermatol 2004; 3: 605–10.

13. Breadon JY, Barnes CA. Comparison of adverse events of laser and light-assisted hair removal systems in skin types IV-VI. J Drugs Dermatol 2007; 6: 40–6.

14. Nouri K, Jimenez G, Trent J. Laser hair removal in patients with Fitzpatrick skin type VI. Cosmetic Dermat 2002; 15(3): 15–6.

15. Adrian RM, Shay KP. 800 nanometer diode laser hair removal in African American patients: a clinical and histologic study. J of Cutan Laser Ther 2000; 2(4): 183–90.

16. Greppi I. Diode laser hair removal of the black patient. Lasers Surg Med 2001; 28(2): 150–5.

17. Alster TS, Bryan H. Williams CM. Long-pulsed Nd:YAG laser-assisted hair removal in pigmented skin: a clinical and histological evaluation. Arch Dermatol 2001; 137(7): 885–9.

18. Ross EV, Cooke LM, Timko AL, Overstreet KA et al. Treatment of pseudofolliculitis barbae in skin types IV, V, and VI with a long-pulsed neodymium: yttrium aluminum garnet laser. J Am Acad Dermatol 2002; 47(2): 263–7.

19. Zelickson BD, Kist D, Bernstein E et al. Histological and ultrastructural evaluation of the effects of a radiofrequency based nonablative dermal remodeling device: a pilot study. Arch Dermatol 2004; 140(2): 204–9.

20. Fitzpatrick R, Geronemus R, Goldberg D et al. Multicenter study of non-invasive radiofrequency for periorbital tissue tightening. Lasers Surg Med 2003; 33: 232–42.

21. Hsu TS, Kaminer MS. The use of nonablative radiofrequency technology to tighten the lower face and neck. Semin Cutan Med Surg 2003; 22: 115–23.

22. Kushikata N, Negishi K, Tezuka Y, Takeuchi K, Wakamatsu S. Non-ablative skin tightening with radiofrequency in Asian skin. Lasers Surg Med 2005; 36(2): 92–7.

23. Bunin LS, Carniol BJ. Cervical facial skin tightening with an infrared device. Facial Plast Surg Clin North Am 2007; 15(2): 179–84.

24. Chua SH, Ang P, Khoo LS, Goh CL. Nonablative infrared skin tightening in Type IV to V Asian skin: a prospective clinical study. Dermatol Surg 2007; 33(2): 146–51.

25. Bryan CP. Ancient Egyptian medicine; The papyrus ebers. Chicago, Il:Ares publishers, 1974.

26. Becker FF, Langford FPJ, Rubin MG, Speelman P. A histological comparison of 50% and 70% glycolic acid peels using solutions with various pHs. Dermatol Surg 1996; 22(5): 463–8.

27. Atzore L, Brundu MA, Orru A et al. Glycolic acid peeling in the treatment of acne. J European Acad Dermatol Venerol 1999; 12: 119–22.

28. Burns RI, Provost-Blank PC, Lawry MA et al. Glycolic acid peels for post inflammatory hyperpigmentation in black patients: a comparative study. Dermatol Surg 1997; 23: 171–4.

29. Smith WP. Epidermal and dermal effects of topical lactic acid. J Am Acad Dermatol 1996; 35: 388–91.

30. Sharquie KE, Al-tikreety MM, AL-Mashandani SA. Lactic acid chemical peels as a new therapeutic modality in melasma in comparison to Jessners solution chemical peels. Dermatol Surg 2006; 32: 1429–36.

31. Urkov JC. Surface defects of the skin treated by controlled exfoliation. III Med J 1946; 89: 75.

32. Grimes PE. Agents for ethnic skin peeling. Dermatol Ther 2000; 13: 159–64.

33. Ueda S, Mitsugi K, Ichige K et al. New formulation of chemical peeling agent: 30% salicylic acid in polyethylene glycol. Absorption and distribution of salicylic acid in polyethelene glycol applied topicallt to skin of hairless mice. J Dermatol Sci 2002; 28: 211–8.

34. Grimes PE. The safety and efficacy of salicylic acid chemical peels in darker racial-ethnic groups. Dermatol Surg 1999; 25: 18–22.

35. Roberts HL. The choloracetic acids. A biochemical study. Br J Dermatol 1926; 38: 323–91.

36. Grimes PE, Rendon ML, Pellerano J. Superficial chemical peels. In: Grimes PE, ed. Aesthetic and Cosmetic Surgery for Darker Skin Types. Lippincott Williams & Wilkins, 2007: 166.

37. Lee WR, Shen SC, Kuo-Hsien W, Hu CH, Fang JY. Lasers and microdermabrasion enhance and control topical delivery of vitamin C. J Inv Dermatol 2003; 121(5): 1118–25.

38. Tsai RY, Wang CN, Chan HL. Aluminium oxide crystal microdermabrasion : a new technique for treating facial scarring. Dermatol Surg 1995; 21: 539–42.

39. Tan MH, Spencer JM, Pires LM et al. The evaluation of aluminium oxide crystal microdermabrasion for photodamage. Dermatol Surg 2001; 27: 943–9.

40. Spencer JM, Kurtz ES. Approaches to document the efficacy and safety of microdermabrasion procedure. Dermatol Surg 2006; 32: 1353–7.

41. America society for Aesthetic plastic surgery. Cosmetic surgery national data bank statistics 2007. Available at http://www.surgery.org/download/2007stats.pdf.

42. Flynn TC, Carruthers JA, Carruthers JA. Botulinum A toxin treatment of the lower eyelid improves infraorbital rhytides and widens the eye. Dermatol Surg 2001; 27: 703–8.

43. Yu CC. Chen PK. Chen YR. Botulinum toxin a for lower facial contouring: a prospective study. Aesthetic Plast Surg 2007; 31(5): 445–51.

44. Hexsel DM, Hexsel CL, Brunetto LT. Botulinum toxin. In: Grimes PE, ed. Aesthetic and cosmetic surgery for darker skin types. Lippincott Williams and Wilkins, 2007; 211–24.

45. Brugges CM. Soft tissue augmentation in skin of color: market growth, available fillers, and successful techniques. J Drugs Dermatol 2007; 6: 51–5.

46. Matory WE. Aging in people of color. In: MatoryWE, ed. Ethnic Considerations in Facial Aesthetic surgery. Philadelphia: Lippincott-Raven, 1998: 151–70.

47. Odunze M, Cohn A, Few JW. Restylane and people of color. Plast Reconstr Surg 2007; 120(7): 2011–6.

19 The treatment of acne scars in different groups
Greg Goodman

INTRODUCTION

Postacne scarring remains a challenge of therapy. The skin behaves as if it has a tremendous memory of the depth and severity of the existing scarring. These scars can require an inordinate amount of therapy to alter and improve their appearance. This chapter will attempt to describe relevant treatment options according to groups defined by different skin colouring, gender and the individuals' acne severity.

PREOPERATIVE PATIENT EDUCATION

The patient needs to be assessed according to the types of scars they have as well as scar severity and extent. This includes assessment from both the psychological and physical points of view.

The practitioner should educate the patient about what type of scars they have and what types of treatment are available for those scar types. There will usually be a number of different treatment possibilities to be explained to the patient, along with their potential adverse effects and complications. Possible risks and likely benefits need to be addressed for every procedure discussed.

As possible he should advise the patient in as much detail as possible about the potential outcomes to be expected from the available treatments. In particular, the patient should be aware that acne scarring is not a condition that usually improves rapidly after therapy (aside from excision and augmentation procedures); instead, there is an incremental improvement over time and often a number of procedures are required, especially when there are to be alterations in collagen.

Often there will be a number of different techniques that will be combined to treat the condition at hand, and the practitioner needs to make sure the patient is aware of the timing and duration of the procedures.

Computer aids such as PowerPoint or similar presentations with embedded videos can be useful educational tools for discussing the different alternatives available for treating the patient's condition.

It is helpful to supply the patient with printed information about discussed techniques and procedures, including the possible risks. If needed, a further appointment can be made to discuss any further questions or concerns that the patient may have.

If the practitioner and patient do not share the same first language, reasonable interpreting efforts must be made. This may mean including family members, an interpreter or printed information in the appropriate language in the consultation.

CONTRAINDICATIONS

The patient should have an appropriate awareness of their disease severity and the outcome likely with treatment. A lack of such awareness should be considered a contraindication to ongoing therapy.

METHODS OF ASSISTING POSTACNE SCARS

There are only a limited number of ways that the scarred skin may be helped. Broadly and simplistically, one can act on the scar by:

Cutting it out. This includes all methods of excising scars. This is necessary in a number of instances, including when the scar is dystrophic, has a white base or is in the middle of a bearded area (Figures 19.1a to 19.1d). This category also includes a variety of "punch" techniques such as punch elevation, punch excision and punch grafting. These techniques are at maximum utility when treating punched-out and "ice pick" scars (Figures 19.2a and 19.2b).

Filling it up. This includes autologous (autologous collagen, dermal and fat grafting) and nonautologous temporary, semi-permanent and permanent augmentation techniques and agents (Figure 19.3).

Altering its color. Sometimes a scar is visible purely because of its color, and sometimes coloring makes an atrophic or hypertrophic scar more visible. The technique used will depend upon the scar's color. Brown coloring or hyperpigmentation in scars often represents postinflammatory hyperpigmentation, and is responsive to medical therapy with bleaching preparations and light chemical skin peeling (Figure 19.4). For erythematous scarring or marking, home care, vascular laser and time may be all that is required (Figure 19.5). Hypopigmented marking is more difficult and may require the use of pigment transfer techniques (Figures 19.6 and 19.7).

Inducing (or reducing) collagen. These are the most commonly used methods, and results can vary. Inducing collagen formation is a common pathway used by all resurfacing techniques, from the most minor home care to superficial treatments such as microdermabrasion and light chemical skin peeling, through to the deeper resurfacing techniques represented by medium and deep chemical peeling, dermabrasion, laser skin resurfacing, plasma skin resurfacing and fractional resurfacing. It is with these techniques, which are the least exact, that patients with darker skin color may experience variable outcomes (Figure 19.8).

All techniques relying on collagen remodeling have several things in common:

- The effect of therapy is often delayed for some months after the treatment.
- There is often a zenith in apparent improvement and then a steady decline of that improvement after any single therapy.
- The degree of collagen remodeling seems to be proportional to the severity of the resurfacing injury.
- There seems to be a reliance on multiple therapies or ongoing treatment to maximize the result.

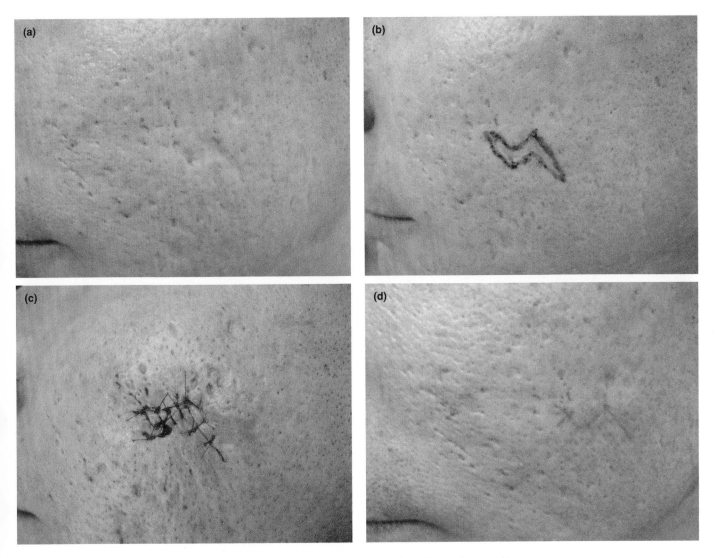

Figure 19.1 (A) W-shaped scar pretreatment, (B) outlined, (C) immediately postexcision and (D) three weeks postexcision.

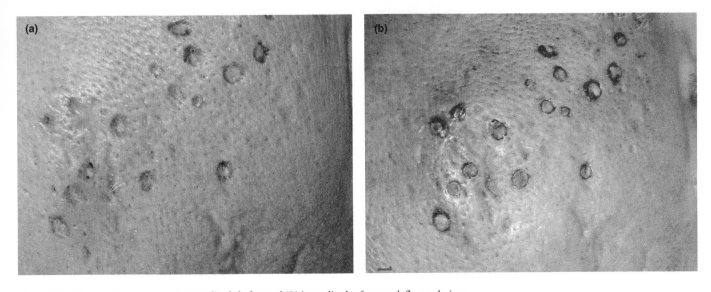

Figure 19.2 Patient with type 4 skin (A) immediately before and (B) immediately after punch float technique.

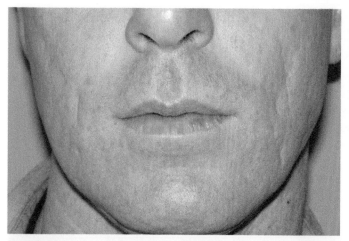

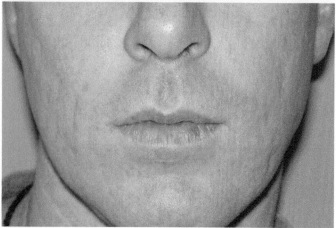

Figure 19.3 Patient before and after subcision, fat transfer and combined CO_2 and erbium laser resurfacing.

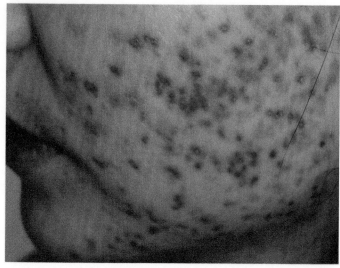

Figure 19.5 Erythematous marking in a patient recovering from active acne.

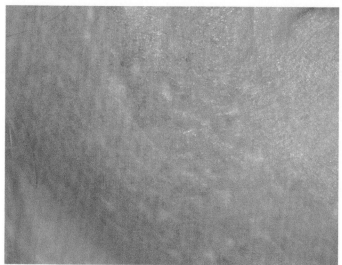

Figure 19.6 Hypopigmented macular scarring.

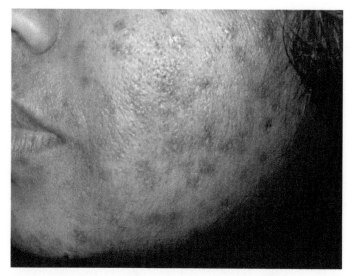

Figure 19.4 Postinflammatory hyperpigmentation following acne misdiagnosed as postacne scarring.

Related but somewhat reversed considerations seem to apply to hypertrophic scars, with multiple and often periodically repeated therapies required to change the apparent 'memory' of the excessive (rather than deficient) fibroblast-produced collagen synthesis.

Relaxing the region. This is occasionally important on the forehead, chin and lower jaw line because of excessive muscle activity on a scarred atrophic and compliant area of skin. Skin puckering from excessive muscle activity amplifies the scarring, a problem which can be remedied (albeit temporarily) by relaxing the puckering with botulinum (Figures 19.9a to d).

GROUP DEFINITIONS

A number of factors influence the skin grouping of any given patient. Table 19.1 summarizes the important points that must be gleaned from the patient's history and examination before proceeding to plan the patient's therapy.

Patients may be grouped by phototyping according to their sun-burning reaction, and their immediate and delayed tanning responses to three minimal erythema doses (MEDs) of skin, as described by Thomas B Fitzpatrick (1) (Table 19.2).

This scale describes sun reactive skin typing based on some inherent genetic traits and one's ability to withstand the ravages

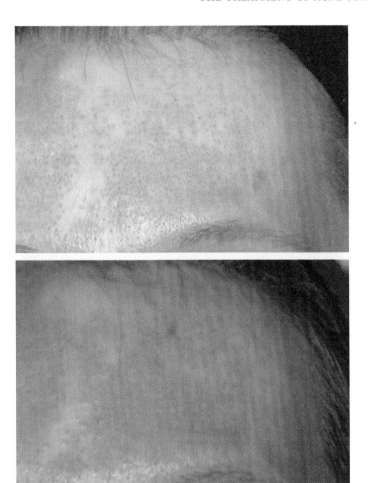

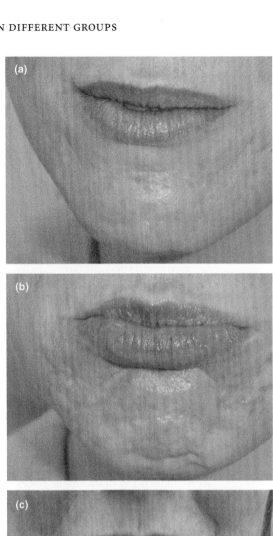

Figure 19.7 Patient before and after autologous automated pigment cell transfer technique (ReCell).

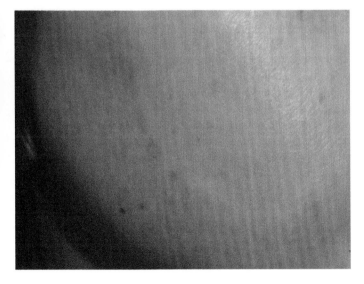

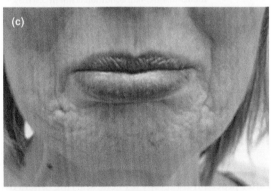

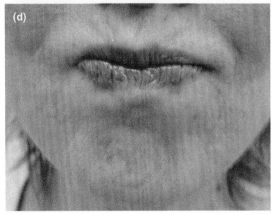

Figure 19.8 Patient with long-term hypopigmentation following laser resurfacing.

Figure 19.9 Patient displaying chin scarring (A) at rest and (B) on animation displaying amplified appearance of scarring. Another patient showing (C) movement-related dimpling and scarring and (D) attempting similar movements two weeks after botulinum toxin and hyaluronic acid injections.

155

Table 19.1 Patient history and examination details.

Parameter	What Needs to be Done
Activity of associated acne	Treat acne before beginning treatment for scarring
Patient's Fitzpatrick skin type	In skin types 3, 4 and 5, one should be concerned about postinflammatory hyperpigmentation. In skin type 6 (black skin) there is usually only a short-term issue with pigment, which seems to be normalized faster than in the less pigmented olive skin types. For darker-skinned patients, procedures with better safety margins are usually chosen.
Gender	When considering the possibilities for treatment, keep in mind that most males do not wear makeup readily, and females do not have beards to hide demarcation lines.
Age	Be concerned about treating the very young (because of emotional maturity) and the very old (because of possibilities for concomitant illness, and questions about motivation for treatment).
Psychological and maturity, physical health	Make sure it is appropriate to proceed with the suggested course of action. Ensure that the patient has an adequate understanding of the limitations of the selected treatment.
Social constraints	Ensure that adequate care is available in the postoperative period, and that the patient is able to attend follow-up appointments. Payment needs to be discussed, especially if there is to be a long process or if expensive equipment is to be used.
Burden of disease	The treatment required will vary according to how much disease load is present. Severe scarring may require a number of procedures and even hospitalization, while with milder disease this is less likely. However, even with milder disease, skin condition is not necessarily assured to reach patient expectations, and the individual may still need multiple (if less morbid) procedures.
Type of scarring	Certain types of scarring (ice pick, gross atrophy, erythematous macular marks, etc) may need their own specific treatments.
Site of scarring	Treatment of certain scarring sites (neck, chest and back) carries more risk of problems such as pigmentation and hypertrophic scarring.

Note: Sun-reactive skin types.

of short-term sun exposure. The ability to produce pigmentary change after procedural therapy for acne scarring differs depending where one sits within the scale.

Individuals with skin types 4 to 6 (and perhaps type 3), mainly those with a deeper coloring, have skin which comes with a collection of benefits related to skin cancers and certain ageing characteristics, but with an increased rate of postinflammatory hyperpigmentation and possibly scarring compared to individuals whose skin is less replete with large melanosomes. Those with fairer colored skin have other issues, especially with respect to their response to resurfacing techniques and the complication of consequent hypopigmentation. It would seem likely that the slowly maturing dermal collagen remodeling following deeper resurfacing procedures (dermabrasion, deep chemical peeling or CO_2 laser resurfacing) is really akin to a slowly increasing fibrosis, becoming paler rather than erythematous as the skin appears in the earlier stages of the wound-healing process.

Those with skin type 2 and perhaps type 3 seem to not have the required epidermal color to adequately camouflage this process. They may also not have complete recovery of the epidermal pigment, and may be at risk of long-term hypopigmentation from deeper resurfacing procedures. Skin type 1 patients are so fair that the hypopigmentation is not readily apparent.

PARTICULAR ADVICE AND PROCEDURES FOR THE PATIENT WITH DARKER SKIN

Scarring is said to be more common in darker-skinned patients, but there are more reliable predictors for a person's risk of scarring than skin colouring. As Grimes and Hunt wrote in 1993, although (as with any elective cosmetic procedure) caution should be exercised, '… [t]he myth that all black patients develop keloids or dyspigmentation after surgery should be dispelled'.(2)

It is said that darker skin types differ from Caucasian skin not only in possessing increased epidermal melanin, but also an increase in the stratum corneum cell layers, increased stratum corneum lipids, increased recovery rate after tape stripping and numerous dermal fibroblasts. Until recently, many of the procedures for the treatment of acne scarring have been particularly difficult for patients with darker skin coloring. Technique-dependent resurfacing procedures (chemical peeling, dermabrasion, laser skin resurfacing, and plasma resurfacing) have all been plagued by substantial morbidity and risk of adverse reactions.

More superficial wounding of the skin in darker individuals, using techniques such as microdermabrasion, superficial skin peeling and nonablative resurfacing, seem to be relatively safe compared to deeper resurfacing techniques. However, significantly deeper treatments such as medical skin rolling and fractional resurfacing seem also to offer a very good comparative safety.

Table 19.2 Reactivity of human skin to solar radiation based on skin phototypes 1 to 6.

Skin Phototype	Constitutive or Unexposed Skin Colour Places (Buttock)	MED Range mJ/cm2 of UVB	Reactivity or Sensitivity to UVR	Sunburn and Tanning History
1	Ivory white (Celtic)	15-30	Very sensitive or reactive ++++	Burns easily, strongly; never tans
2	White (Celtic)	25-40	Very sensitive or reactive +++/++++	Burns easily, and tans minimally with difficulty
3	White (Scandinavian, Mediterranean)	30-50	Quite reactive or sensitive +++	Burns moderately; tans moderately and uniformly
4	Beige or lightly tanned (Asian, Hispanic)	40-60	Moderately reactive ++	Burns minimally; tans easily and moderately
5	Moderate brown or tanned (Asian, Indian)	60-90	Minimally sensitive +	Rarely burns; tans profusely (dark brown)
6	Dark brown or black (Afro American, Australian Aboriginal)	90-150	Least sensitive 0. +	Never burns; tans profusely (deep brown or black)

The particular problems for a darker-skinned patient undergoing treatment for postacne scarring revolve around the probability of prolonged erythema and pigmentary change, and a higher risk of hypertrophic scarring. The patient needs to be made aware of this so that they can weigh up the benefits and risks, and prepare themselves for a prolonged postoperative recovery. Procedures such as dermal and subcutaneous autologous and nonautologous fillers and subcision carry no further risk, independent of photoreactive skin type. Some procedures, such as light skin peels, microdermabrasion, skin rolling and fractional resurfacing, carry minimally more risk. The procedures that require special explanations to the patient are the technique-dependent resurfacing procedures such as dermabrasion, laser skin resurfacing and medium and deep chemical peeling.

Gender

At the risk of generalizing and over-simplifying gender differences, it is true to say that acne-scarred males can be more problematic to treat than females. Males usually are not willing to use makeup; they have beard and body hair to contend with, making dressings difficult; and often they are less accepting of procedures with downtime and/or requiring multiple attendances.

Postoperative makeup is very important if one is considering treating the face in a regional or localized fashion with resurfacing procedures. However, sometimes the beard hair is an ally if one is leaving a demarcation line at the jaw line: simply allowing stubble growth will camouflage such a line well. If resurfacing with any modality (aside from fractional devices) is performed on a male, it should be full-facial to minimize embarrassment and maximize merging.

Postacne scars in beard hair areas may be superficial, with beard hair unaffected or deeper, in which case beard hair may be absent, requiring a surgical approach to that scar. A bald atrophic scarred area in the middle of an otherwise hair-bearing region may look very obvious, but leveling the scar and leaving it bald looks little better. Often there will be multifistulous sinus tracts distorting hair growth and further producing foreign body inflammation from the wayward growth of these hairs into the skin. Treatment options may include punch or wider elliptical excision, or occasionally hair-bearing punch grafts.

From my experience (and with notable exceptions), males may tend to struggle more than females through multiple painful treatments such as fractional resurfacing or therapies requiring staging of different treatments, partly because of the pain they experience and partly because of the patience required for an outcome. Be sure to adequately explain these factors to the patient before embarking on these types of management options.

Age

Age is not a major determinant of therapy, but a few points need to be stressed. The very young, such as teenagers, need to be guided towards the lowest risk, least invasive and least daunting procedures where possible. Before treating teenagers for acne scars it is important to have their acne under good control. Parents or guardians need to be brought into the management process. One must determine whether the patient has the decision-making maturity required and will be able to cope with the procedure and whatever complications may ensue.

Table 19.3 Graded severity or burden of disease of postacne scarring.

Grade	Characteristics
1) Macular disease	Erythematous, hyper- or hypopigmented flat marks visible to the patient or observer at any distance
2) Mild disease	Mild atrophy or hypertrophy that may not be obvious at social distances of 50 cm or greater and may be covered adequately by makeup, the normal shadow of shaved beard hair (in males) or normal body hair (if the scarring is extrafacial)
3) Moderate disease	Moderate atrophic or hypertrophic scarring that is obvious at social distances of 50 cm or greater and is not covered adequately by makeup, the normal shadow of shaved beard hair (in males) or normal body hair (if the scarring is extrafacial), but can still be flattened by manual stretching of the skin (if atrophic)
4) Severe disease	Severe atrophic or hypertrophic scarring that is obvious at social distances >50 cm, is not covered adequately by makeup, the normal shadow of shaved beard hair (in males) or normal body hair (if the scarring is extrafacial), and cannot be flattened by manual stretching of the skin

Middle age is a time that may require a different approach to just remedying acne scars. If the initial activity has been severe enough, middle age may see the ageing process catching up with the patient. The shrinking face of age and the tissue destruction as a result of cystic acne lead to a cascading effect of the skin. However, this effect is interrupted by the scarring that catches the tissues, producing an irregular 'hanging curtain' effect. Patients with this problem will need more than routine resurfacing procedures. They require all the skills of the treating dermatologist to implement therapy that involves some restructuring of the ageing face as well as treatment directed more specifically at the scarring.

Old age brings with it other potential issues, notably the health of the patient and questions about their motivations for seeking treatment at this stage of life. If these factors are not problematic, the elderly age of a patient should not be necessarily influence treatment.

BURDEN OR SEVERITY OF DISEASE

When seeing a patient with postacne scarring for the first time, it is most useful to determine both the severity of their disease (see Table 19.3) and the type of scarring present (see Tables 19.4a to 19.4d).

After determining the severity of disease, the first rule, I feel, is to give patients hope that their condition can be improved, but not to give false hope that their scars can be completely removed. Patients require treatment plans together with an understanding that their condition will take time and patience, and possibly multiple therapies, to settle.

OVERVIEW OF THE EVIDENCE FOR MANAGING POSTACNE SCARRING

Existing evidence

Postacne scarring is a reasonably common disease and the treatment of this condition should start well before the scars are evident. One of the few epidemiology studies on the prevalence of postacne scarring suggests that the type and extent of scarring

Table 19.4a Grade 1: Abnormally colored macular disease.

Definition	Examples of Scars	Treatment Plan
Erythematous, hyper- or hypopigmented flat marks visible to the patient or observer at any distance	Erythematous flat marks (Figure 19.5)	Time and optimized home care (retinoids, topical antiinflammatories), often supplemented by vascular lasers
	Hyperpigmented flat marks (postinflammatory marks) (Figure 19.4)	Optimized home care (bleaching, sun protection etc) and light strength peels +/- microdermabrasion
		Supplemented by pigment lesion lasers or intense pulsed light (IPL) only if required
	Hypopigmented macular scars (Figures 19.6 and 19.7)	Pigment transfer procedures (blister grafting, autologous cell transfer), maybe fractional resurfacing

Note: Safe treatment modalities for olive and dark-skinned patients.
Acceptable treatment modalities for olive and dark-skinned patients.
Relatively less safe treatment modalities.

Table 19.4b Grade 2: Mildly abnormally contoured disease.

Definition	Examples of Scars	Treatment Plan
Mild atrophy or hypertrophy that may not be obvious at social distances of 50 cm or greater and may be covered adequately by makeup, the normal shadow of shaved beard hair (in males) or normal body hair (if the scarring is extrafacial)	Mild, rolling, atrophic scars (Figures 19.10 and 19.11)	If localized: Consider combination of blood transfer, skin needling or rolling or microdermabrasion and/or superficial dermal fillers If generalized: Multiple treatments of nonablative lasers, fractional resurfacing often complemented by the localized treatment modalities either simultaneous or as follow-up treatments
	Small, soft, papular scars (Figure 19.12)	Fine wire diathermy (FWD); maybe fluorouracil injections if FWD unsuccessful

Note: Safe treatment modalities for olive and dark-skinned patients.
Acceptable treatment modalities for olive and dark-skinned patients.
Relatively less safe treatment modalities.

Table 19.4c Grade 3: Moderately abnormally contoured disease.

Grade 3	Examples of Scars	Treatment Plan
Moderate atrophic or hypertrophic scarring that is obvious at social distances of 50 cm or greater and is not covered adequately by makeup, the normal shadow of shaved beard hair (in males) or normal body hair (if the scarring is extrafacial), but can still be flattened by manual stretching of the skin (if atrophic)	ablative lasers or dermabrasion	If generalized: Medical skin rolling or fractionated resurfacing If these are unavailable, consider ablative lasers or dermabrasion or plasma skin resurfacing If localized: Dermal fillers or subcision Intralesional corticosteroids and/or fluorouracil and/or vascular laser; combine with silicon sheeting
	Mild to moderate hypertrophic or papular scars (Figure 19.15)	

Note: Safe treatment modalities for olive and dark-skinned patients.
Acceptable treatment modalities for olive and dark-skinned patients.
Relatively less safe treatment modalities.

Table 19.4d Grade 4: Severely abnormally contoured disease.

Definition	Examples of Scars	Treatment Plan
Severe atrophic or hypertrophic scarring that is obvious at social distances >50 cm, is not covered adequately by makeup, the normal shadow of shaved beard hair (in males) or normal body hair (if the scarring is extrafacial), and cannot be flattened by manual stretching of the skin	Punched out atrophic (deep 'boxcar') and 'ice pick' scars (Figures 19.16, 19.17 and 19.18)	If numerous, deep and small, consider focal trichloroacetic acid (CROSS technique), maybe combined with fractional resurfacing If fewer and broader but still <4 mm in diameter consider punch techniques (float, excision grafting), with or without subsequent fractional resurfacing or ablative resurfacing techniques
	Bridges and tunnels, dystrophic scars (Figure 19.1a–d)	Excision
	Marked atrophic scars (Figures 19.3, 19.19 and 19.20)	Fat transfer, stimulatory fillers such as PLA, hydroxyapatite, silicon (if fat transfer is not feasible), occasionally rhytidectomy if acquired cutis laxa
	Significant hypertrophic or keloid scars (Figure 19.21)	Intralesional corticosteroids steroids or fluorouracil and / or vascular laser

Note: Safe treatment modalities for olive and dark-skinned patients.
Acceptable treatment modalities for olive and dark-skinned patients.
Relatively less safe treatment modalities.

was in part correlated with the site of the acne, the acne severity and the time that had elapsed before adequate treatment. Facial scarring affected both sexes equally and occurred in 95% of cases. A delay up to three years between acne onset and adequate treatment related to the ultimate degree of scarring.(3) As with many procedure-based topics in dermatology, there are not many clinical trials either on acne scarring generally or on acne scarring across different skin groups.

There is a body of peer-reviewed data on acne scarring and a smaller amount that more specifically discusses different skin groups and their respective problems. The intersection between these two topics is less well covered; however, it is probably the quality rather than the quantity that is at issue.

Critical reviews and meta-analysis studies are generally lacking in the acne scarring literature.

No truly randomized prospective comparative (level A) studies exist. Studies tend to lack validity due to flawed design (for example, having no severity data, no emphasis on intention to treat, uncertainty about blinding observers/patients or inadequate power).

Some articles are prospective and some retrospective, but they are usually descriptive case reports and case series; (4, 5) that is,

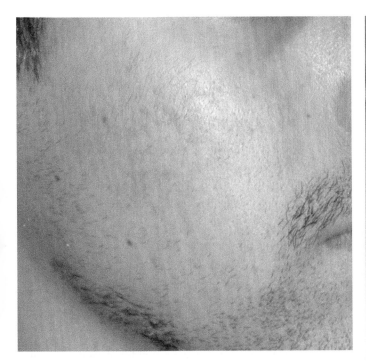

Figure 19.10 Patient with grade 2 subtle and focal atrophic postacne scarring on the mid-right cheek.

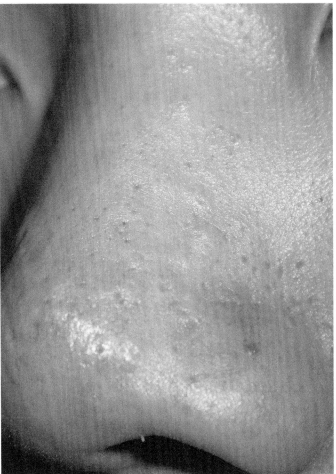

Figure 19.12 Patient with mild papular (grade 2) nasal acne scars.

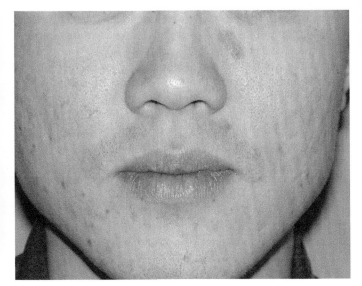

Figure 19.11 Patient with generalized mildly atrophic (grade 2) postacne scarring.

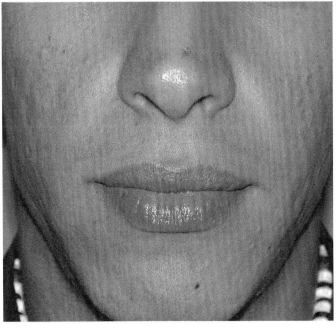

Figure 19.13 Fitzpatrick skin type 4 patient with grade 3 moderate atrophic acne scarring.

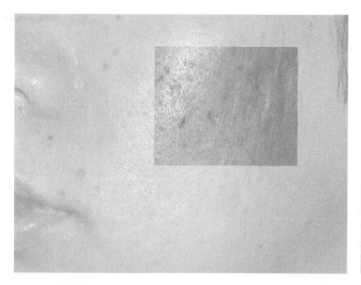

Figure 19.14 Patient with focal (outlined) grade 3 moderate atrophic acne scarring.

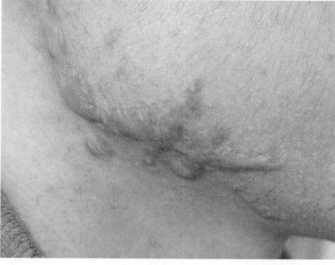

Figure 19.15 Patient with grade 3 moderate to severe right jaw line hypertrophic scar.

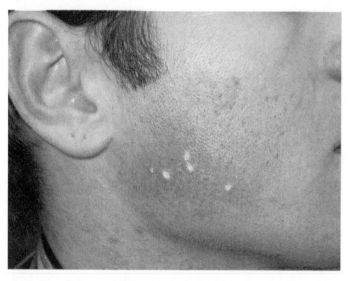

Figure 19.16 Focal trichloroacetic acid to ice pick scars are close to 100% concentration.

descriptions of procedures without formal studies conducted (level C evidence). Most studies on postacne scarring have been uncontrolled, nonblinded and not randomized even if prospective.

Some limited comparative studies have been described for lasers and acne scarring (level B).

OBSTACLES TO OBTAINING EVIDENCE

The difficulties in evaluating acne scarring are manifold.

There is no simple clinically reproducible method for evaluating the volume of deficiency or excess of a single acne scar or an acne scarred area.

Techniques to measure specific lesion volume, such as silicon profilometry or three-dimensional photography, confocal microscopy or cutaneous ultrasound, are outside the abilities of usual practice. Some techniques cannot measure more than limited areas, with some difficulty in reproducibility. Others are cumbersome, difficult to use, impractical or too expensive.

Photography has often been a poor measure with respect to uniformity of the normal camera variables of using the same camera, same settings, same backdrop, same lighting, same patient angle distance and same magnification. Even if these parameters are standardized, photography, which is inherently a two-dimensional technique, presents difficulties for estimating the volume of scarring, which is a three-dimensional issue. Turning the patient's profile ever so slightly between one photograph and the next will completely alter the ability of the observer, no matter how blinded the study, to determine improvement.

Often studies resort to analyzing patients over time to try to estimate a percentage of subjective or objective improvement. Baseline and posttreatment ('before and after') photographs may be compared subjectively or objectively, or patients may be asked to estimate their improvement percentage. Often a relatively simple grading system is used, such as a scale of no improvement (0%), mild improvement (25%), moderate improvement (50%), excellent improvement (75%) and complete eradication (100%). What this improvement percentage refers to is often ill-defined; 'improvement' might mean to the depth of scars, the number of scars, changes in scar type or global cosmetic improvement.

Patient satisfaction rating is another scale used. It has been arguably as accurate as and perhaps more important than any objective method utilized, yet it is open to many biases, making it a less than desirable benchmark.

Long-term follow-up studies are required on many of the ablative technologies to determine long-term efficacy and complications such as hypopigmentation; these studies are largely missing from the literature.

Adequate classifications exist for acne morphology and severity, but unfortunately there is no agreed classification for the morphology or severity of postacne scarring. Limited inroads have occurred over recent years, with various attempts made at describing different scar types. However, the lack of consensus in morphological description remains concerning, as it interferes with one's ability to compare articles discussing scar type and response to therapy.

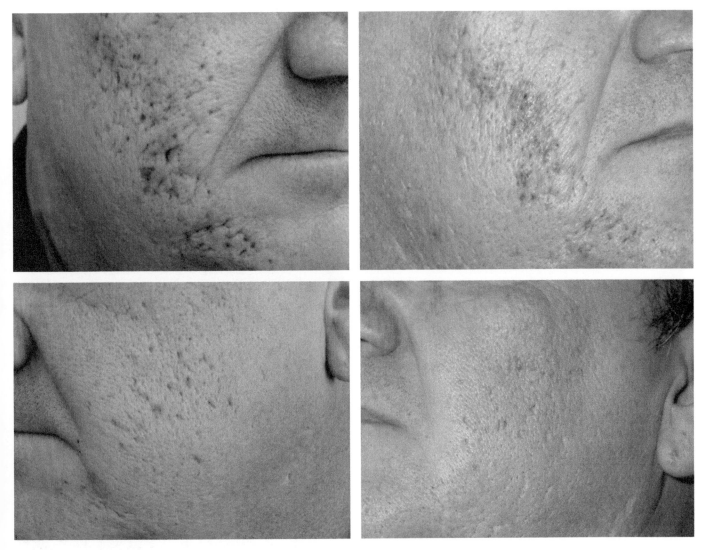

Figure 19.17 Patient with Fitzpatrick skin type 4 showing improvement in severe (grade 4) ice pick and dystrophic scarring with fractional resurfacing.

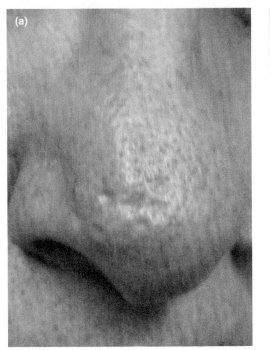

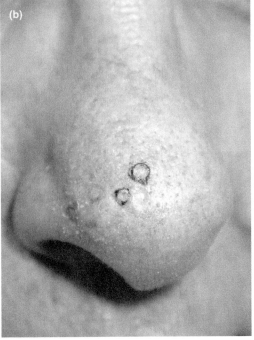

Figure 19.18 Patient with grade 4 atrophic scarring before and one week after punch float technique to the nose.

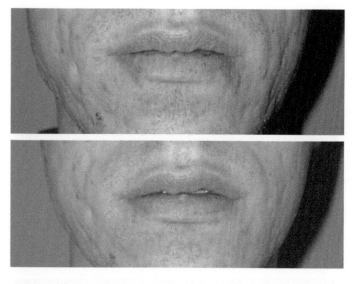

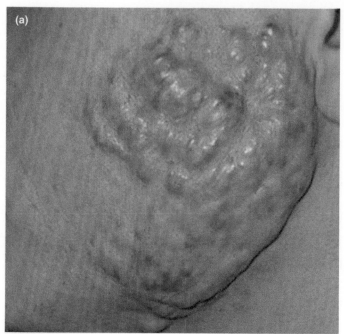

Figure 19.19 Patient with grade 3 atrophic scarring before and after two treatments of polylactic acid injections.

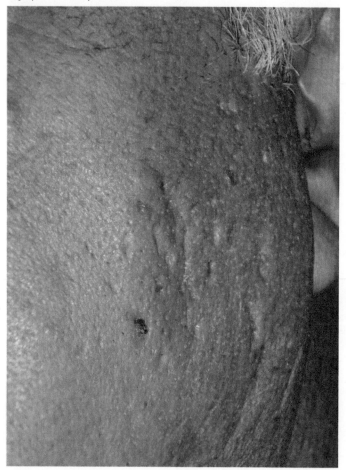

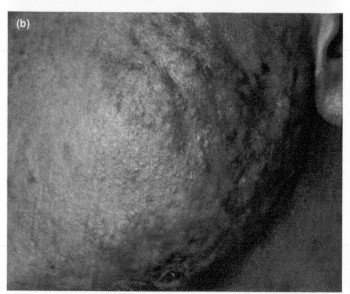

Figure 19.21 Patient with very severe (grade 4) keloidal postacne scarring on the left jaw line (A) before and (B) after multiple fluorouracil treatments.

Figure 19.20 Fitzpatrick skin type 5 patient with grade 4 punched out atrophic postacne scars.

Even less defined is any attempt in the literature to define the burden of disease of postacne scarring. There has been no agreed objective quantitative or qualitative scoring system of global severity to allow discussion and comparison of patients and their response to therapy (or that of a cohort) and for the purposes of further comparative studies.

Without adequate classification and measure of disease it is hard to perceive how we may compare different patients, their response to treatments and studies performed by different practitioners or investigating units.

Evidence on ablative and fractionated resurfacing technologies for various acne-scarring groups

Laser skin resurfacing

Despite the above general comments, there has been an excellent systematic review of the treatment of postacne scarring by laser resurfacing (see Figures 19.3 and 19.22).(6) In this analysis the authors identified no controlled studies and only 16 case series illustrating the effects of CO_2, (7–19) erbium YAG lasers (20, 21) or a combination of CO_2 and erbium lasers (22) for the treatment

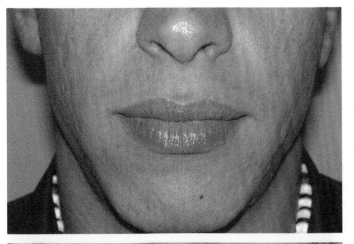

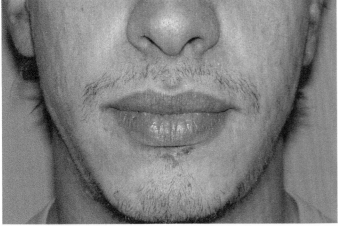

Figure 19.22 Thin-type 4 patient before and three weeks after CO_2 and erbium laser resurfacing, showing typical delayed resurrection of pigmentation.

of postacne scarring patients. The authors could find no studies of reasonable quality. In terms of temporary morbidity, they did find that pigmentation as a side-effect was common, being evident, even transiently, in up to 44% of patients. The duration of pigmentary change was said to range between one and six months with CO_2 laser and two to three weeks with erbium laser. The length and erythema in the 14 studies averaged out for CO_2 laser at six to 16 weeks and for erbium laser at one to three months. The mean improvement in scarring varied between 25 and 81% for the CO_2 laser and between 50 and 70% for the erbium YAG laser. Measurements of improvement will usually photography with disparate attempts at blinding observers.

Two of these studies, (13, 18) and one subsequently, (5) have discussed the use of ablative lasers in dark-colored skin. In one of these studies, (18) 36 patients with skin types 2 through 5 underwent resurfacing with CO_2 laser and were followed up for six months. Although nine patients developed hyperpigmentation, this had completely settled by the three-month postoperative visit. Two patients developed focal erythema, but no scarring developed. Although this was termed a prospective study, the improvement was graded by the patients at the six-month follow-up visit.

Another study of 25 patients of Asian and Hispanic background included patients treated primarily for acne scarring.(13) Again, hyperpigmentation maximal at six weeks and present in some patients for three to four months appear to be the main

postoperative concerns. The authors stated that acne scar treatment with the lasers appeared less effective than that for rhytides and improvement appeared to average out at about 25%.

In a third small study (5) of 16 patients (13 of whom had acne scarring) of predominantly skin types 3 and 4, erythema was present in all patients but gradually faded over 6 months. Pigmentation was present at three months in 33% of patients. At six months, one patient had residual pigmentation. Only one patient developed mild minimal hypopigmentation at six months, which cleared by 12 months. Another patient developed hypopigmentation at 12 months.

Dermabrasion
Although a number of authors have suggested that dermabrasion is less likely to cause pigmentary sequelae, (23, 24) I could find no actual prospective or retrospective studies or case series to illustrate effect of dermabrasion on darker-colored skin. Since it was suggested that the cold injury caused by cryoanesthesia was partly at issue in causing pigmentary abnormalities, a case series considering sequential patients utilizing tumescent anesthesia were presented in an attempt to limit this injury (Figure 19.23).(25) There were experiential reports from experienced physicians suggesting that morbidity associated with dermabrasion is predictable in all skin types.(26, 27)

Chemical peeling
A number of case series have been presented on the use of medium and deep chemical peeling in the treatment of postacne scarring. (28, 29) Again, a portion of patients develop postinflammatory hyperpigmentation following treatment with this technique, which seems to settle in most patients over the first 3 months postoperatively. One paper utilizing a modified phenol peel on 46 Asian patients (28) (11 of whom had acne scarring as their prime indication) suggested that this treatment was effective, with seven of these patients improving by 51% or more. Over 74% of all patients developed postinflammatory hyperpigmentation. In 11% of patients, postoperative erythema lasted longer than three months and there was also one case each of scar formation and long-term hypopigmentation.

Another paper utilizing a medium strength trichloroacetic acid peel in 15 dark skinned patients with acne scarring showed improvement in all but one patient and moderate or marked improvement in nine of the patients.(29) Seventy-three percent of the patients suffered from transient hyperpigmentation. The authors concluded that the peel is a safe and effective modality for the treatment of postacne scarring in dark-skinned patients.

A variation of chemical peeling involving the use of 60 to 100% trichloroacetic acid (30, 31) (termed the CROSS technique, Figure 19.16) has excited interest of in the treatment of smaller 'ice pick' and poral type scars which have always been difficult to treat. Basically, this modality scars the inside of the cylindrical scar, making it cosmetically more appealing. A similar concept has been discussed with the use of high-energy CO_2 laser.(32) A very well-conducted study of 65 patients initially used to describe this technique (31) divided patients into two treatment groups of 65% and close to 100% trichloroacetic acid in dark-skinned patients of skin types 4 to 6. The study showed no significant incidence of complications.

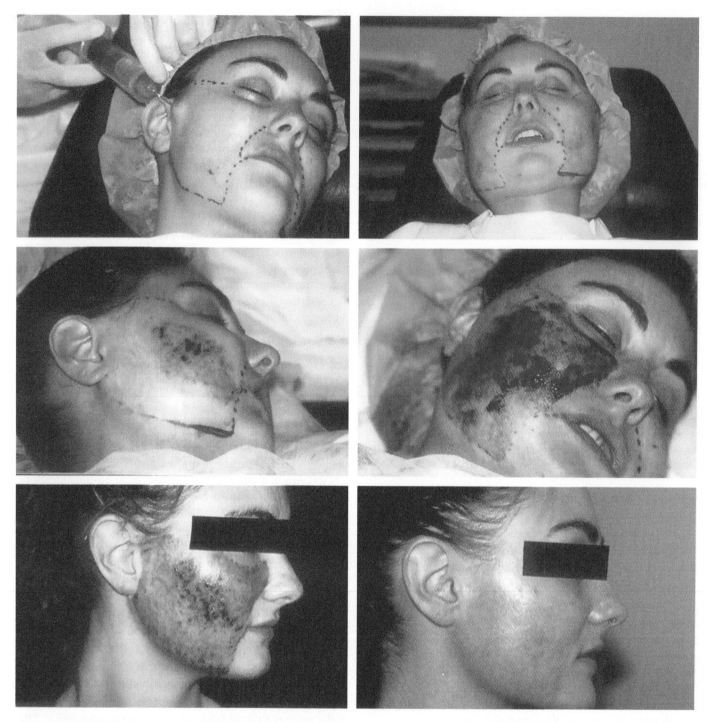

Figure 19.23 Patient undergoing tumescent dermabrasion illustrating infiltration, procedure, day one and day five postoperative appearance.

Plasma skin resurfacing

At the time of writing, there is no manuscript in the literature on this new method of resurfacing in regard to acne scarring. This technology utilizes a plasma cloud of electrons originating from nitrogen atoms and radiofrequency stimulation of these atoms. It appears to have utility for postacne scarring, and we can expect to see such use in the literature in the near future. Anecdotally, it appears that postinflammatory hyperpigmentation in darker-skinned patents may be a feature of this technology.

Fractional resurfacing

A recently introduced laser technology employing the concept of 'fractionated photothermolysis' produces small vertical zones of full-thickness thermal damage from a mid-infrared laser (Figures 19.17 and 19.24).(33) This is akin to sinking posts or drilling holes of thermal damage, with areas surrounding these posts left free of damage. This is a method of ablative resurfacing without the patient having to experience a pronounced healing phase.

There have been a number of recent studies suggesting its efficacy in postacne scarring. One important recent study on treatment of Asian skin (34) showed that increased densities of the small vertical zones of damage cause more swelling, redness and hyperpigmentation compared to higher fluences or energy of these zones. Patient satisfaction was higher when treated with higher fluences but not higher densities.

An excellent prospective case series of 53 patients (35) with atrophic acne scarring using blinded observers showed 51 to 75% improvement in 90% of patients. Adverse events included no incidence of dyspigmentation or scarring. Importantly, clinical response rates were independent of age, gender and Fitzpatrick skin type.

A number of smaller studies and case reports looking at acne scarring, hypopigmented and postsurgical scarring (36–38) have also suggested satisfactory outcomes.

This technology may allow treatment of extra-facial scarring, which has not been accessible with other resurfacing technologies. It would appear that other fractionated wavelengths may be useful, especially CO_2 laser (10 600 nm) and erbium laser (2934 nm) (Figure 19.24). We may anticipate that other fractionated wavelengths (such as 532 nm) may have efficacy in the treatment of other aspects of scarring, such as the red or brown coloring seen in more recent scars. However, literature is lacking at the present time to confirm these possibilities.

EVIDENCE ON NONABLATIVE TECHNOLOGIES FOR ATROPHIC ACNE SCARRING

Manual skin needling or rolling

A concept not dissimilar to fractionated resurfacing, manual needling or skin rolling may be used when expensive machinery is not available. In its simplest form one may employ a 30-gauge needle, introduced into the skin to a controlled depth with the aid of a small artery forceps held at about 2 to 3 mm from the tip, to stab the skin repeatedly, but this is only appropriate for small areas of scarring. For larger areas, a tattoo gun without pigment may be used or a needle studded rolling pin (39) may be rolled over the face or extra-facial area. The dermal trauma heals with collagen remodeling, and this is responsible for any improvement in atrophic scarring (Figure 19.25). Needling or rolling can be readily added to other procedures such as dermal augmentation or fat transfer.

ADEQUATE STUDIES INTO THIS TECHNOLOGY ARE ENTIRELY LACKING AT THIS POINT IN TIME

Nonablative resurfacing

Nonablative lasers appear to have a role in the treatment of minor atrophic acne scarring. This topic seems to have been studied more methodically than treatment with ablative lasers. Although prospectively based case series still dominate the literature, there seems to be more thought put into the outcome measurements. Some true comparative studies between laser systems have been performed (40) and different conditions utilizing the same laser system have also been compared. (41, 42) The major lasers for this purpose have been the mid-infrared lasers at wavelengths of 1320 nm, 1450 nm and 1540 nm, appropriately cooled to protect

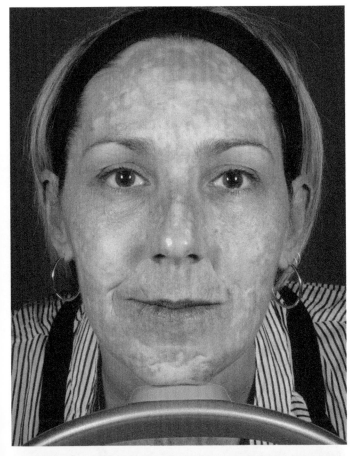
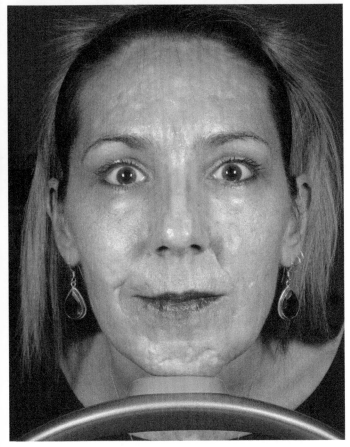

Figure 19.24 Fractional resurfacing illustrating blue tracking optical guide.

165

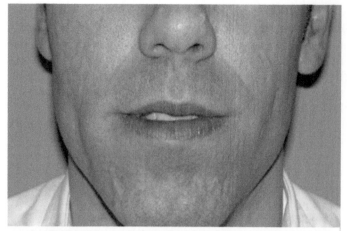
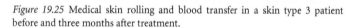
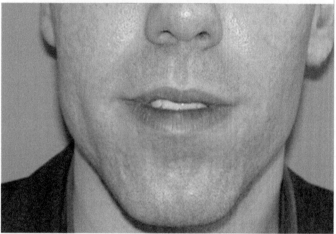

Figure 19.25 Medical skin rolling and blood transfer in a skin type 3 patient before and three months after treatment.

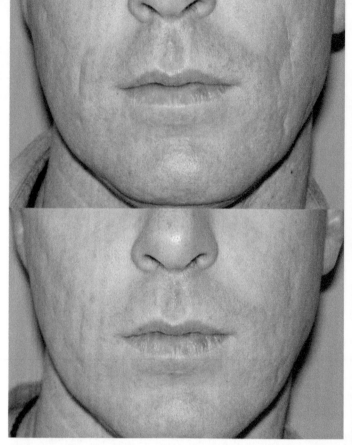

Figure 19.26 Patient before and three weeks after combined treatment with blood transfer, fat transfer and subcision.

the epidermis whilst targeting dermal water.(40–45) These lasers use conducted heat from the chromophore to produce a diffuse dermal injury, heating to above 50 degrees Celsius and inducing collagen remodeling. Repeated treatments are required and longevity of the result is still largely unknown.

This technology seems safe when it has been studied in Asian skin (41, 45) although postinflammatory hyperpigmentation can be seen if blistering occurs. There appears to have been a reasonable level of patient satisfaction and perception of efficacy, (42) but objectively and on the basis of histology there may be somewhat less efficacy.(41)

EVIDENCE ON AUGMENTATION AND SIMILAR PROCEDURES FOR ATROPHIC POSTACNE SCARRING

Autologous blood transfer

Amongst autologous agents blood transfer is a possible option for patients with milder atrophic acne scarring. It relies on stimulation of the implanted chromophore (autologous blood) by relatively low-level vascular laser or intense pulsed light. Blood is injected immediately after drawing by simple injection with a 1 ml syringe and attached 30-gauge needle high up in the dermis, distending the scar and giving a bleb with a bruised appearance. This bruise is then targeted as any blood vessel would

be, but with approximately 50 to 75% of the usual fluence. A single case series suggested that treatment may be repeated at monthly intervals until adequate correction is attained.(46) This treatment is most often performed in combination with other procedures such as fat transfer and subcision of deeper scars (Figure 19.26).

Fat transfer

For grossly atrophic disease with destruction of the deeper tissues, fat remains the optimal replacement agent (Figures 19.3 and 19.26). Fat is an excellent deeper augmentation material. It is cheap, readily available, and will not be rejected nor induce allergic reactions. It is easy to work with and is without risk of communicable disease. The issue of permanence has gradually been resolved (47) and it is just as effective and safe in any skin coloring. However, despite some anecdotal reports of its efficacy, (48, 49) at this time there are no adequate studies to illustrate its efficacy in postacne scarring.

Subcision

Subcision of scars appears to work by breaking up the attachments of atrophic acne scars, releasing the surface from the deeper structures. Successive treatments appear to produce further improvement. (50, 51) The technique usually involves the insertion of a sharp hypodermic needle. The depth of the probe insertion depends on the type of scar being treated, with intradermal insertion for small superficial scars, but deeper dermal undermining for more severely bound down scars. It has become a first-line treatment for many isolated moderately bound down atrophic scars. This is despite a lack of controlled studies. One interesting split-face designed study utilizing subcision on one side alone compared to a nonablative laser combined with subcision on the other side was used to show the relative efficacy of the combined side, (52) suggesting a synergistic effect between these two modalities.

Dermal grafting

Dermal grafting may be used for recent deep focal or linear scars. (53–55) Aside from some case series, there have been no controlled studies or comparative studies reported in the literature. This technique is somewhat limited by cyst formation and the requirement for a donor site to be prepared by either dermabrasion or laser skin resurfacing and the dermis harvested.

Punch techniques

Punch techniques such as punch excision, (56) grafting (57) and elevation or float techniques (58) have been useful and probably remain the golden standard for punched out scars up to approximately 3 to 4 mm in width (deep 'boxcar' and larger 'ice pick' scars). These techniques are all old ones and have not been studied with any scientific rigor (Figure 19.18).

Nonautologous tissue augmentation

For patients with few atrophic scars, there is now quite an array of injectable fillers, including human collagen and hyaluronic acid amongst the short-term agents, and many agents of a longer term nature, including the reintroduction of silicon and variations of polyacrylamides for longer correction. However, there are no controlled trials on use of these to treat acne scarring. A very elegant prospective, double-blinded, randomized, placebo-controlled study of 145 evaluated patients treated with autologous cultured fibroblasts in a phase three clinical trial showed particularly good results in the 50 patients treated for acne scarring. The response rate at six months was 48.4% compared to 7.7% for placebo.(59) Unfortunately, it would appear that this type of product is no longer available.

Evidence on cytotoxic and vascular laser therapy for hypertrophic postacne scarring

Cytotoxics

Traditionally, high-strength corticosteroids have been used for the intralesional drugs of choice in the treatment of hypertrophic and keloidal acne scars. However, there has been recent interest in the intralesional use of the cytotoxics fluorouracil (60–62), bleomycin (63, 64) and mitomycin (65, 66) as treatments for hypertrophic and keloidal scars. Fluorouracil is usually utilized at a concentration of 50mg/ml and has been mixed 80:20 with low-strength intralesional steroid (Figure 19.18). It may also be used alone.(67) Usually about 1 ml is utilized in each session and often 0.1 to 0.3 ml is all that is required for an individual scar. Recently, the molecular basis of the action of fluorouracil (5-FU) has been elucidated.(68) 5-FU appears to be a potent inhibitor of TGF-beta/SMAD signalling, capable of blocking TGF-beta-induced, SMAD-driven up-regulation of COL1A2 gene expression in a JNK-dependent manner.

Vascular lasers

In 1995, it was reported that flashlamp-pumped pulsed dye tunable laser was useful in the treatment of keloid sternotomy scars, with improvement in scar height, skin texture, erythema and pruritus in the laser-treated scars.(69) This initial work has been borne out by more recent studies.(70, 71)

A procedural guide for the perplexed

There is a continuing battle to balance the safety of the patient and the efficacy of the procedure in many cases of postacne scarring. There are no methods capable of totally removing acne scarring; every treatment is a compromise. Hence, it behooves the physician to do a number of things when addressing the problem of postacne scarring.

Manufacture a set of realistic expectations for the patient. It is vital that the patient realizes the impossibility of completely removing the scars.

Listen to the patient. Try to understand the relative importance of a temporary but useful and maybe very accurate result, produced by such agents as temporary fillers, compared to a more permanent but perhaps less accurate result using procedures such as excision or punch techniques. Understand the limitations of the patient's budget, intellect, social circumstances, work requirements (including the ability to stay out of the sun during any required healing phase) and capacity for accepting complications if they were to occur. Even predictable morbidity can be difficult for a patient who is not anticipating it, and often (even when information is given in both written and verbal forms) patients underestimate the postoperative phase of even relatively mild procedures.

Educate the patient about the nature of acne scarring, the apparent 'memory' of the skin for the position and severity of scarring, and its seeming reluctance to alter with therapy. Point out that this skin memory is most apparent with techniques that rely upon 'collagen remodeling', a group of techniques that includes almost all active skincare, space surface treatments

Table 19.5a Methods of scar improvement not relying on collagen remodeling – excisional and filler technologies.

	Morbidity	Longevity of Result	Relative Cost	Efficacy	General Safety	Safety for Darker Skin
Temporary dermal augmentation	+	+	++	+++	+++	+++
Fat transfer	+	+++	++	+++	+++	+++
Semipermanent/ permanent filler	+	++/+++	++/+++	+++	+	+
Excision of scar, including punch techniques	++	+++	+	+++	++	++

Table 19.5b Scar revision techniques reliant on resurfacing or similar technologies of collagen remodeling.

	Morbidity	Longevity of Result	Relative Cost	Efficacy	General Safety	Safety for Darker Skin
Dermabrasion	+++	+++		++	++	+
Deep and medium chemical peeling	+++	++/+++	++	++	+/++	+
Laser skin resurfacing	+++	++/+++	++/+++	++	++	+
Fractionated resurfacing	+	?+++	+++	+++	+++	?+++

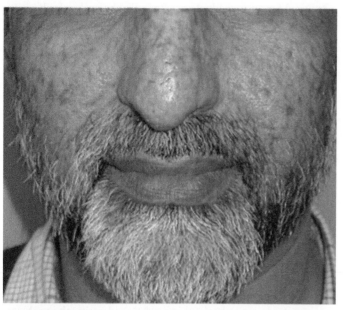

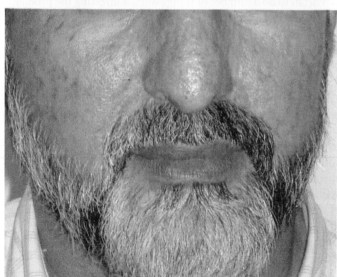

Figure 19.27 Patient with small pox scarring before and after laser skin resurfacing and multiple fractional resurfacings.

such as microdermabrasion and light skin peels, and nonablative and ablative resurfacing techniques. The patient needs to be aware that the possibility of incomplete results and the requirement for multiple treatments and ongoing therapies categories this group of techniques and processes. Some patients will desire a single therapeutic intervention to 'fix' their problem, and often this is unachievable for a condition such as acne scarring. Instead the patient should be educated to accept a number of therapeutic interventions to achieve optimal results. A carefully mapped-out plan of action is required for most patients, with an understanding that a 'one size fits all' model is not satisfactory for most cases. This requirement for ongoing treatment increases with the complexity of the scar types and the disease burden of the patient.

It is particularly relevant for this chapter to note that the most efficacious procedure may not be practical or may be too likely to produce unsatisfactory complications or excess morbidity. This procedure may therefore have to be passed over in favor of a less effective treatment with a lower level of risk.

It is also important for the physician to realize his or her own limitations. If the patient's condition requires expertise in an operation that is outside the physician's capability or requires equipment that the physician cannot access, the physician should refer the patient to a more appropriate clinic.

Tables 19.5a and 19.5b give comparisons of different techniques according to the practical parameters of cost, longevity, efficacy and safety which the patient should appreciate before embarking on treatment.

DIRECTIONS FOR THE FUTURE AND CONCLUSIONS

The treatment of acne scarring is evolving in a way that is comforting to both the patient and the practitioner, becoming safer for a wide range of skin types. As useful as they have been, ablative technologies are on the wane due to a relative intolerance to the twin 'evils' of downtime and adverse events. For a short while, attempts to replace these technologies resulted in treatments whose results may have obeyed Hippocrates' first rule, but gave no meaningful improvement to the patient. The advents of manual skin rolling, focal TCA peeling and then fractional resurfacing have been major advances but one should not forget very useful techniques from the past such as punch techniques, excisional surgery, and subcision.

Mildly ablative resurfacing is making a comeback in the form of plasma skin resurfacing and mid range erbium laser resurfacing. These ablative technologies are trying to occupy the 'halfway house' between downtime and complications on one hand and efficacy on the other. They offer more rapid healing and more limited morbidity and may have a place in the future.

Fractional resurfacing without doubt seems to be the most useful new technology, and new fractional wavelengths will be added over the coming years. We will probably see a convergence between these technologies pushing the boundaries of patient tolerance and efficacy. This type of treatment has also added an ability to treat unusual forms of scarring using knowledge gleaned from the experience of treating postacne scarring Figure 19.27).

Dermal augmentation and our understanding of what can be achieved with it is now increasing exponentially and we can envisage safer, longer term and more elegant materials and techniques to work with in the future for the correction of focal atrophic acne scarring disease.

The treatment of hyperplastic postacne scarring continues to be disappointing and we await an improved understanding of its pathogenesis. Some improvements have been made in this treatment (such as new cytotoxic therapies) but we still have a long way to go.

The future always looks brighter than the past, and this is certainly true when one looks at this hitherto very difficult disease of postacne scarring, especially its treatment in the wide range of skin types encountered by the practitioner.

REFERENCES

1. Fitzpatrick TB. The validity and practicality of sun-reactive skin types I through VI. Arch Dermatol 1988; 124: 869–71.
2. Grimes PE, Hunt SG. Considerations for cosmetic surgery in the black population. Clin Plast Surg 1993; 20: 27–34.
3. Layton AM, Henderson CA, Cunliffe WJ. A clinical evaluation of acne scarring and its incidence. Clin Exp Dermatol 1994; 19: 303–8.
4. Chua SH, Ang P, Khoo LS, Goh CL. Nonablative 1450-nm diode laser in the treatment of facial atrophic acne scars in type IV to V Asian skin: a prospective clinical study. Dermatol Surg 2004; 30: 1287–91.
5. Goh CL, Khoo L. Laser skin resurfacing treatment outcome of facial scars and wrinkles in Asians with skin type III/IV with the Unipulse CO_2 laser system. Singapore Med J 2002; 43(1): 28–32.
6. Jordan R, Cummins C, Burls A. Laser resurfacing of the skin for the improvement of facial acne scarring: a systematic review of the evidence. Br J Dermatol 2000; 142: 413–23.
7. Bernstein LJ, Kauvar AN, Grossman MC, Geronemus RG. The short- and long-term side effects of carbon dioxide laser resurfacing. Dermatol Surg 1997; 23: 519–25.
8. Alster TS, West TB. Resurfacing of atrophic facial acne scars with a high-energy, pulsed carbon dioxide laser. Dermatol Surg 1996; 22: 151–5.
9. Apfelberg DB. Ultrapulse carbon dioxide laser with CPG scanner for full-face resurfacing for rhytids, photoaging, and acne scars. Plast Reconstr Surg 1997; 99: 1817–25.
10. Apfelberg DB. A critical appraisal of high-energy pulsed carbon dioxide laser facial resurfacing for acne scars. Ann Plast Surg 1997; 38: 95–100.
11. Apfelberg DB. The Ultrapulse carbon dioxide laser with computer pattern generator automatic scanner for facial cosmetic surgery and resurfacing. Ann Plast Surg 1996; 36: 522–9.
12. Bernstein LJ, Kauvar AN, Grossman MC, Geronemus RG. Scar resurfacing with high-energy, short-pulsed and flashscanning carbon dioxide lasers. Dermatol Surg 1998; 24: 101.
13. Ho C, Nguyen Q, Lowe NJ, Griffin ME, Lask G. Laser resurfacing in pigmented skin, Dermatol Surg 1995; 21: 1035–7.
14. Rubach BW, Schoenrock LD. Histological and clinical evaluation of facial resurfacing using a carbon dioxide laser with the computer pattern generator. Arch Otolaryngol Head Neck Surg 1997; 123: 929–34.
15. Shim E, West TB, Velazquez E et al. Short-pulse carbon dioxide laser resurfacing in the treatment of rhytides and scars: a clinical and histopathological study. Dermatol Surg 1998; 24: 113–7.
16. David LM, Sarne AJ, Unger WP. Rapid laser scanning for facial resurfacing. Dermatol Surg 1995; 21: 1031–3.
17. Garrett AB, Dufresne RGJ, Ratz JL, Berlin AJ. Carbon dioxide laser treatment of pitted acne scarring. J Dermatol Surg Oncol 1990; 16: 737–40.
18. Ruiz-Esparza J, Barba GJ, Gomez de la Torre OL, Huerta FB, Parga VE. UltraPulse laser skin resurfacing in Hispanic patients. A prospective study of 36 individuals. Dermatol Surg 1998; 24: 59–62.
19. Ting JC. 'Carbon dioxide laser treatment of facial scars', in ISCLS Abstracts. American Society for Dermatologic Surgery, 1998: 118.
20. Kye YC. Resurfacing of pitted facial scars with a pulsed Er:YAG laser. Dermatol Surg 1997; 23: 880–3.
21. Drnovsek-Olup B, Vedlin B. Use of Er:YAG laser for benign skin disorders. Lasers Surg Med 1997; 21: 13–9.
22. Weinstein C. Computerized scanning erbium:YAG laser for skin resurfacing. Dermatol Surg 1998; 24: 83–9.
23. Jackson BA. Lasers in ethnic skin: a review. J Am Acad Dermatol 2003; 48(6 Suppl): S134–8.
24. Harmon CB, Mandy SH. Dermabrasion. In: K Nouri, S Leal-Khouri, eds. Techniques in Dermatologic Surgery. Mosby: New York, 2003.
25. Goodman GJ. Dermabrasion using tumescent anaesthesia. J Dermatol Surg Oncol 1994; 20: 802–7.
26. Pierce HE. Cosmetic surgery of black skin. Derm Clin 1988; 6: 377–85.
27. Yarborough JM. Dermabrasive surgery: state of the art. Clin Dematol 1987; 4: 75–80.
28. Park JH, Choi YD, Kim SW, Kim YC, Park SW. Effectiveness of modified phenol peel (Exoderm) on facial wrinkles, acne scars and other skin problems of Asian patients. J Dermatol 2007; 34: 17–24.
29. Al-Waiz MM, Al-Sharqi AI. Medium-depth chemical peels in the treatment of acne scars in dark-skinned individuals. Dermatol Surg 2002; 28: 383–7.
30. Yug A, Lane JE, Howard MS, Kent DE. Histologic study of depressed acne scars treated with serial high-concentration (95%) trichloroacetic acid. Dermatol Surg 2006; 32: 985–90.
31. Lee JB, Chung WG, Kwahck H, Lee KH. Focal treatment of acne scars with trichloroacetic acid: chemical reconstruction of skin scars method. Dermatol Surg 2002; 28: 1017–21.
32. Koo SH, Yoon ES, Ahn DS, Park SH. Laser punch-out for acne scars. Aesthetic Plast Surg 2001; 25: 46–51.
33. Manstein D, Herron GS, Sink RK, Tanner H, Anderson RR. Fractional photothermolysis: a new concept for cutaneous remodeling using microscopic patterns of thermal injury. Lasers Surg Med 2004; 34: 426–38.
34. Kono T, Chan HH, Groff WF et al. Prospective direct comparison study of fractional resurfacing using different fluences and densities for skin rejuvenation in Asians. Lasers Surg Med 2007; 39: 311–4.
35. Alster TS, Tanzi EL, Lazarus M. The use of fractional laser photothermolysis for the treatment of atrophic scars. Dermatol Surg 2007; 33: 295–99.
36. Hasegawa T, Matsukura T, Mizuno Y et al. Clinical trial of a laser device called fractional photothermolysis system for acne scars. J Dermatol 2006; 33: 623–7.
37. Glaich AS, Rahman Z, Goldberg LH, Friedman PM. Fractional resurfacing for the treatment of hypopigmented scars: a pilot study. Dermatol Surg 2007; 33: 289–94.
38. Behroozan DS, Goldberg LH, Dai T, Geronemus RG, Friedman PM. Fractional photothermolysis for the treatment of surgical scars: a case report. J Cosmet Laser Ther 2006; 8: 35–8.
39. Fernandes D. Skin needling as an alternative to laser. Paper delivered at IPRAS, San Francisco; 1999.
40. Tanzi EL, Alster TS. Comparison of a 1450-nm diode laser and a 1320-nm Nd:YAG laser in the treatment of atrophic facial scars: a prospective clinical and histologic study. Dermatol Surg 2004; 30: 152–7.
41. Chan HH, Lam LK, Wong DS, Kono T, Trendell-Smith N. Use of 1320 nm Nd:YAG laser for wrinkle reduction and the treatment of atrophic acne scarring in Asians. Lasers Surg Med 2004; 34: 98–103.
42. Bhatia AC, Dover JS, Arndt KA, Stewart B, Alam M. Patient satisfaction and reported long-term therapeutic efficacy associated with 1320 nm Nd:YAG laser treatment of acne scarring and photoaging. Dermatol Surg 2006; 32: 346–52.
43. Kim KH, Geronemus RG. Nonablative laser and light therapies for skin rejuvenation, Arch Facial Plast Surg 2004; 6: 398–409.
44. Sadick NS, Schecter AK. A preliminary study of utilization of the 1320-nm Nd:YAG laser for the treatment of acne scarring. Dermatol Surg 2004; 30: 995–1000.
45. Chua SH, Ang P, Khoo LS, Goh CL. Nonablative 1450 nm diode laser in the treatment of facial atrophic acne scars in type IV to V Asian skin: a prospective clinical study. Dermatol Surg 2004; 30: 1287–91.
46. Goodman GJ. Blood transfer: the use of autologous blood as a chromophore and tissue augmentation agent. Dermatol Surg 2001; 27: 857–62.
47. Coleman SR. Long-term survival of fat transplants: controlled demonstrations. Aesth Plast Surg 1995; 19: 421–5.
48. Goodman GJ. Post-acne scarring: a review. J Cosmet Laser Ther 2003; 5: 77–95.
49. Goodman GJ. Autologous fat transfer and dermal grafting for the correction of facial scars. In: M Harahap, ed. Surgical techniques for cutaneous scar revision. Marcel Dekker: New York, 2000: 311–49.
50. Orentreich DS. Subcutaneous incisionless (subcision) surgery for the correction of depressed scars and wrinkles. Derm Surg 1995; 21: 543–9.

51. Branson DF. Dermal undermining (scarification) of active rhytids and scars: enhancing the results of CO2 laser skin resurfacing. Aesthetic Surg 1998; 18: 36–7.

52. Fulchiero GJ, Parham-Vetter PC, Obagi S. Subcision and 1320-nm Nd:YAG nonablative laser resurfacing for the treatment of acne scars: a simultaneous split-face single patient trial. Dermatol Surg 2004; 30: 1356–9.

53. Swinehart JM. Pocket grafting with dermal grafts: autologous collagen implants for permanent correction of cutaneous depressions. Am J Cosmet Surg 1995; 12(4): 321–31.

54. Abergel RP, Schlaak CM, Garcia LD. The laser dermal implant: a new technique for preparation and implantation of autologous dermal grafts for the correction of depressed scars, lip augmentation, and nasolabial folds using silk touch laser technology. Am J Cosmet Surg 1996; 13(1): 15–8.

55. Goodman GJ. Laser assisted dermal grafting for the correction of cutaneous contour defects. Derm Surg 1997; 23(2): 95–9.

56. Grevelink JM, White VR. Concurrent use of laser skin resurfacing and punch excision in the treatment of facial acne scarring. Dermatol Surg 1998; 24: 527–30.

57. Johnson W. Treatment of pitted scars: punch transplant technique. J Dermatol Surg Oncol 1986; 12: 260.

58. Orentreich N, Durr NP. Rehabilitation of acne scarring. Dermatol Clinics 1983; 1: 405–13.

59. Weiss RA, Weiss MA, Beasley KL, Munavalli G. Autologous cultured fibroblast injection for facial contour deformities: a prospective, placebo-controlled, phase iii clinical trial. Derm Surg 2007; 33: 263–8.

60. Fitzpatrick RE. Treatment of inflamed hypertrophic scars using intralesional 5-FU. Dermatol Surg 1999; 25: 224–32.

61. Lebwohl M. From the literature: intralesional 5-FU in the treatment of hypertrophic scars and keloids: clinical experience. J*Am Acad Dermatol 2000; 42: 677.

62. Uppal RS, Khan U, Kakar S et al. The effects of a single dose of 5-fluorouracil on keloid scars: a clinical trial of timed wound irrigation after extralesional excision. Plast Reconstr Surg 2001; 108: 1218–24.

63. Bodokh I, Brun P. Treatment of keloid with intralesional bleomycin. Ann Dermatol Venereol 1996; 123(12): 791–4.

64. Espana A, Solano T, Quintanilla E. Bleomycin in the treatment of keloids and hypertrophic scars by multiple needle punctures. Dermatol Surg 2001; 27: 23–7.

65. Bailey JN, Waite AE, Clayton WJ, Rustin MH. Application of topical mitomycin C to the base of shave-removed keloid scars to prevent their recurrence. Br J Dermatol 2007; 156: 682–6.

66. Stewart CE, Kim JY. Application of mitomycin-C for head and neck keloids. Otolaryngol Head Neck Surg 2006; 135: 946–50.

67. Gupta S, Kalra A. Efficacy and safety of intralesional 5-fluorouracil in the treatment of keloids. Dermatology 2002; 204: 130–2.

68. Wendling J, Marchand A, Mauviel A, Verrecchia F. 5-fluorouracil blocks transforming growth factor-beta-induced alpha 2 type I collagen gene (COL1A2) expression in human fibroblasts via c-Jun NH2-terminal kinase/activator protein-1 activation. Mol Pharmacol 2003; 64: 707–13.

69. Alster TS, Williams CM. Treatment of keloid sternotomy scars with 585 nm flashlamp-pumped pulsed-dye laser. Lancet 1995; 345(8959): 1198–2000.

70. Manuskiatti W, Fitzpatrick RE. Treatment response of keloidal and hypertrophic sternotomy scars: comparison among intralesional corticosteroid, 5-fluorouracil, and 585-nm flashlamp-pumped pulsed-dye laser treatments. Arch Dermatol 2002; 138: 1149–55.

71. Manuskiatti W, Fitzpatrick RE, Goldman MP. Energy density and numbers of treatment affect response of keloidal and hypertrophic sternotomy scars to the 585-nm flashlamp-pumped pulsed-dye laser. J Am Acad Dermatol 2001; 45: 557–65.

20 Hair transplantation
Alfonso Barrera

Over the past two decades the author has dedicated a significant part (60%) of my Aesthetic Plastic Surgery practice to hair transplantation.

With the advances in technique available today we can truly provide natural and aesthetically pleasing results, by the using 1–2 hair follicular unit grafts (Micrografts) and 3–4 hair follicular unit grafts (Minigrafts).

There has been a very significant evolution from the "punch graft" technique to the current follicular unit graft technique.

The original hair plugs or punch grafts were described by Orentrech in 1959 (1) for the treatment of male pattern baldness (MPB) and were the standard of care for some 20–25 years. We learned a lot from the use of hair plugs, especially the donor "dominance concept" that is the fact that the longevity of hair growth is dependent on the genetic programming of the hair follicles of the donor area.

This concept is the foundation to the success of hair transplantation; the transplanted hair will continue to grow on the transplanted site as long as it was going to do so in the donor area.

Unfortunately the hair plugs (10–20 hairs per graft) resulted in an artificial corn row appearance. As the use of smaller and more numerous grafts were introduced truly natural and aesthetically pleasing results were finally predictably obtained.

How did this happen? The use of single hair grafts on the scalp was first reported by Nordstrom (2) in 1980. He described the benefit of such grafts camouflaging the scarring and unnatural appearance of hair plugs, finally allowing for natural looking results. It was very time consuming to work at the front hairline and it didn't seem feasible at the time that the entire area of baldness could be treated with such small grafts.

Uebel (3) in 1991 reported his ingenious idea of what we call today the "stick and place" technique using of micrografts (1–2 hair grafts) and minigrafts (3–4 hair grafts) in large numbers (1,000–1,200 grafts) to graft large areas of hair loss such as the entire top of the head in cases of MPB.

Since the 1990s gradually these techniques of large number of very small grafts have become the standard of care. Minor refinements continue today and primarily consist of denser packing of smaller grafts.

Based on Uebel's work reported in 1991, I introduced hair transplantation into my practice, I have been able to further increase the number of grafts transplanted in a single session up to 2,900 for MPB patients. Over the past 14 years performing hair transplantation for MPB. Furthermore, I have found additional applications restoring natural looking hair in reconstructive cases of scalp and facial hair loss from various causes. Such as: accidents, burns, tumor resections, congenital deformities, etc. including restoring eyebrows, moustaches beard (4–10) and more recently other body areas including pubic area lower legs.(11)

Also for historical interest, the use of single hair grafts was originally described by Tumura (12) in 1943 when he reported use of single hair grafts to restore pubic hair. Subsequently Fujita (13) in 1953 used hair transplantation for reconstructing eyebrows.

In 1984 Headington (14) described a very important concept in hair anatomy, the "Follicular Unit". When we study the histology of skin (scalp) traditionally we see vertical sections. He studied transverse microscopic sections of the human scalp and noticed that hair grows in follicular units with 1, 2,3 or 4 hairs with their independent neurovascular, sebaceous glands, sweat glands, and pilo-erectile muscle surrounded by a sheath of collagen (Figure 20.1). These follicular units appear to be true physiologic units. Maintaining these intact units appears to increase the survival and ultimate hair growth of the grafts.

The genetic information for hair growth is located at the hair follicle level. Male patients who are genetically programmed to develop MPB will end up with a variety of patterns, either losing the hair only at the front hairline, only at the crown or the whole top. See the Norwood classification (15) in Figure 20.2. The areas that go bald have different genetic programming than the areas of scalp that do not. MPB usually occurs primarily on the top of the head and not on the occipital or temporal areas. The hair follicles on the top of the head are genetically sensitive to Dehydrotestosterone (DHT) and the hair follicles on the occipital and temporal areas are not.

As mentioned above the donor hair once transplanted to the top part of the head and hairline is going to continue growing on the transplanted area for as long as it was going to grow on the donor site, this is the so called "donor dominance" concept. Thanks to this we can successfully perform hair transplantation and have results that last a long time.

Female patients normally also have dehydrotestosterone in their system, although at lower levels. Those females who develop Female Pattern Alopecia have genetic trait consisting of hypersensitivity at the hair follicle levels to the presence of DHT. Women have a different thinning pattern than men. Usually this presents as a diffuse thinning throughout most of the scalp. Luckily sometimes it spares the low occipital area, allowing some women to be candidates for hair transplantation.

As to the physiology of hair, it is worth mentioning that hair grows in cycles as follows: Anagen is the actively growing phase. In this phase the follicular cells are actively multiplying and keratinizing. In a non-balding scalp, normally about 90% of the hairs are in this phase, which lasts about 3 years. During the Catagen phase the base of the hair becomes keratinized, forming a club, and separates itself from the dermal papilla. It then moves toward the surface and is eventually connected to the dermal papilla only by a connective tissue strand. This phase lasts 2 to 3 weeks. During the Telogen phase, also called the resting phase, the attachment at the base of the follicle becomes weaker until the hair finally sheds. During this period the follicle is inactive and hair growth ceases. This phase lasts 3–4 months and it is frequently triggered after hair transplantation.

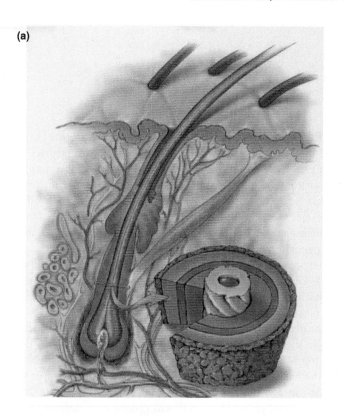

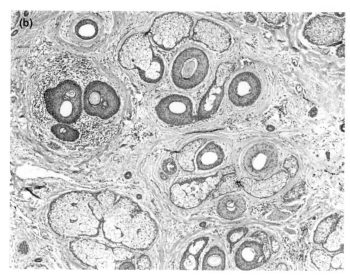

Figure 20.1 (A) Illustration of a hair follicle. (B) Transverse hystologic H&E Stain demonstrating 1-2-3 and 4 hair follicular units.

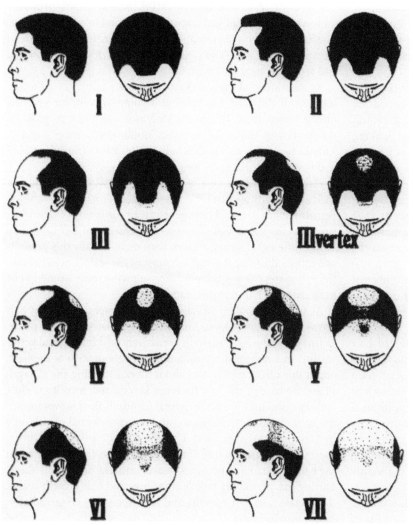

Figure 20.2 (A) Noorwood Classification of male pattern Baldness.

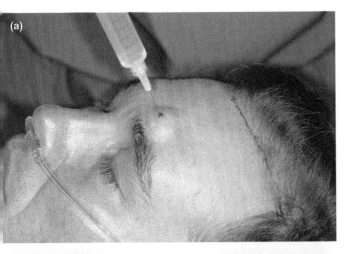

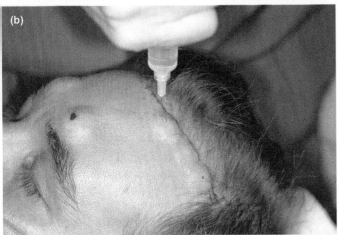

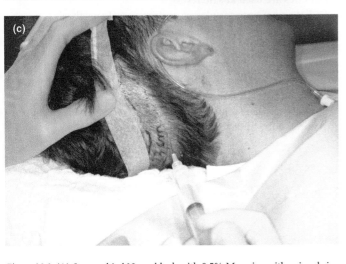

Figure 20.3 (A) Supraorbital Nerve block with 0.5% Marcaine with epinephrine 1:200,000. (B) Ring block with 0.5% Marcaine with epinephrine 1:200,000. (C) Occipital nerve block and local infiltration with 0.5% Marcaine with epinephrine 1:200,000.

It is important to keep this in mind and explain it to patients before a hair transplantation procedure. This is important as post-transplantation the catagen and telogen phases occur almost invariably. Normally for about 2 weeks the transplanted hair may continue to grow and then a large percentage of it and some of the native hair will shed temporarily. The hair goes into the telogen phase triggered by the trauma of so many little incisions and perhaps the temporary loss of blood supply to the transplanted hair follicles. This is called telogen effluvium . It takes about 3 months before it shifts into gear on to the Anagen phase in which the hair starts to grow again.

Therefore for the first 3 to 4 months after hair transplantation there is normally no visible improvement, in fact the patient's hair may even look thinner than before the procedure.

Once the grafts shift into the Anagen phase, fine villous hair appears and gradually thickens into terminal hair. Visually significant increase in hair density and growth does not occur until approximately 5–6 months postoperatively and often takes 10–12 months for the final result. In female patients it may take a little longer.

PATIENT SELECTION

Current techniques in hair transplantation are quite successful on patients of any and all racial backgrounds and provide aesthetically pleasing results consistently. Naturally patient selection is important as well as an accurate and artistically performed surgical technique.

To date, we have no method to create new hair. All current techniques for hair restoration involve redistributing the patient's existing hair. Therefore candidates for hair transplantation are limited to those who have a favorable donor site surface area and density relative to the size of the area to be transplanted. The better candidates for this procedure are those who have denser and larger donor area (occipital and temporal areas) and proportionally smaller bald areas.

Several centers worldwide are working on tissue engineering in an attempt to clone hair follicles or culture and multiply hair follicles in the laboratory. When successful, we will be able to treat patients with limited donor hair (the follicular challenged patient). At that time we will need only harvest a sample of hair follicles, and then grow additional follicles in the laboratory. This will eliminate donor site morbidity and discomfort almost completely.

Unfortunately MPB is a progressive condition. The rate of hair loss may slow down after the age of 40 years, but it never stops completely. Therefore the preoperative plan must insure natural results both short and long-term. Good communication with patients is essential to establish realistic expectations.

Be conservative as to the new hairline design, think short term but also long term, design a mature hairline and leave a reasonable degree of frontotemporal recession even in the younger patient.

There is no magic number as to the distance from the eyebrows to the ideal hairline, as there is a huge variety of head dimensions and craniofacial proportions. It is best to draw a planned hairline in advance that seems appropriate and aesthetically pleasing. A natural appearance is enhanced by creating irregularity at the hairline border, to better mimic nature.

The appearance of fullness has to do with hair mass, which is related to the number of hairs, the thickness of the individual hair shafts, the texture and color of the hair, as well as the curliness of the hair. In addition, the contrast of colors between the scalp and the hair also has a significant influence on the optical illusion of fullness. Most experts today agree that the average healthy non balding patient has a density of about 200 hairs/cm2 (range 130 to 280) and that only 50% of this number is needed to give an appearance of normal density, which is ideally about 100 hairs/cm2 (range 65 to140). Generally, about 70–80 hairs/cm^2 looks reasonably good. Realistically this number can be transplanted in two sessions of micrografting and minigrafting.

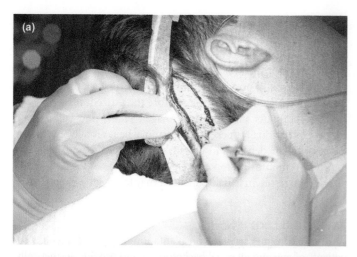

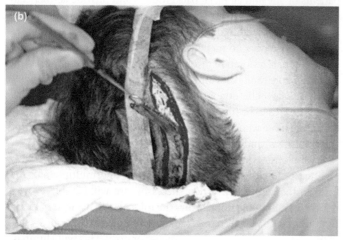

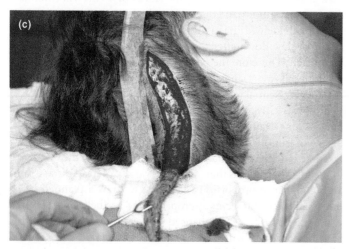

Figure 20.4 Typical donor site. Length will vary depending on the number of grafts planned and the density of the donor area. Generally I take 1 cm width and 15–28 cm in horizontal length. (A, B, C) Harvesting the right side of the donor ellipse.

In addition to hair transplantation for the correction of male or female pattern baldness, the author has found many reconstructive applications as well:

1) Postsurical conditions as the lost sideburn and temporal hairline after Facelift and forehead lifting procedures
2) Revision of unfavorable results from previous hair transplantation procedures

(i.e., the plug look, corn field rows and hairline scars). Here I do plug removal and recycling.
3) Correction of hair loss burn injuries.
4) Posttraumatic injuries.
5) Certain congenital conditions may also result on hair loss such as is the absence of hair as in the prolabium in cases of bilateral cleft lips, Hairloss due to excision of congenital lesions such as Hairy Nevus, Arterio-Venous Malformations, or after involution of strawberry hemangiomas, etc.

TECHNIQUE:

For cases of MPB, the author typically does perform 1,000 and 2,500 grafts per session depending on the degree of hair loss. This labor-intensive procedure requires an organized and efficient surgical team.

My surgical team consists of three surgical assistants and myself. He remains in the operating room for the duration of the procedure and insert all grafts. Efficiency is key when transplanting large number of grafts in a single session.

The author performs the procedure with the patient in the supine position. He prefers mildly sedated with Midzolam (Versed) and Sublimaze (fentanyl), which are titrated for each patient. The patient's vital signs, EKG rhythm, and O2 saturation are monitored throughout the procedure.

Supraorbital and occipital nerve blocks are established with 0.5% bupivacaine with 1:200,000 epinephine (approximately 30 ml). This includes a ring block just below the proposed hairline. A tumescent solution of 0.5% lidocaine with 1:200,000 epinephrine is then infiltrated in the donor site, Figure 20.3. As always, care must be taken to insure that the both any sedation and local anesthetics are used at safe levels.

Pediatric patients are placed under general anesthesia.

The patient's head is turned to the left Using a # 10 scalpel blade the author harvests the right half of the donor ellipse.(Figure 20.4) Under 3.5X loupe magnification with Personna Prep Blades immediately thin slices 1.5 to 2.0 mm in thickness are dissected from the donor ellipse over a sterile wooden board and handed to the assistants. The author prefers a wooden board because it provides a non slippery firm surface, Figure 20.5.

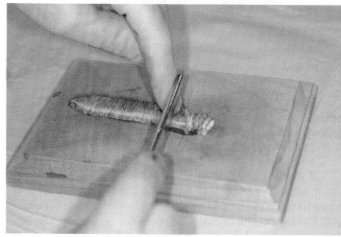

Figure 20.5 Making 2-mm thick slices, parallel to the hair follicles, using a Personna Prep Blade. On hard autoclaved wood.

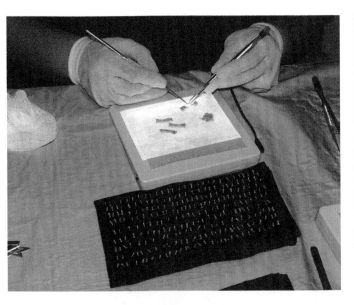

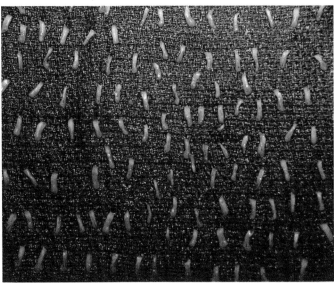

Figure 20.6 Dissection of the 2-mm slices of scalp into the individual follicular units (under magnification) using background lighting for translucency.

Figure 20.9 View of follicular units.

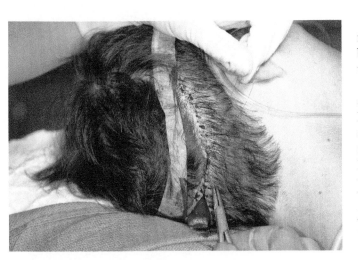

Figure 20.7 Closure of right half of donor site.

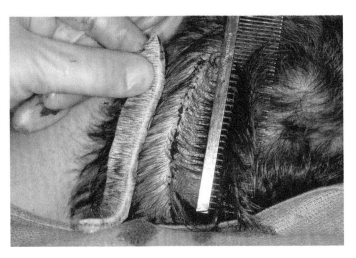

Figure 20.8 After harvest and closure of left side (half) of donor ellipse.

The assistants under magnification prepare the final grafts from these slices with background lighting and using # 10 scalpel blades. (Figure 20.6). While the surgeon closes the right half of the donor strip (Figure 20.7).

The dissection of the grafts is the most tedious part of the procedure and one of the most important steps, the grafts obviously need to be handled gently and atraumatically. As described this is performed on a wooden board that has been autoclaved. The darker and thicker the individual hair shafts the easier it is to dissect the grafts. The ideal grafts have intact hair shafts all the way from the subcutaneous fatty tissue to the scalp surface, and contain from one to four hairs. Again they must be handled as atraumatically as possible. The grafts are handled with jeweller's forceps by the fatty tissue under the hair bulbs or by the tissue around them, not by the hair bulb or dermal hair papilla itself.

In cases of very light-colored or white hair we use microscopes (10X) for a safe dissection of the grafts. The author prefers the Mantis Microscope.

The incisions must be made precisely parallel to the hair shafts at all times to minimize the loss of hair follicles. The harvested scalp and all grafts are kept chilled in normal saline until transplanted.

The surgeon then turns the patient's head to the right for harvesting the left half of the donor ellipse. The surgeon subsequently closes the left side donor site and then finishes slicing the remaining segment of the donor ellipse.(Figure 20.8).

Several hundred grafts will have been dissected at this point. They are lined up in rows on a wet green or blue surgical towel and are now ready for insertion. The process of graft dissection and insertion continues until all the grafts are transplanted (Figure 20.9).It is imperative to keep the grafts wet, desiccation damages the hair bulbs.

Key points to remember in graft dissection are:

1. Maintain the follicular units as intact as feasible.
2. In patients with dark hair 3.5X loupe magnification is sufficient to dissect most grafts as follicular units.
3. In patients with light hair or gray hair surgical microscopes and background lighting may be needed for more accurate dissection.

Graft Insertion: Infiltration of tumescent solution into the recipient area is important for several reasons, the most important of which is to promote hemostasis and to produce temporary edema of the scalp, which facilitates graft insertion. The safe volume of lidocaine which can be used varies depending on the patient's body mass. In larger men the author may use 150 ml of 0.5% lidocaine with 1:200,000 epinephrine when transplanting 1,000 grafts or more.

If good hemostasis is not obtained with this solution, the author increases the epinephrine strength to 1:100,000. Optimal hemostasis is often achieved if the tumescent solution is infiltrated in thirds. First inject the anterior region. Once a large number of grafts has been inserted there, proceed posteriorly doing the same for the middle third and finally the posterior third. Doing this sequentially allows us to take advantage of the peak times of epinephrine effect.

Over time in the graft recipient sites the fibrinogen turns into fibrin. Once this occurs the grafts adhere better to the recipient slits. Then repetitively return anteriorly to insert more grafts placing them densely, minimizing the risk of "popping out" of neighboring grafts. The epinephrine effect is often still adequate when returning to the anterior region to place additional grafts otherwise re-inject, as long as the local anesthetic does not exceed safe doses.

The author uses a "stick and place" technique. A slit is created and immediately a graft is inserted, using 22.5 Sharp point blades at and 1cm in front of the hairline, Figure 20.10. This too creates a nice transition zone, intentionally making a slight irregularity to mimic nature. With these blades, the scars are undetectable every time, posterior to that the author preferred to use No. 11 Feather Personna blades Figure 20.11.

On the face the technique of graft insertion is similar but more difficult as there is a much more tendency for grafts to pop out as others are inserted In the author's experience in restoring the eyebrows, moustache, or beard has he has found that that it is best to make most or all of the slits initially (in a preliminary fashion) and insert the grafts later to minimize this problem.

On small cases the grafts are harvested from a small donor ellipse from the occipital area posterior to the mastoid prominence and dissected as for scalp transplantation. The size of the donor strip will clearly vary from very small to a large one depending on the number of grafts needed and the donor site hair density.

The slits on the face are made with a No. 22.5 Sharpoint blade you can also use an 18gauge needle always inserting the blade at the angle of the desired direction of hair growth, laterally and upward following the direction of the natural eyebrows when doing that, in the case of sideburns or temporal hair line, moustache or beard we then also angle the blade with which we are making the slits so it orients the hair growth in the proper direction.

For dressings the author generally uses one or two layers of Adaptic, Kerlex and 3"elastic Ace bandage for the scalp.

with scars from the lip repair. Shown before and after a single session of follicular unit grafts. Notice how a few moustache hairs camouflage the scarring significantly.

Discussion: The presented technique provides superior results compared to previously described hair restoration techniques.

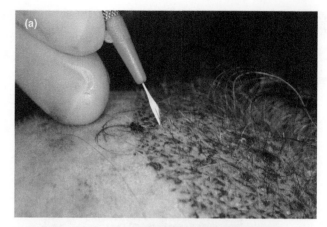
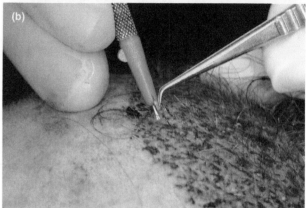
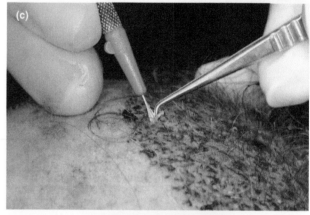
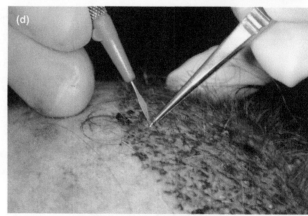

Figure 20.10 (A) Using a 22.5 Sharpoint blade for graft insertion. Try to orient the blade in a natural hair direction. (B, C, D) Blade inserted and grafts being placed into the incision using the blade as a shoe horn.

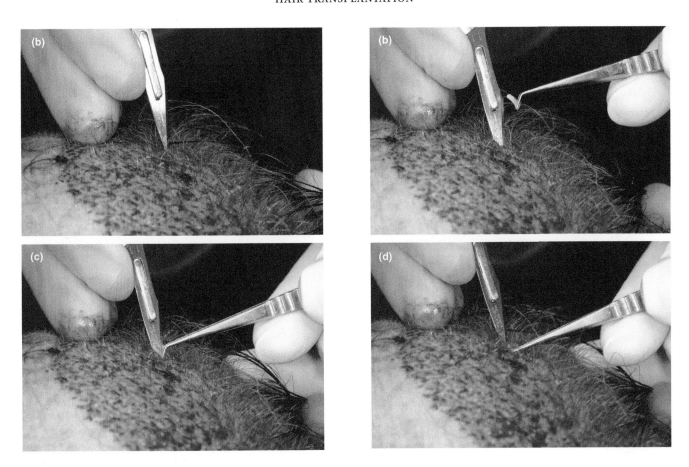

Figure 20.11 (A, B, C, D) Use of the Feather 11 blade further posteriorly.

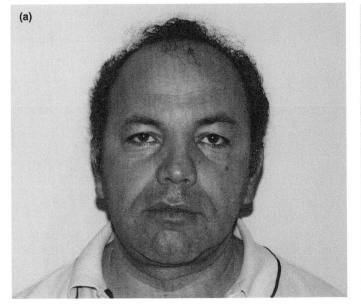

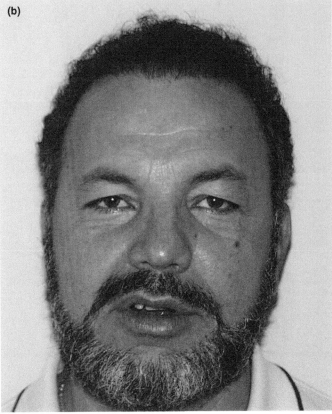

Figure 20.12 (Continued).

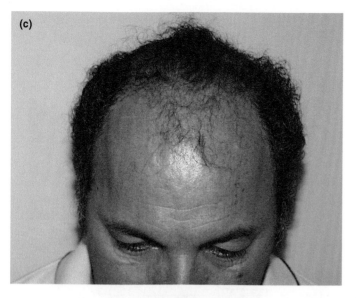

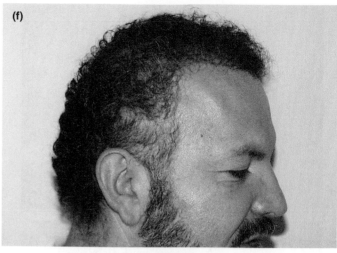

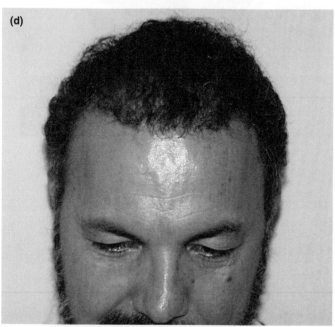

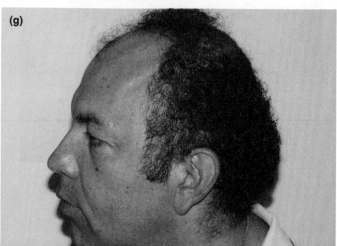

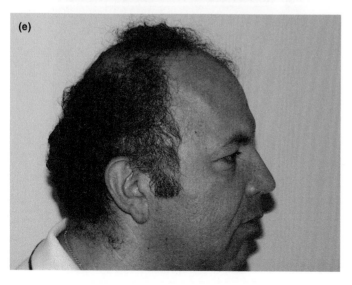

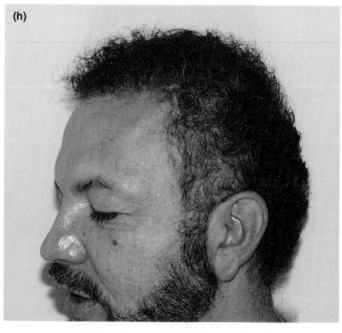

Figure 20.12 (Continued).

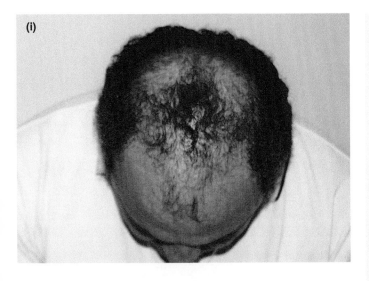

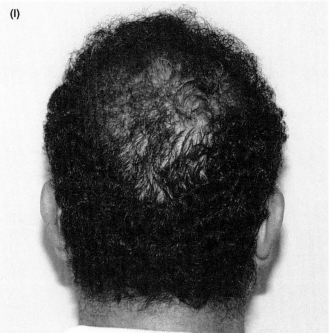

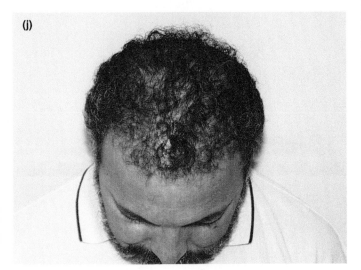

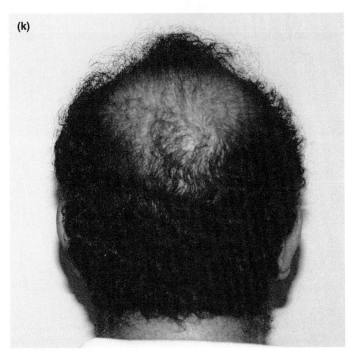

Figure 20.12 46-year-old man with MPB VII, before and one year after 2,040 follicular unit grafts, single session. Notice the significant rejuvenation and overall aesthetic improvement.

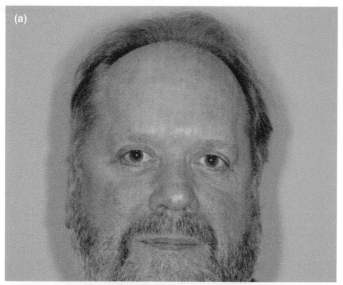

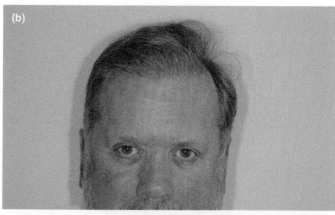

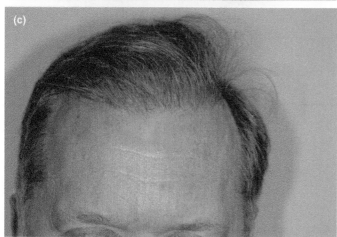

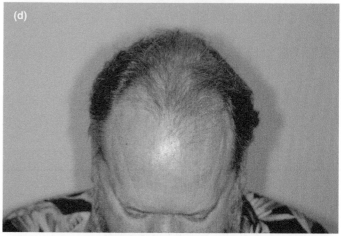

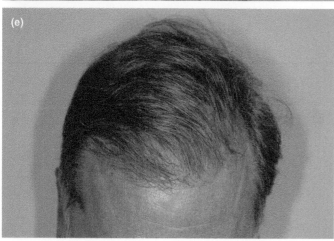

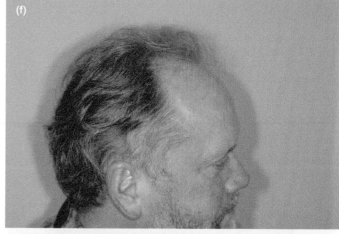

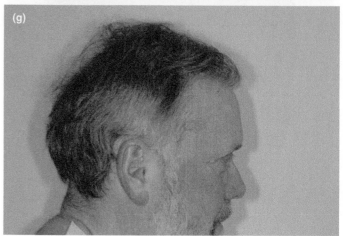

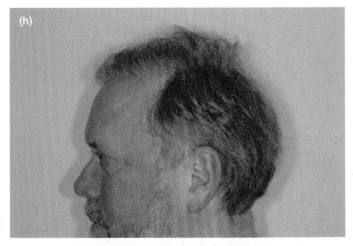

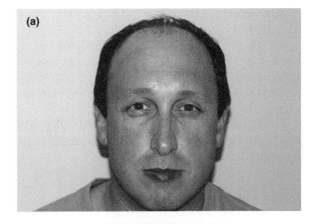

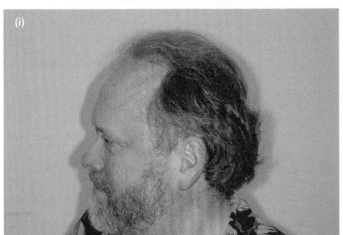

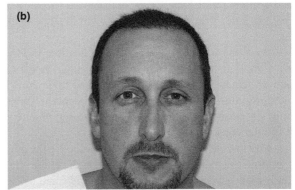

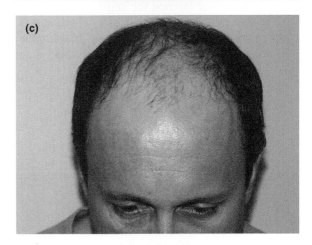

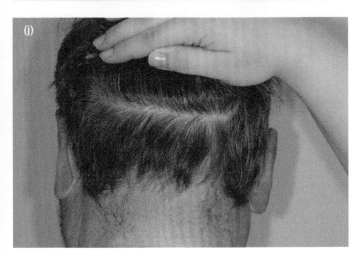

Figure 20.13 56-Year-old man with Male Pattern Baldness VII, before and one year after 2,400 follicular unit grafts, single session.

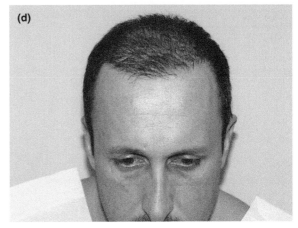

Figure 20.14 42-year-old man with Male Pattern Baldness VII. Before and one year after a single session of 2,450 in a single session.

181

1. A natural result both short term and long term
2. Minimal scarring, usually undetectable
3. Minimal down time can often be accomplished in just one session or two sessions (It is not uncommon to do a second session to achieve higher hair density).
4. The direction of the hair can usually be controlled by angling the surgical blade
5. The desired hairline design can be controlled with precision.
6. "Safety", there are no worries about flaps ischemia, tip necrosis or expander exposures and extrusion.

PROBLEMS AND COMPLICATIONS

As with a face-lift procedure, patients are told to temporarily expect dysesthesia and hypesthesia cephalad to the horizontal donor site closure. This, however, resolves within a few weeks to months.

The author has encountered very few complications in 14 years treating more than 1,000 patients without a single incidence of infection or hematoma. In one patient who had undergone four hair plug procedures elsewhere a minor dehiscence occurred at the donor site closure (less than an inch) but this granulated and healed spontaneously.

In two patients, one who was African-American and the other of Mediterranean origin, keloid scars developed at the donor site.

Initially many patients had ingrown hairs and small inclusion cysts because the author inserted the grafts too deep. By altering his technique the author has been able to prevent this by leaving the epidermis of the grafts slightly superficial to the epidermis of the recipient scalp. This also prevents small-diameter pitting.

Conclusion: In properly selected patients of all ethnic backgrounds the use of follicular unit grafts micrografts and minigrafts as described provides safe and predictable results and a high level of patient satisfaction.

REFERENCES

1. Orentreich N. Autografts in alopecias and other selected dermatological conditions. Ann NY Acad Sci 1959; 83: 463–79.
2. Nordstrom REA. Micrigrafts for improvement of the frontal hairline after hair transplantation. Aesthetic Plast Surg 1981; 5: 97.
3. Uebel CO. Micrografts and minigrafts: a new approach to baldnes surgery. Ann Plast Surg 1991; 27: 476.
4. Barrera A. Micrograft and minigraft megasession hair transplantation: review of 100 Consecutive Cases. Aesthet Surg J 1997; 17(3): 165.
5. Barrera A. Micrograft and minigraft megasession hair transplantation results after a single session. Plast Reconstr Surg 1997; 100(6): 1524.
6. Barrera, A. Refinements in hair transplantation: micro and minigraft megasession. Perspectives in Plast Surg 1998; 11(1): 53.
7. Barrera A. The use of micrografts and minigrafts for the correction of the postrhytidectomy lost sideburn. Plast Reconstr Surg 1998; 102(6): 2273.
8. Barrera A. The use of micrografts and minigrafts for the treatment of burn alopecia. Plast Reconstr Surg 1999; 103(2): 581.
9. Barrera A. Hair grafting tips and techniques. Perspectives in Plast Surg 2001; 15(2): 147–58.
10. Barrera A. Hair transplantation: The Art of Micrografting and Minigrafting Quality Medical Publishing. First Edition; 2002.
11. Barrera A, Phillips LG, Barrera FF. Hair grafts in lower leg reconstruction. Plast Reconstr Surg 2007; 120(2): 22e–5e.
12. Tamura H. Pubic hair transplantation. Jpn J Dermatol 1943; 53: 76.
13. Fujita K. Reconstruction of eyebrows. La Lepr 1953; 22: 364.
14. Headington JT. Transverse microscopic anatomy of the human scalp. Arch Dermatol 1984; 120: 449.
15. Norwood OT, Shiell R. Eds Hair Transplantation, 2nd Ed. Sringfield ILL: Charles C. Thomas; 1984.

21 Aesthetic procedures for patients with medical problems
Chad L Prather

INTRODUCTION

In the gap between cosmetic treatments for aesthetic improvement and medical treatments for human disease lay the aesthetic procedures for medical problems—those procedures that were pioneered for, or are primarily used for, cosmetic improvement, yet have been extended to treat cutaneous and subcutaneous medical conditions. Certainly, surgical and procedural treatments have long been utilized by dermatologists to treat medical conditions. However, those treatments such as surgical excision and cryotherapy, which have historically been a mainstay of medical treatment though they may also be used for aesthetic rejuvenation, are not considered here. Rather, the most popular of those modalities that have been established primarily as cosmetic procedures, but may also benefit patients with medical problems, will be emphasized.

As aesthetic clinicians established and developed expertise in various cosmetic dermasurgical procedures, these modalities naturally became tools in the arsenal for cutaneous medical problems as well, particularly in those without satisfactory oral or topical remedies. Injectable toxins, soft tissue augmenting agents, chemical peels, laser and light therapies, liposuction, dermabrasion, and sclerotherapy have all proven useful in the purely medical arena, and their applications for cutaneous human disease continue to grow. Indeed, in many instances, procedures developed for aesthetic conditions have become the most efficacious therapies for medical cutaneous problems. The most widely used of these modalities are botulinum toxins, soft tissue fillers, chemical peels, and laser and light therapy, and the medical, rather than aesthetic, uses of these modalities are considered here.

BOTULINUM TOXIN

Botulinum toxins are unique in their progression to therapeutic use, moving from historical "poison" to isolated medical use for strabismus in the 1970s, and then exploding in popularity for aesthetic employment beginning in the 1990s.(1, 2) Extensive aesthetic use and cultural popularity have fostered widespread availability of botulinum toxins, which has since led to attempts at treating various medical conditions that involve muscle or exocrine gland hyperactivity, many of which are cutaneous.(3)

Botulinum toxins have become an important treatment modality for primary **hyperhidrosis**, or excessive sweating of the axillae, palms, soles, and inguinal areas without discernable cause.(4, 5) When injected intradermally, botulinum toxin acts upon local cholinergic nerve endings causing local chemodenervation and decreased perspiration.(6) Significant decreases in sweating have been achieved with **axillary hyperhidrosis**, where 100 units of Type A botulinum toxin (Botox™, Allergan, Irvine, CA) per axilla injected superficially may provide improvement of hyperhidrosis for 4–6 months.(7–11) Likewise, several authors have described successful techniques for **palmar hyperhidrosis**, typically using

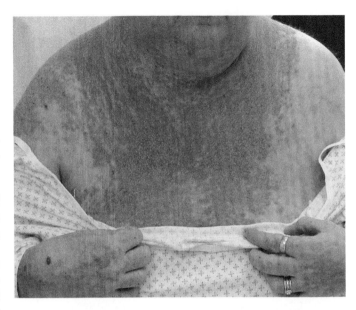

Figure 21.1 Darier's Disease. (Photo courtesy of Scott M. Jackson, MD).

100 units of Botox™ or 5,000 units of Myobloc™ (botulinum toxin Type B) (Elan Pharmaceuticals, San Diego, CA) superficially in each palm.(12–15) Iodine starch or paper tests may be used to assess the degree of hyperhidrosis, and topical amide anesthetics and median and ulnar nerve blocks may help provide comfort during palmar and finger injection.

Cases of improvement in **Darier's Disease** (Figure 21.1) (16, 17), **Hailey Hailey disease** (Figure 21.2) (18, 19), **pitted keratolysis** (20), **bromhidrosis** (21), **chromhidrosis** (22, 23), and **dyshidrotic hand dermatitis (pompholyx)** (Figure 21.3) (24) have also been reported with botulinum toxin injection. Relief in these disorders is likely secondary to a decrease in eccrine, apocrine, or apo-eccrine glandular activity, or a combination of these.(25)

Aphthous ulcers have also been reported to respond well to botulinum toxin. Yang and Jang reported a significant decrease in pain at the site of ulceration after 3 days compared to the 1–2 weeks normally necessary with aphthous ulcers. Furthermore, they observed prevention of recurrence in the same site for 4–6 months following the injection of 1 unit of Botox™.(26)

Raynaud's phenomenon, or episodic vasospasm of the digital arteries, may lead to pain, dysesthesia, digital ulceration, and even digital infarction. Several investigators have effectively used botulinum toxin Type A, injected into the hand and fingers at a dose of 100 units/hand, to achieve significant pain reduction and healing of digital ulcers in both primary idiopathic (**Raynaud's disease**) and secondary (**Raynaud's syndrome**) forms of this disease, such as secondary to scleroderma (Figure 21.4).(27–29) Van Beek and colleagues treated 11 patients and found that all reported significant pain reduction 1–2 days after injection that persisted for months after injection, and that 9 with nonhealing

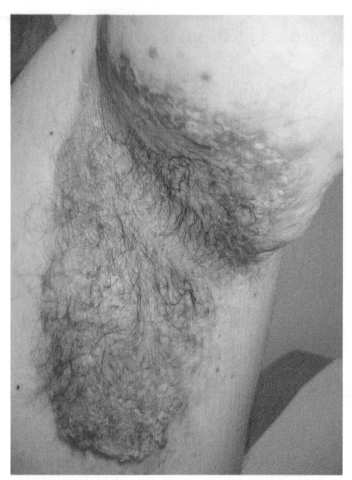

Figure 21.2 Darier's Disease. (Photo courtesy of Scott M. Jackson, MD).

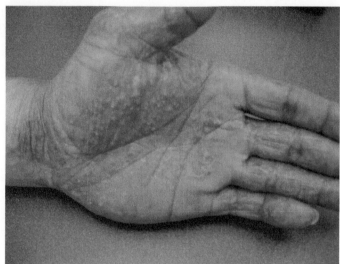

Figure 21.3 Pompholyx. (Photo courtesy of Scott M. Jackson, MD).

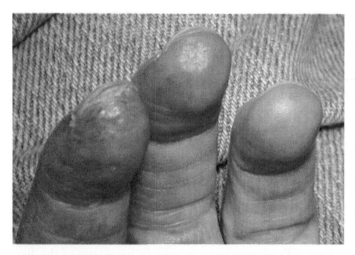

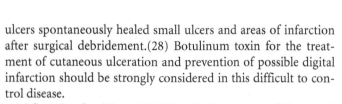

Figure 21.4 Raynaud's syndrome secondary to scleroderma.

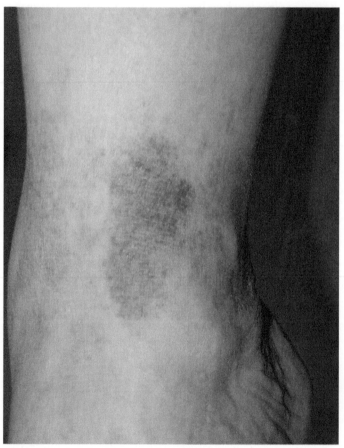

Figure 21.5 Lichen simplex chronicus. (Photo courtesy of Scott M. Jackson, MD).

ulcers spontaneously healed small ulcers and areas of infarction after surgical debridement.(28) Botulinum toxin for the treatment of cutaneous ulceration and prevention of possible digital infarction should be strongly considered in this difficult to control disease.

Lichen simplex (Figure 21.5) has also been successfully treated with botulinum toxin. Heckmann and colleagues reported

successful treatment in four patients with lesions on the legs. (30) Lyophilized Type A botulinum toxin (Dysport, Ipsen Ltd, Beaufort, France) was injected intradermally into the lesions, with 3 of 4 patients achieving disappearance of pruritus and one patient achieving a 50% decrease in pruritus after 1 week. 5 of 6 lesions cleared completely, and 3 of 4 patients were still clear at 3 months. Likewise, Weinfield reported the successful treatment of two patients with **notalgia paresthetica** of the back with botulinum toxin.(31) One patient treated with 18 units to the area remained symptom free after 18 months, and the second patient achieved complete relief with a 24 unit dose and a 48 unit dose 18 months later. The mechanism of clearance in both lichen simplex and notalgia paresthetica is hypothesized to be due to, as in other diseases, the toxin's potent inhibition of acetylcholine, but also its potential inhibition of substance P and glutamate. Thus botulinum toxin Type A may be considered an antipruritic modality as well.(32) Similarly, chronic, persistent **thelalgia** (nipple pain) has also been successfully treated with botulinum toxin.(33)

Numerous non-cutaneous medical conditions have been reported to respond to botulinum toxins as well, including the original conditions of blepharospasm, strabismus, and cervical dystonia for which botulinum toxin was used prior to widespread aesthetic adoption. Although beyond the scope of this publication, the use of injectable toxins for the treatment of headache, urinary incontinence, constipation, chronic anal fissure, chronic prostatitis, allergic rhinitis, sialorrhea, Frey's syndrome, chronic osteoarthritic pain, trigeminal neuralgia, and epiphora continue to be investigated. And as injectable toxins increase in scope, topically applied botulinum toxin is reportedly poised to arrive on the international market as well, and will likely further expand the usefulness of this historical "poison". Perhaps more than any other aesthetic modality, botulinum toxin has the potential to leap far beyond its most current popular use in the aesthetic arena.

SOFT TISSUE AUGMENTATION

Although fillers such as fat, paraffin, and silicone have been used for various cutaneous defects since the late 19th century (34), modern soft tissue augmenting agents for aesthetic use have exploded in popularity over the past decade. Numerous injectable products are now on market for the correction of rhytides and for cosmetic facial revolumization. Fillers, however, are not restricted to purely cosmetic applications.

Both the *en coup de sabre* linear variant and **Parry-Romberg** hemi-facial variant of **scleroderma** have been successfully treated with liquid silicone and autologous fat transplants.(35–38) Lapiere and colleagues reported the correction of a forehead defect with a single stage autologous fat transplant from the hip, with sustained correction at 1 year.(36) These variants of scleroderma are particularly difficult to treat, and autologous fat has become the filler of choice for such facial defects. These deformities may also respond very well to newer semipermanent and permanent fillers coming to market, and future studies are warranted.

Insensitive foot ulcers, as seen in **diabetes mellitus** and **Hansen's disease**, may also benefit from soft tissue augmentation with liquid injectable silicone.(39–41) Although injectable silicone for this purpose is not widely employed due to its controversial nature, Balkin long advocated its use as a fluid prosthesis and demonstrated its excellent safety profile when utilized for this purpose.(42, 43) Liquid silicone serves as a soft prosthetic device and can relieve corns and calluses, reduce pain in weight bearing scars, reduce the incidence of recurring neuropathic ulcers, and protect skin at points of bony pressure.

Finally, **HIV-associated facial lipoatrophy**, a medical condition that may stigmatize affected individuals and severely impact quality of life, is best treated with longer duration tissue augmenting agents.(44) Poly-L-lactic acid and highly purified liquid injectable silicone administered in small doses by the microdroplet serial puncture technique have proven to be the most practical and efficacious fillers to date for this manifestation of HIV-associated lipodystrophy.(45)

CHEMICAL PEELS

Aside from the many cosmetic benefits of chemical peeling, patients with cutaneous medical problems may also benefit from light and medium depth peeling procedures. **Acne, melasma**, and chronic actinic damage with or without **actinic keratoses** all benefit from various types of chemical peels.

Chemical peeling for the improvement of **acne** is a well-established modality.(46–49) Very light or light peels with glycolic acid 20–70%, trichloroacetic acid 10–35%, Jessner's solution, salicylic acid, pyruvic acid, resorcinol 30–50% preparations, and solid carbon dioxide (CO_2) improve acne vulgaris by corneocyte desquamation and a subsequent decrease in comedonal and inflammatory lesions. Beta hydroxy acids such as salicylic acid are theorized to work best for acne due to their lipophilic nature, which leads to enhanced pilosebaceous unit penetration. Kessler and colleagues recently compared 30% glycolic acid peels to 30% salicylic acid peels in a double-blind, randomized, controlled study.(46) While both were equally efficacious, the 30% salicylic acid peels showed a greater sustained effectiveness at 2 months.

Melasma, or hyperpigmented patches of the face that are worsened by estrogens and sun exposure, may show pathology at the epidermal or dermal level, or both. While notoriously difficult to treat, melasma may also be improved with very light or light chemical peels.(50–52) Glycolic acid, trichloroacetic acid (TCA), 1% tretinoin, salicylic acid, and kojic acid peels have all demonstrated efficacy in lightening the hyperpigmentation, particularly with repeated application. Melasma is particularly prone to occur in patients with higher Fitzpatrick skin types, and Grimes has demonstrated that 20% and 30% salicylic acid peels are particularly safe in ethnic groups with darker skin.(51)

Chemical peeling also efficaciously treats **chronic actinic damage** and **actinic keratoses**. For the treatment of actinic damage and precancerous lesions, the medium depth chemical peel is considered the practitioner's peel of choice, as it demonstrates the greatest measure of efficacy without compromising an adequate degree of safety. By definition, full-thickness destruction of the epidermis and partial or full thickness destruction of the papillary dermis constitutes a medium depth peel. Although there are various ways to achieve a medium depth peel, such as the Brody solid CO2 ice with 35% TCA combination (53), the Monheit combination of Jessner's solution and 35% TCA (54), and the Coleman combination of glycolic acid and 35% TCA (55), the author's preferred method is the Monheit peel with Jessner's/35% TCA.(56) Multiple actinic keratoses, or keratoses on a background of significant solar damage, respond very well to medium depth peels, and typically show a clearance of existing lesions and a delay in new lesion formation for several months to several years. The procedure is particularly well suited for the male with actinic keratoses that have required repeated removal with either cryosurgery or 5-fluorouracil chemoexfoliation. The entire face can be treated as a unit, or subfacial cosmetic unit such as forehead, temples, cheeks, or chin can be treated independently. Active lesions can be removed, and as yet undetected growths will also be removed as the epidermis is sloughed. Medium depth peeling is a reliable treatment for full epidermal destruction, and can be combined with cryosurgery and/or dermasanding for thicker resistant solitary lesions.

LASER AND LIGHT THERAPIES

Laser and light-based therapies encompass a wide range of devices that deliver energy to various chromophores and molecular targets in the cutaneous and subcutaneous tissues, including hemoglobin, melanin, water, and DNA, to affect histologic structures in the integumentary system such as vessels, hair follicles and associated glandular structures, collagen, and rapidly dividing cells.

Several pilosebaceous and glandular disorders may be treated and improved by laser devices. Goldman reported significant improvement in 17 patients with **axillary hyperhidrosis** using a subdermal 1,064-nm Nd:YAG laser in a minimally invasive fashion.(57) Kim and colleagues reported marked improvement in 88 patients with **osmidrosis** (hyperhidrosis and excessive odor) using subcutaneous curettage combined with CO_2 laser, although 4 patients had partial skin necrosis and delayed wound healing.(58) **Hidradenitis suppuritiva** may also be treated with the CO_2 laser, but requires deep tissue removal and secondary healing.(59, 60)

Acne vulgaris may benefit from several laser and light-based therapies.(61, 62) Although large scale randomized controlled studies are lacking for many laser devices, Munavalli and Weiss found in their review that the 1450 nm diode laser did show promise of benefit, but that the 585-nm pulsed dye laser had mixed results.(63) Treatment success with combined 585/1,064-nm lasers has also been reported.(64) On the other hand, several studies have demonstrated the efficacy of photodynamic therapy (PDT) in the treatment of acne with 5-aminolevulanic acid combined with a blue light or broadband intense pulsed light (IPL). (65, 66) Photo-excitation of the Proprionibacterium acnes porphyrins after exposure to the appropriate light source in the blue or red visible spectrum causes singlet oxygen radicals to occur within the microorganism, resulting in the selective destruction of the bacteria.(67) For this reason, PDT works best to alleviate inflammatory lesions rather than comedones.

Vascular disorders are also a superb target for laser and light-based therapies because hemoglobin serves as a chromophore in the absorption spectrum of several laser wavelengths. The treatment of congenital vascular malformations, including **hemangiomas** and **port wine stains**, is well described with several laser types, including the argon, argon-pumped tunable dye, potassium titanyl phosphate (KTP), copper vapor and bromide, krypton lasers.(68) The flashlamp-pumped pulsed dye laser (PDL) is considered the most efficacious laser for such lesions, however. (69) As laser treatment of these somewhat common lesions has been extensively addressed in the literature, further review is beyond the scope of this chapter.

The prominent erythematous and vascular components of **rosacea** are effectively treated with both the PDL at purpuric and subpurpuric settings and IPL with a 515-nm filter.(70–73)

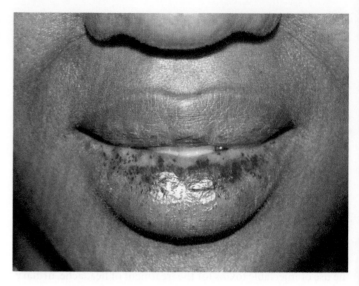

Figure 21.6 Hereditary hemorrhagic telangiectasia (Osler Weber Rendu).

Rhinophyma, a form of rosacea characterized by hypertrophic sebaceous glands, has likewise been treated with a 1450-nm diode laser in mild to moderate forms (74), but requires treatment with a CO_2 laser in more severe forms.(75) **Hereditary hemorrhagic telangiectasia**, or Osler Weber Rendu syndrome (Figure 21.6), presents with characteristic telangiectasias at multiple sites, including the lips, oral cavity, fingers, and nose. The cutaneous lesions may be effectively treated with the PDL (76), but the more problematic intranasal or gastrointestinal lesions that often result in epistaxis must be treated by infrared coagulation, radiofrequency, argon laser, or the Nd:YAG laser.(77) **Angiokeratoma of Fordyce**, asymptomatic vascular lesions of the genitalia and lower abdomen, may also be successfully treated with PDL (78), or the long pulsed Nd:YAG.(79)

Keratinizing disorders may also be improved with laser devices. **Hailey Hailey** disease benefits from both CO_2 and Nd:YAG lasers. (80, 81) Likewise, **Darier's Disease** may be improved with the CO_2 and Nd:YAG lasers as well.(81, 82) Although multiple lasers have been utilized to treat **psoriasis** (Figure 21.7), including the CO_2, Er:YAG, PDL, and 1320 nm Nd:YAG lasers, the 308-nm excimer laser has proven most efficacious outside of narrowband ultraviolet B light.(83)

Medical disorders involving collagen and connective tissues may also benefit from laser therapy. Monchromatic, coherent Low-Level Laser Therapy (LLLT) has anecdotally been found to improve healing time in **chronic cutaneous ulcerations**, but a recent review by Sobanko and Alster found evidence lacking to recommend its use for wound healing at this time.(84) 670-nm continuous-wave red light emitting diode (LED) light has also shown promise in speeding incisional **wound healing**, but further human studies are warranted.(85) **Keloids** (Figure 21.8) may benefit from 585 or 595-nm flashlamp PDL as an adjunct to excisional cold steel or CO_2 surgery.(86–88) **Morphea** (Figure 21.9) has also been reported to respond to PDL, although the mechanism of action remains unknown.(89) **Sarcoidosis** in various forms has also been successfully treated with laser therapy—**scar sarcoidosis** with the PDL (90) and the Q-switched ruby laser (91), and **lupus pernio** with the flashlamp PDL.(92) **Elastosis**

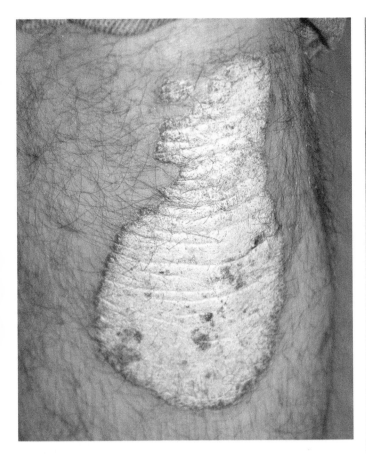

Figure 21.7 Psoriasis.

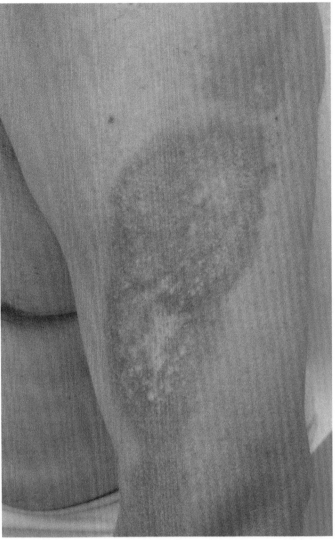

Figure 21.9 Morphea. (Photo courtesy of Scott M. Jackson, MD).

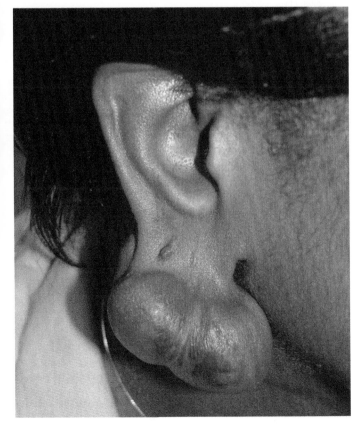

Figure 21.8 Keloid.

perforans serpiginosa has been reported to respond to PDL (93), although treatment failure with PDL and other lasers has also been reported.(94) Both **trichoepitheliomas** (Figure 21.10) and facial **angiofibromas** (adenoma sebaceum) of **tuberous sclerosis** (Figure 21.11) may be treated with both CO_2 and argon devices, although these lesions will likely recur with time.(95, 96)

Pigmentary disorders of a medical nature may also be treated by laser and light-based devices, particularly when melanin is the target chromophore. **Melasma** has shown improvement with Er:YAG, CO_2, and Q-Switched Alexandrite laser.(97, 98) It has also shown benefit with fractional photothermolysis, which, like the CO_2 laser targets collagen rather than pigment.(99) **Dermal melanocytosis**, such as that seen with **nevus of Ota** and **nevus of Ito** may be successfully treated with the Q-switched Nd:YAG or Q-switched Alexandrite lasers.(100) Pigmentary depositions caused by medications or other exposure may also be improved. **Argyria** responds to the Q-switched Nd:YAG (101), and **minocycline induced hyperpigmentation** (Figure 21.12) responds to both the Q-switched ruby and Q-switched Alexandrite devices. (102, 103)

187

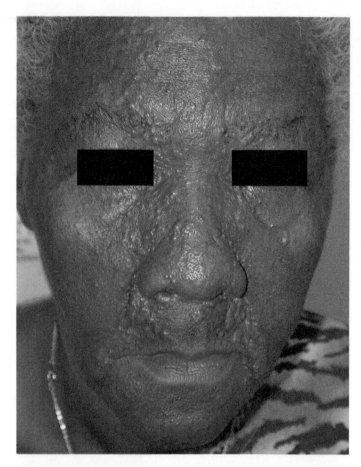

Figure 21.10 Trichepitheliomas.

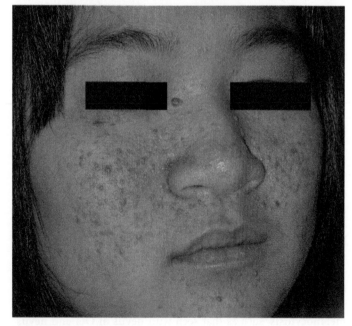

Figure 21.11 Tuberous Sclerosis.

SUMMARY

Although four of the most popular cutaneous procedures—botulinum toxins, fillers, chemical peels, and laser- and light-based therapies—are primarily considered aesthetic modalities, they also have myriad uses for treating medical conditions.

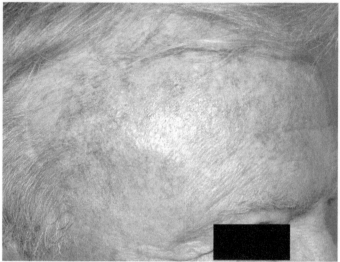

Figure 21.12 Hyperpigmentation secondary to chronic minocycline.

Indeed, the borders between aesthetic treatments and medical treatments are often very loosely drawn. As procedural aesthetic treatments continue to expand, they scope of medical problems to which they may be applied will likely also grow.

REFERENCES

1. Erbguth FJ. From poison to remedy: the chequered history of botulinum toxin. J Neural Transm 2008; 115(4): 559–65.
2. Carruthers A, Carruthers J. History of the cosmetic use of botulinum A exotoxin. Dermatol Surg 1998; 24(11): 1168–70.
3. Dressler D. Botulinum toxin drugs: future developments. J Neural Transm 2008; 115(4): 575–7.
4. Hornberger J, Grimes K, Naumann M et al. Recognition, diagnosis, and treatment of primary focal hyperhidrosis. J Am Acad Dermatol 2004; 51(2): 274–86.
5. Absar MS, Onwudike M. Efficacy of botulinum toxin type A in the treatment of focal axillary hyperhidrosis. Dermatol Surg 2008; 34(6): 751–5.
6. Whelchel DD, Brehmer TM, Brooks PM et al. Molecular targets of botulinum toxin at the mammalian neuromuscular junction. Mov Disord 2004; 9(Suppl 8): S7–S16.
7. Odderson IR. Long-term quantitative benefits of botulinum toxin type A in the treatment of axillary hyperhidrosis. Dermatol Surg 2002; 28(6): 480–3.
8. Heckmann M, Ceballos-Baumann AO, Plewig G. Botulinum toxin A for axillary hyperhidrosis (excessive sweating). N Engl J Med 2001; 344: 488–93.
9. Glogau RG. Botulinum A neurotoxin for axillary hyperhidrosis: no sweat Botox. Dermatol Surg 1998; 24: 817–9.
10. Tan SR, Solish N. Long-term efficacy and quality of life in the treatment of focal hyperhidrosis with botulinum toxin A. Dermatol Surg 2002; 28(6): 495–9.
11. Solish N, Bertucci V, Dansereau A et al. A Comprehensive approach to the recognition, diagnosis, and severity-based treatment of focal hyperhidrosis: Recommendations of the Canadian Hyperhidrosis Advisory Committee. Dermatol Surg 2007; 33(8): 908–23.
12. Lowe NJ, Yamauchi PS, Lask GP et al. Efficacy and safety of Botulinum toxin type A in the treatment of palmar hyperhidrosis: a double-blind, randomized, placebo-controlled study. Dermatol Surg 2002; 28(9): 822–7.
13. Zaiac M, Weiss E, Elgart G. Botulinum toxin therapy for palmar hyperhidrosis with ADG needle. Dermatol Surg 2000; 26(3): 230.
14. Shelley WB, Talanin NY, Shelley ED. Botulinum toxin therapy for palmar hyperhidrosis. J Am Acad Dermatol 1998; 38: 227–9.
15. Baumann L, Slezinger A, Halem M et al. Double-blind, randomized, placebo-controlled pilot study of the safety and efficacy of Myobloc (Botulinum Toxin Type B) for the treatment of palmar hyperhidrosis. Dermatol Surg 2005; 31(3): 263–70.

16. Santiago-Et-Sánchez-Mateos JL, Beà S, Fernández M et al. Botulinum toxin type A for the preventive treatment of intertrigo in a patient with Darier's disease and Inguinal hyperhidrosis. Dermatol Surg 2008; 34(12): 1733–7.

17. Kontochristopoulos G, Katsavou AN, Kalogirou O et al. Letter: botulinum toxin type A: an alternative symptomatic management of darier's disease. Dermatol Surg 2007; 33(7): 882–3.

18. Lapiere JC, Hirsh A, Gordon KB et al. Botulinum toxin type A for the treatment of Axillary Hailey–Hailey Disease. Dermatol Surg 2000; 26(4): 371–4.

19. Kang NG, Yoon TJ, Kim TH. Botulinum toxin type A as an effective adjuvant therapy for Hailey–Hailey Disease. Dermatol Surg 2002; 28(6): 543–4.

20. Tamura BM, Cucé LC, Souza RL, Levites J. Plantar hyperhidrosis and pitted keratolysis treated with botulinum toxin injection. Dermatol Surg 2004; 30: 1510–14.

21. Lee JB, Kim BS, Kim MB et al. A case of foul genital odor treated with botulinum toxin A. Dermatol Surg 2004; 30(9): 1233–5.

22. Wu JM, Mamelak AJ, Nussbaum R, McElgunn PSJ. Botulinum toxin A in the treatment of chromhidrosis. Dermatol Surg 2005; 31(8): 963–5.

23. Matarasso SL. Treatment of facial chromhidrosis with botulinum toxin type A. J Am Acad Dermatol 2005; 52(1): 89–91.

24. Kontochristopoulos G, Gregoriou S, Agiasofitou E et al. Letter: regression of relapsing dyshidrotic eczema after treatment of concomitant hyperhidrosis with botulinum toxin-A. Dermatol Surg 2007; 33(10): 1289–90.

25. Lonsdale-Eccles A, Leonard N, Lawrence C. Axillary hyperhidrosis: eccrine or apocrine? Clin Exp Dermatol 2003; 28(1): 2–7.

26. Yang TY, Jang TY. The value of local botulinum toxin A injection in the treatment of the pain of aphthous ulcer. Eur Arch Otorhinolaryngol 2009; 266(3): 445–8.

27. Sycha T, Graninger M, Auff E, Schnider P. Botulinum toxin in the treatment of Raynaud's phenomenon: a pilot study. Eur J Clin Invest 2004; 34(4): 312–3.

28. Van Beek AL, Lim PK, Gear AJ, Pritzker MR. Management of vasospastic disorders with botulinum toxin A. Plast Reconstr Surg 2007; 119(1): 217–26.

29. Kossintseva I, Barankin B. Improvement in both Raynaud disease and hyperhidrosis in response to botulinum toxin type A treatment. J Cutan Med Surg 2008; 12(4): 189–93.

30. Heckmann M, Heyer G, Brunner B, Plewig G. Botulinum toxin type A injection in the treatment of lichen simplex: an open pilot study. J Am Acad Dermatol 2002; 46(4): 617–9.

31. Weinfeld PK. Successful treatment of notalgia paresthetica with botulinum toxin type A. Arch Dermatol 2007; 143(8): 980–2.

32. Wollina U, Konrad H, Petersen S. Botulinum toxin in dermatology - beyond wrinkles and sweat. J Cosmet Dermatol 2005; 4(4): 223–7.

33. Eigelshoven S, Kruse R, Rauch L et al. Thelalgia in man: successful treatment with botulinum toxin. Arch Dermatol 2006; 142(9): 1242–3.

34. Klein AW, Elson ML. The history of substances for soft tissue augmentation. Dermatol Surg 2000; 26(12): 1096–105.

35. Milan MF, Bennett JE. Scleroderma en coup de sabre. Ann Plast Surg 1983; 10(5): 364–70.

36. Lapiere JC, Aasi S, Cook B, Montalvo A. Successful correction of depressed scars of the forehead secondary to trauma and morphea en coup de sabre by en bloc autologous dermal fat graft. Dermatol Surg 2000; 26(8): 793–7.

37. Sterodimas A, Huanquipaco JC, de Souza Filho S et al. Autologous fat transplantation for the treatment of Parry-Romberg syndrome. J Plast Reconstr Aesthet Surg 2008; [Epub ahead of print].

38. Stone J. Parry-Romberg syndrome: a global survey of 205 patients using the internet. Neurology 2003; 61(5): 674–6.

39. Wallace WD, Balkin SW, Kaplan L, Nelson S. The histologic host response to liquid silicone injections for prevention of pressure-related ulcers of the foot: a 38-year study. J Am Podiatr Med Assoc 2004; 94(6): 550–7.

40. van Schie CH, Whalley A, Vileikyte L et al. Efficacy of injected liquid silicone in the diabetic foot to reduce risk factors for ulceration: a randomized double-blind placebo-controlled trial. Diabetes Care 2000; 23(5): 634–8.

41. Balkin SW, Rea TH, Kaplan L. Silicone oil prevention of insensitive pressure ulcers. Int J Lepr Other Mycobact Dis 1997; 65(3): 372–4.

42. Balkin SW. Injectable silicone and the foot: a 41-year clinical and histologic history. Dermatol Surg 2005; 31: 1555–9.

43. Balkin SW. The fluid silicone prosthesis. Clin Podiatry 1984; 1(1): 145–64.

44. Jones D. HIV facial lipoatrophy: causes and treatment options. Dermatol Surg 2005; 31: 1519–29.

45. Prather CL, Jones DH. Liquid injectable silicone for soft tissue augmentation. Dermatol Ther 2006; 19(3): 159–68.

46. Kessler E, Flanagan K, Chia C et al. Comparison of alpha- and beta-hydroxy acid chemical peels in the treatment of mild to moderately severe facial acne vulgaris. Dermatol Surg 2008; 1: 45–50.

47. Zakopoulou N, Kontochristopoulos G. Superficial chemical peels. J Cosmet Dermatol 2006; 5(3): 246–53.

48. Robertson KM. Acne vulgaris. Facial Plast Surg Clin North Am 2004; 12(3): 347–55.

49. Briden ME. Alpha-hydroxyacid chemical peeling agents: case studies and rationale for safe and effective use. Cutis 2004; 73(2 Suppl): 18–24.

50. Lim JTE. Treatment of melasma using kojic acid in a gel containing hydroquinone and glycolic acid. Dermatol Surg 1999; 25(4): 282–4.

51. Grimes PE. The safety and efficacy of salicylic acid chemical peels in darker racial-ethnic groups. Dermatol Surg 1999; 25(1): 18–22.

52. Moy LS, Murad H, Moy RL. Glycolic acid peels for the treatment of wrinkles and photoaging. J Dermatol Surg Oncol 1993; 19(3): 243–6.

53. Brody HJ. Variations and comparisons in medium depth chemical peeling. J Dermatol Surg Oncol 1989; 15: 953–63.

54. Monheit GD. The Jessner's + TCA peel: a medium depth chemical peel. J Dermatol Surg Oncol 1989; 15: 945–50.

55. Coleman WP, Futrell JM. The glycolic acid trichloroacetic acid peel. J Dermatol Surg Oncol 1994; 20: 76–80.

56. Monheit GD, Prather CL. Chemical peels for precancerous skin lesions. In: MacFarlane DF, ed. A Practical Approach to Skin Cancer Management. New York: Springer, forthcoming edition, 2009.

57. Goldman A, Wollina U. Subdermal Nd-YAG Laser for axillary hyperhidrosis. Dermatol Surg 2008; 34(6): 756–62.

58. Kim IH, Seo SL, Oh CH. Minimally invasive surgery for axillary osmidrosis: combined operation with CO2 Laser and subcutaneous tissue remover. Dermatol Surg 1999; 25(11): 875–9.

59. Lapins J, Sartorius K, Emtestam L. Scanner-assisted carbon dioxide laser surgery: a retrospective follow-up study of patients with hidradenitis suppurativa. J Am Acad Dermatol 2002; 47(2): 280–5.

60. Finley EM, Ratz JL. Treatment of hidradenitis suppurativa with carbon dioxide laser excision and second-intention healing. J Am Acad Dermatol 1996; 34(3): 465–9.

61. Bernstein EF. Double-pass, low-fluence laser treatment using a large spot-size 1,450 nm laser improves acne. Lasers Surg Med 2009; 41(2): 116–21.

62. Laubach HJ, Astner S, Watanabe K et al. Effects of a 1,450 nm diode laser on facial sebum excretion. Lasers Surg Med 2009; 41(2): 110–5.

63. Munavalli GS, Weiss RA. Evidence for laser- and light-based treatment of acne vulgaris. Semin Cutan Med Surg 2008; 27(3): 207–11.

64. Jung JY, Choi YS, Yoon MY et al. Comparison of a pulsed dye laser and a combined 585/1,064-nm laser in the treatment of acne vulgaris. Dermatol Surg 2009; [Epub ahead of print].

65. Michael HG, Mitchel PG. 5-Aminolevulinic acid photodynamic therapy: where we have been and where we are going. Dermatol Surg 2004; 30(8): 1077–84.

66. Santos MA, Belo VG, Santos G. Effectiveness of photodynamic therapy with topical 5-Aminolevulinic acid and intense pulsed light versus intense pulsed light alone in the treatment of acne vulgaris: comparative study. Dermatol Surg 2005; 31(8): 910–5.

67. Sigurdsson V, Knulst AC, van Weelden H. Phototherapy of acne vulgaris with visible light. Dermatology 1997; 194(3): 256–60.

68. Tanzi EL, Lupton JR, Alster TS. Lasers in dermatology: four decades of progress. J Am Acad Dermatol 2003; 49(1): 1–31.

69. Woo SH, Ahn HH, Kim SN, Kye YC. Treatment of vascular skin lesions with the variable pulse 595 nm pulsed dye laser. Dermatol Surg 2006; 32(1): 41–8.

70. Schroeter CA, von Below SH, Neumann HAM. Effective treatment of rosacea using intense pulsed light systems. Dermatol Surg 2005; 31(10): 1285–9.

71. Jasim ZF, Woo WK, Handley JM. Long-pulsed (6-ms) pulsed dye laser treatment of rosacea-associated telangiectasia using subpurpuric clinical threshold. Dermatol Surg 2004; 30(1): 37–40.

72. Mark KA, Sparacio RM, Voigt A et al. Objective and quantitative improvement of rosacea-associated erythema after intense pulsed light treatment. Dermatol Surg 2003; 29(6): 600–4.

73. Laube S, Lanigan SW. Laser treatment of rosacea. J Cosmet Dermatol 2002; 1(4): 188–95.

74. Apikian M, Goodman GJ, Roberts S. Management of mild to moderate rhinophyma with a 1,450-nm diode laser: report of five patients. Dermatol Surg 2007; 33(7): 847–50.

75. Haas A, Wheeland RG. Treatment of massive rhinophyma with the carbon dioxide laser. J Dermatol Surg Oncol 1990; 16(7): 645–9.

76. Harries PG, Brockbank MJ, Shakespeare PG, Carruth JA. Treatment of hereditary haemorrhagic telangiectasia by the pulsed dye laser. J Laryngol Otol 1997; 111(11): 1038–41.

77. Grover S, Grewal RS, Verma R et al. Osler-Weber-Rendu syndrome: a case report with familial clustering. Indian J Dermatol Venereol Leprol 2009; 75: 100.

78. Lapidoth M, Ad-El D, David M, Azaria R. Treatment of angiokeratoma of fordyce with pulsed dye laser. Dermatol Surg 2006; 32(9): 1147–50.

79. Özdemir M, Baysal I, Engin B, Özdemir S. Treatment of angiokeratoma of fordyce with long-pulse neodymium-doped yttrium aluminium garnet laser. Dermatol Surg 2009; 35(1): 92–7.

80. Christian MM, Moy RL. Treatment of Hailey–Hailey Disease (or Benign Familial Pemphigus) using short pulsed and short dwell time carbon dioxide lasers. Dermatol Surg 1999; 25(8): 661–3.

81. Beier C, Kaufmann R. Efficacy of erbium: YAG laser ablation in Darier disease and Hailey-Hailey disease. Arch Dermatol 1999; 135: 423–7.

82. Chen TM, Wanitphakdeedecha R, Nguyen TH. Carbon dioxide laser ablation and adjunctive destruction for Darier-White Disease (Keratosis Follicularis). Dermatol Surg 2008; 34(10): 1431–4.

83. Raulin C, Grema H. Psoriasis vulgaris. An indication for lasers? Hautarzt 2003; 54(3): 242–7.

84. Sobanko JF, Alster TS. Efficacy of low-level laser therapy for chronic cutaneous ulceration in humans: a review and discussion. Dermatol Surg 2008; 34(8): 991–1000.

85. Erdle BJ, Brouxhon S, Kaplan M et al. Effects of continuous-wave (670-nm) red light on wound healing. Dermatol Surg 2008; 34(3): 320–5.

86. Alster TS. Laser treatment of hypertrophic scars, keloids and striae. Dermatol Clin 1997; 15: 419–29.

87. Alster TS. Improvement of erythematous and hypertrophic scars by the 585 nm flashlamp-pumped pulse dye laser. Ann Plast Surg 1994; 32: 186–90.

88. Goldman MP, Fitzpatrick RE. Laser treatment of scars. Dermatol Surg 1995; 21: 685–7.

89. Eisen D, Alster TS. Use of a 585 nm Pulsed Dye Laser for the Treatment of Morphea. Dermatol Surg 2002; 28(7): 615–6.

90. Holzmann RD, Astner S, Forschner T, Sterry G. Scar sarcoidosis in a child: case report of successful treatment with the pulsed dye laser. Dermatol Surg 2008; 34(3): 393–6.

91. Grema H, Greve B, Raulin C. Scar sarcoidosis treatment with the Q-switched ruby laser. Lasers Surg Med 2002; 30: 398–400.

92. Cliff S, Felix RH, Singh L et al. The successful treatment of lupus pernio with the flashlamp pulsed dye laser. J Cutan Laser Ther 1999; 1: 49–52.

93. Kaufman AJ. Treatment of elastosis perforans serpiginosa with the flashlamp pulsed dye laser. Dermatol Surg 2000; 26(11): 1060–2.

94. Saxena M, Tope WD. Response of elastosis perforans serpiginosa to pulsed CO2, Er:YAG, and dye lasers. Dermatol Surg 2003; 29(6): 677–8.

95. Song MG, Park KB, Lee ES. Resurfacing of facial angiofibromas in tuberous sclerosis patients using CO2 laser with flashscanner. Dermatol Surg 1999; 25(12): 970–3.

96. Arndt KA. Adenoma sebaceum: successful treatment with the argon laser. Plast Reconstruct Surg 1982; 70: 91–3.

97. Manaloto RMP, Tina Alster. Erbium: YAG laser resurfacing for refractory melasma. Dermatol Surg 1999; 25(2): 121–3.

98. Nouri K, Bowes L, Chartier T et al. Combination treatment of melasma with pulsed CO2 laser followed by Q-Switched alexandrite laser: a pilot study. Dermatol Surg 1999; 25(6): 494–7.

99. Rokhsar CK, Fitzpatrick RE. The treatment of melasma with fractional photothermolysis: a pilot study. Dermatol Surg 2005; 31(12): 1645–50.

100. Chan HH, Alam M, Kono T, Dover JS. Clinical application of lasers in Asians. Dermatol Surg 2002; 28(7): 556–63.

101. Rhee DY, Chang SE, Lee MW et al. Treatment of argyria after colloidal silver ingestion using Q-Switched 1,064-nm Nd:YAG laser. Dermatol Surg 2008; 34(10): 1427–30.

102. Friedman IS, Shelton RM, Phelps RG. Minocycline-induced hyperpigmentation of the tongue: successful treatment with the Q-Switched Ruby laser. Dermatol Surg 2002; 28(3): 205–9.

103. Alster TS, Gupta SN. Minocycline-induced hyperpigmentation treated with a 755-nm Q-Switched alexandrite laser. Dermatol Surg 2004; 30(9): 1201–4.

22 Secondary rhytidectomy and revision procedures
Seth A Yellin and Anita B Sethna

UNDERSTANDING YOUR PATIENT

Like all aesthetic interventions, the goal of secondary surgical facial enhancement should be to make the patient look better while not telegraphing that something has been done; an unoperated, natural appearance is always the desired outcome. However, for some patients a realistic opportunity for success may be compromised due to previous procedures. Creating a face that is harmonious, vibrant, youthful and natural may be more difficult and in some cases, unachievable. Most often, however, secondary aesthetic facial surgery simply requires that excellent surgical and aesthetic judgment and skill be applied, in a routine fashion, to achieve the desired outcome.

Though the initial surgical concepts are the same regardless of whether you are performing a primary or secondary operation, the timing of intervention, the choice of techniques and possibly, the need to address aesthetic issues created by previous procedures makes secondary facial aesthetic surgery unique.

The initial patient consultation is an important first step in establishing a strategy for success. For patients presenting for secondary facial surgery, the tone of the discussion may be influenced by their previous experience, which may have been a negative one. This makes creating an initial positive experience for the patient even more critical. As the surgeon, you should provide a comfortable, nonthreatening environment, which will encourage openness with your patient. Avoid barriers between you and your patient such as a desk and instead, sit next to them in front of a mirror.(1) This is perhaps the easiest way to put your patient at ease. Remember that it is often uncomfortable for the patient to discuss their concerns, especially if they were unhappy with their initial cosmetic surgery. By listening and valuing the patient's input, you reinforce the point that you respect their opinions and understand their issues. As with primary surgery, when discussing secondary procedures, the patient's motivations and desires remain paramount to the discussion. Don't neglect their concerns in favor of what you feel are more pressing aesthetic problems. Of course, if the patient is receptive, you should point out all of the aesthetic issues you deem to be important, but not to the exclusion of the patient's chief concerns. A basic rule to keep in mind is if you correct what bothers the patient rather than what bothers you, your patient will be happy and satisfied. However, if you push the patient into correcting a facial feature that was not really a concern of theirs, and you have a surgical complication, the patient will be much less understanding and will most likely be quite unhappy. As the surgeon, your goal should be to create happy patients, which ultimately is a formula for your own happiness.

Though the consultation is a time to listen, assess the problems at hand, formulate a plan for correction and educate, just as importantly, it is a time to bond with your patient. It is also a time to determine if you are compatible, share a similar aesthetic vision and to decide if you are willing to assume the care of the patient. Be cautious if the patient is concerned with problems that you don't appreciate, is overtly hostile toward the previous surgeon or if the patient is overly flattering to you. If you decide to offer the patient surgery, a frank discussion must be had regarding the achievable goals and limitations that may exist due to the patient's current state of aging and consequences of the previous procedures. An honest discussion must occur in order to establish realistic expectations. This is critical if your goal is to satisfy the patient and maintain professional credibility.

To help guide you in your assessment, several issues need to be considered that make a secondary consultation unique. In addition to your routine aesthetic assessment, several questions need to be clarified. If you were not the initial surgeon, what are the reasons the patient is not returning to that physician? What exactly was done for the patient? Does the patient feel that their initial concerns were satisfactorily addressed? Were they happy with the results? When was the previous surgery? Is secondary surgery intended to be corrective of primary surgical intervention or a separate aesthetic issue altogether? Were the incisions used appropriate for your purposes? Finally, was the previous experience positive? If not, your preoperative discussion must not only educate the patient but may have to debunk preconceived notions they have regarding the procedure(s) you will need to perform. Patient may be less anxious of surgery if things went well the first time, but more anxious than they would otherwise be if things did not. These issues may require more hand holding for the patient and you need to be prepared for this both before and after surgery.

Additionally, understanding the patient's satisfaction with their previous surgical experience provides insight into their expectations and ability to achieve happiness from aesthetic surgical enhancement. It is important to keep in mind that as cosmetic surgeons, though we operate on the face, our ultimate goal should be to improve our patients' inner sense of well being. For some individuals, though they are focused on improving their external appearance with the hope of improving their self-esteem, their problems are more than skin deep. Ideally, these patients are identified during the initial consultation and are guided in a different direction rather than towards secondary surgery.

To better understand the patient's "natural look" when they were younger, to gain insight into the patient's assessment of their previous surgical result and to determine realistic goals for surgical rejuvenation, it is helpful to study old photographs of the patient from several angles and ages when available. Review photographs of the patient when they were about 10 years younger (a realistic goal for rejuvenation) and ideally when they were much younger (20s and 30s). This will help you understand the patient's "look" when they were at the peak of their adult attractiveness. This will also help guide your aesthetic judgment. Nothing makes a patient look less like them self than, for example, over lifting a brow when, as a younger individual, their brows were low and full. If you can recreate the anatomy of their youth, you will create a happy patient. Of course, if the patient has a particular aesthetic issue that they never liked, then by all means, address it. But if the patient was generally proud of their appearance when they were younger, your goal should be to re-establish that look as reasonably as possible.

PREOPERATIVE CONSIDERATIONS IN SECONDARY FACIAL REJUVENATION

Be sensitive to the general aging of the patient. If the body and hands look very old, facial rejuvenation may create aesthetic disharmony and these observations should be discussed. This may be particularly relevant in secondary surgery patients as they are more often older individuals. Another consideration should be the general health of the patient. Even if a patient has significant aesthetic issues that are amenable to surgical correction, under no circumstance should you suspend your good medical judgment and be pressured to operate on a patient unless they are medically sound. The good news is that the risk of postoperative complication from face-lift procedures are similar in patients older than 75 years compared to a younger cohort, when matched for American Society of Anesthesiologists (ASA) physical class. In properly selected patients who are active and whose ASA class is either 1 (a normal healthy patient) or 2 (a patient with mild systemic disease), a face-lift is just as safe in older individuals as it is in middle-aged patients.(2) To reduce the risk of complications for all of your patients seeking facial rejuvenation, regardless of age, there are several issues that must be addressed before surgery. Since hematoma formation is the most common complication from face-lift surgery, with a reported incidence of between 1% and 15% (3–9) and has been correlated with a preoperative systolic blood pressure above 150 mm Hg (10), it is critical that the patient's primary care physician control their blood pressure, well before the planned procedure. Since antihypertensive medications are frequently prescribed in the age group of patients seeking secondary rhytidectomy, it is important to counsel them to take their medications the morning of surgery with a small sip of water and to have the medications with them for after surgery. Additionally, aspirin, nonsteroidal antiinflammatory medications (NSAIDs), vitamin E, ginko biloba, ginseng, and garlic and ginger supplements have all been shown to have adverse clotting effects and are to be avoided for 2 weeks before and after surgery. (11) As a matter of routine, all herbal and vitamin supplements should be stopped for 2 weeks before and after surgery. The use of tobacco products causes a 12-fold increase in the risk of skin flap necrosis.(12) To reduce this risk, all tobacco products (including nicotine patches) must be stopped for a minimum of at least 2 weeks before and after surgery. Even with smoking cessation, the incidence of skin flap necrosis is still higher in previous smokers when compared with those who have never smoked (13) and this must be explained to the patient preoperatively. Furthermore, a complete medical history must be obtained prior to surgery to identify conditions that may negatively impact the patient's postoperative course such as Raynaud's disease, which has been correlated with skin flap necrosis (14) and Ehlers-Danlos syndrome,

which predisposes to widened scars. Finally, a detailed discussion of the risks of surgery must be reviewed with the patient, even if they have had the procedure done before.

As the surgeon, be cognizant of underlying facial asymmetries and proportions and point them out to the patient preoperatively. The patient will always study their face carefully after surgery and may detect subtle asymmetries that they did not notice preoperatively. If you point them out before surgery and discuss the aesthetic implications of these structural issues, it is an explanation. Postoperatively, if the patient is the first to point out these asymmetries, your response will be interpreted as an excuse.

Finally, photo-document all patients before aesthetic surgery. It is not only considered to be the standard-of care, but is a critical record of the patient's preoperative condition and will be crucial when assessing the patient's results postoperatively.

Be as meticulous with your photographs as you are with surgery. Control for focal distance, lighting, eye, head and body position, distance from the background and exposure. Reproducibility and consistency should be your goal.

REASONS FOR SECONDARY FACIAL AESTHETIC SURGERY

There are many different clinical scenarios that call for either revision surgery or a planned second procedure. It is helpful to examine the motivations of the patient, as they will guide your clinical management. If you were the initial surgeon and your patient is dissatisfied with their results because they feel that their concerns were not fully corrected you must not be defensive but instead take the time to understand the patient's objections. Leave your ego at the door. If the patient is unhappy with the initial surgery, regardless of whether you or anyone else feels that the results were good, the operation was not successful.(1) That doesn't mean that anything was done incorrectly or that in your opinion, anything more could have been done to correct the problem. If, in fact that is the case, you need to explain your assessment to the patient, while being sympathetic to their concerns. However, if there is room for improvement it is often a good idea to address the issue in a forthright, nonevasive manner. To maintain a positive patient relationship, addressing the issue with a revision procedure in a timely manner, dictated by good surgical judgment, is advised.

If the secondary procedure is intended to correct a problem created by previous surgery performed either by you or another surgeon, emotional support and an understanding, supportive, nonjudgmental attitude are essential. As with all soft tissue procedures, tincture of time will often allow the problem to "fix" itself. However, with time, some problems can be exacerbated due to scar contracture, abnormal scar deposition or scar widening. If conservative measures such as serial steroid injections and massage fail to address the issue, and the patient is concerned, revision surgery is indicated. It is generally recommended that any revision procedure be delayed for at least 1 year from surgery. However, if in your surgical judgment the problem is not going to resolve with time, then earlier intervention is indicated. It is important to stress that any revision procedure should only be undertaken if the patient is bothered by the problem. Even if you, as the surgeon, feel that a better result is achievable and are willing to do the revision at no cost to the patient, additional complications can occur which may make the situation worse. Therefore, the patient must appreciate the value of revision and be willing to assume the additional risk and recovery.

When patients present with aesthetic issues that either were not addressed initially or developed over time as they continued to age, there is no urgency or emotional overtones to the discussion. This makes communication much more comfortable for both parties. However, if the procedure(s) were successful but did not "last" as long as they had been told or expected, some additional time and discussion may be necessary so that realistic expectations for the next procedure can be established. Overall, in these clinical circumstances, the timing of surgery will depend on more mundane concerns such as mutual convenience, downtime and cost.

AESTHETIC INTERVENTIONS

The surgical goals and concepts are the same regardless of whether you are performing primary or secondary facial rejuvenation. Skin is the material with which the surgeon works and it must look its best to make the patient look their best. Therefore, sun related skin changes such as rhytids, hyperpigmentation and spider veins are treated with either ablative or nonablative skin therapy. Preoperative Botox® is helpful as a biological dressing, keeping the skin resting while it is healing after ablative treatment for facial rhytidosis in areas such as the forehead, glabella, crow's feet and white lip. Ongoing Botox® therapy may be indicated to prolong the effects of resurfacing. Additionally, to optimize results and maintain improvement, topical daily skin care is recommended and should include exfoliation, hydration, collagen stimulation, color correction and broad-spectrum sun protection. Gravitational changes, i.e., skin and muscle laxity, must be addressed with surgical soft tissue repositioning and skin resection. Finally, volumetric loss, deficiency or redistribution, particularly in the mid-face, naso-jugal fold (tear trough), and cheek highlight areas, may be corrected with surgical repositioning of deep tissues (e.g., a mid-face, sub-periosteal lift), implants, and/or the use of injectable fillers (e.g., hyaluronic acid), collagen stimulants (e.g., Sculptra), or fat injections. These interventions will help to reestablish a natural heart shape to the female face, with the mid-face being the widest vertical third of the face, counteracting the elongation and squaring off of the lower face that occurs with age. Properly placed mid-facial volume will also create a smooth transition from the lower eyelid to the cheek, creating a unified aesthetic unit. This creates a vertically short lower eyelid, volumized medial cheek and a lateral cheek highlight, all of which lend a youthful appearance to the face. Realize that as surgeons, we tend to divide the face into isolated aesthetic units so that we may discuss and correct various problem areas on the face. However, most people view the face and neck as one unified aesthetic unit. Therefore, it is critical that when rejuvenating a face we recognize this fact and, when possible, correct skin textural changes, laxity and volume loss to create a harmonious and natural facial appearance.

Additionally, if the patient is receptive, lip architecture should be reestablished. When altering the lips, unless the patient specifically requests a fuller look, your goal should be to reestablish the anatomy of their youth, not necessarily to create an idealized lip aesthetic. When volumizing the lip area, several points can be made. Proportionate lip volume with the lower lip being about one third fuller than the upper lip, particularly in the central one third, looks most attractive. If lacking, the vermillion border and philtral columns should be strengthened. An excessively full white upper lip, which can occur due to over zealous filling of vertical lip rhytids, should be avoided, as it can lend a simian appearance to the face. Additionally, the labial-mandibular grooves, a.k.a. the marionette lines, should be volumized and the corners of the lip made to curl upward slightly.

Another important consideration is to reestablish a pleasing neck contour. When patients present for secondary cervicofacial rhytidectomy, recrudescence of neck skin laxity and platysmal bands or cervical irregularities following previous surgery are frequent complaints. This often necessitates a secondary face-lift with wide cervical skin undermining and muscle plication to correct skin and muscle issues. To address contour irregularities fat sculpting, fat repositioning or fat grafting may be indicated.

Older patients requesting secondary facial rejuvenation often have skin that has lost a substantial amount of elasticity, which has both favorable and unfavorable consequences. Less elasticity often leads to very thin and aesthetically acceptable scars, as there is less intrinsic tension on the closure. However, inelastic skin that has undergone previous face-lift surgery has a propensity to reveal misdirection of the lateral cheek skin rhytids, which should follow the relaxed skin tension lines. This gives an upward sweep appearance to the cheek, which is very unnatural. Thus, in revision rhytidectomy surgery, to avoid this problem, a less vertical, more posterior redirection of the cheek skin or composite flap is indicated. The surgeon must also decide if incision placement from previous surgery is appropriate, and may be used again or, if it needs to be modified. To assess this, one must consider personal preferences, the current hairline, ear lobule position, tragal architecture, how well the scars healed previously and the degree of cervical skin laxity, which will dictate the length of the posterior cervical scars. Under most circumstance, it is preferred in men and women, for both primary and secondary rhytidectomy procedures, to use a retro-tragal incision design. For most men, it is even more important to maintain surgical anonymity than it is for women and in most cases after presenting both pretragal and posttragal options to male patients, men prefer to shave the tragus or get laser hair removal rather than have a visible scar in front of their ear. Even if the incision curves inward just above the tragus and follows a natural crease, a pretragal incision can always be seen. It is important to remind your patients that they are trading skin laxity for a scar. As the surgeon, it is your job to hide the scars and close them meticulously and of course, it is the patients "job" to heal well. In most cases, the trade off is well worth it. Of course, in secondary face-lift surgery, scars already exist so the risk-reward ratio is even more favorable.

When performing a secondary cervicofacial rhytidectomy, it is recommended to execute each surgical maneuver as you would with a primary procedure, only modify the direction and tension of tissue repositioning and the amount of tissue to be excised. However, it is also important to have a surgical fall back position. That is, if things are not going well, for example during submuscular aponeurotic system (SMAS) elevation, the tissue plane may be scarred by previous surgery or atrophic due to the patient's

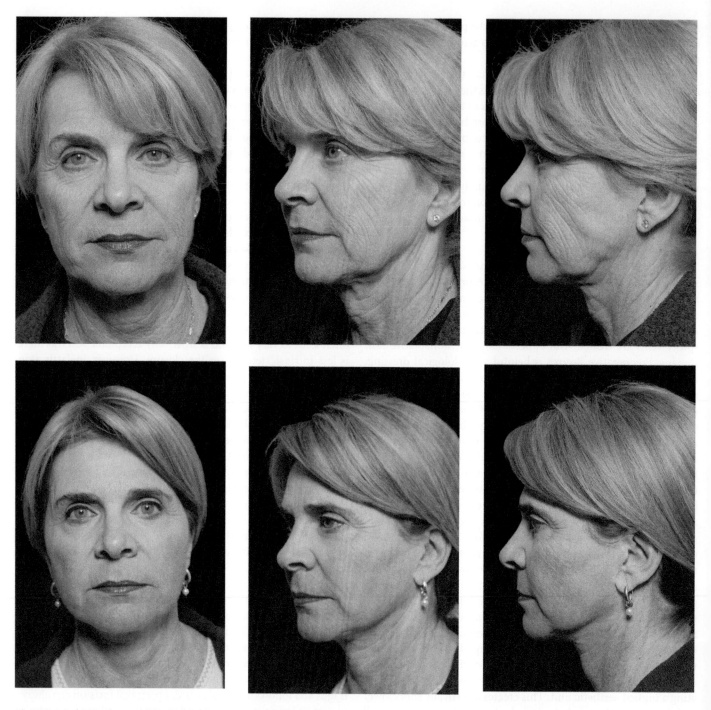

Figure 22.1 Before & after secondary facelift, blepharoplasty & laser resurfacing.

age and you may need to convert to a SMASectomy plication technique rather than a SMAS flap and imbrication procedure. Remember, this is cosmetic surgery. Patient safety comes first.(1)

SECONDARY CERVICOFACIAL RHYTIDECTOMY TECHNIQUE, PEARLS & DETAILS

For patients who are focused on recurrence of skin laxity of the lateral cheek and jowl only, a lateral cheek lift using a SMAS flap and imbrication technique is routinely done. If the SMAS is atrophic or significantly adherent due to previous surgery, a plication technique with or without a SMASectomy is recommended.

However, for patients who present with some degree of recurrent cervical laxity with or without cervical fat excess, a complete secondary cervicofacial rhytidectomy is indicated.(Figure 22.1)

The operation begins by marking the patient in the upright position in the preoperative holding area, which allows you to determine the effects of gravity on the facial tissues. (Figure 22.2) The incision is marked to begin about 3 cm above the ear in the temple hairline and curve inferiorly to the helical root. It follows the contours of the ear in a retro-tragal fashion, falls into the facial-lobule junction and then onto the conchal bowl, not in the postauricular sulcus as the scar tends to migrate onto the mastoid over time. It makes a right angle turn at the level of the common

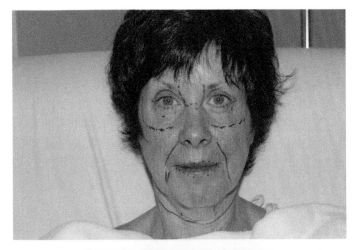

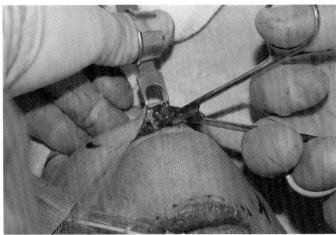

Figure 22.3 Cervical dissection, subcutaneous plane developed.

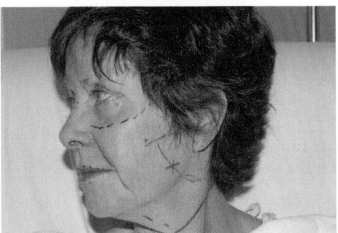

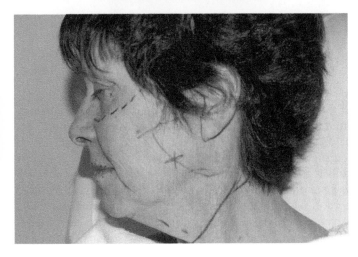

Figure 22.2 Preoperative facial markings.

crus and then follows the posterior hairline for a distance determined by cervical laxity, typically between 3 and 6 centimeters. When actually making the incision in this area, a trichophytic technique is employed; that is, the skin is incised at an extreme bevel just inside the hairline to preserve hair follicles and encourage hair growth through the scar. Rarely is it recommended or desirable to create a pretragal incision, even for men, or follow the temple tuft to preserve the sideburn, as the scar can often be seen, even with the most careful closure. The temple hair-line can be

kept at the same level by redirecting the temple flap more posteriorly and less vertically. If a sideburn incision is utilized, a trichophytic incision is performed. If the scar is visible postoperatively, micro-follicular hair unit transfer can be used to camouflage the scar. To correct an excessively high temporal hairline or to repair an area of alopecia from previous surgery, hair grafts can be harvested, divided and placed at the time of secondary facelift surgery or as a separate procedure.

During surgery, the patient is intubated and an intravenous antibiotic, which covers gram-positive bacteria, is administered. To eliminate the risk of bladder distension, the patient is catheterized for any procedure lasting more than 3 hours, which should make the patient more comfortable resulting in lower perioperative blood pressure. This will reduce the risk of postoperative hematoma, which appears to be most closely linked to perioperative hypertension.(11)

Approximately 20 cc of lidocaine 0.75% with epinephrine 1:150,000 is routinely injected in the neck and then the face and neck are prepped and draped in a sterile fashion. As an alternative, one may choose to use plain 0.5% lidocaine. This is supported by Jones and Grover (9) who reviewed more than 900 patients undergoing cervicofacial rhytidectomies, and concluded that the elimination of adrenaline from the injection fluid is the only factor that correlates in a statistically significant manner with hematoma reduction. It is felt that one avoids the rebound effect after the adrenaline effect wears off, which can lead to delayed bleeding that was not detected and controlled during surgery. The authors also claim that operative time does not increase more than 5 minutes per side.

An incision is made in the submental crease and a subcutaneous plane developed. (Figure 22.3) Wide pretunneling using a 2.7 mm blunt tipped liposuction cannula, without suction, between the anterior borders of the sternocleidomastoid (SCM) muscles is performed and the dissection carried inferiorly to the level of the thyroid cartilage. (Figure 22.4) If indicated, liposuction is then performed with the same cannula. A thin layer of fat must be left on the skin flap to maintain a natural appearance of the neck. Wide subcutaneous undermining is then accomplished using scissor dissection with care taken to preserve the marginal mandibular nerve.(Figure 22.5) Patients undergoing secondary

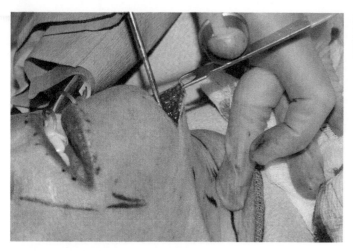

Figure 22.4 Cervical dissection, pretunneling with cannula.

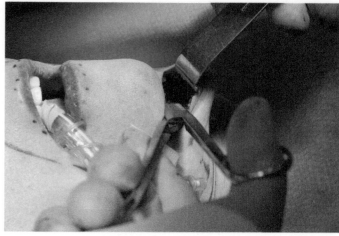

Figure 22.5 Cervical dissection, wide undermining.

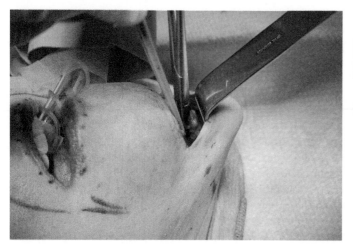

Figure 22.6 Interplatysmal fat removal.

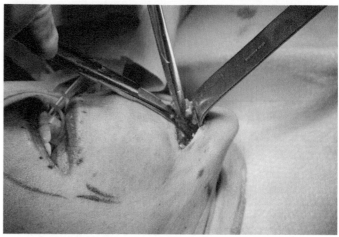

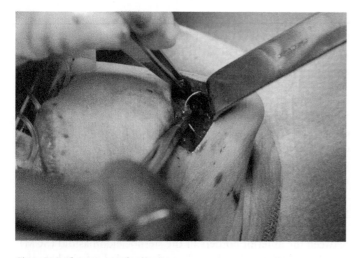

Figure 22.7 Platysma muscle plication.

facelifts may be at particular risk for marginal mandibular nerve injury due to fibrosis and adherence of the subcutaneous tissues to the platysma. Furthermore, older individuals may have a very thin, atrophic platysma, which will afford little protection to the

nerve. The "danger zone" for injury to this nerve is from the angle of the mandible to its crossing by the facial artery and extends from the inferior border of the mandible to a parallel line 3 cm below.(15) After the cervical skin is elevated, additional fat contouring may be done under direct vision. The interplatysmal fat is then grasped, clamped with a Kelly clamp, bipolar cauterized and excised.(Figure 22.6) This helps to clearly identify the medial borders of the platysma and debulks sub-platysmal soft tissue centrally, which facilitates the creation of a pleasing cervicomental angle. Transverse cutting of the platysma is nonanatomic and unnecessary. The medial platysmal borders are then plicated with multiple, buried 3–0 PDS sutures. (Figure 22.7) Hemostasis is confirmed using a lighted retractor (Figure 22.8) and the submental incision closed with interrupted, 5–0 plain gut sutures in a vertical mattress fashion to prevent depression of the scar, which can accentuate chin ptosis.

If the chin appears ptotic, which gives the lower face a very aged look, as a consequence of previous face-lift surgery or advanced age, a fat flip-flop-flap may be an appropriate remedy. To execute this flap, there must be adequate subcutaneous fat in the central neck; otherwise free fat transfer may be indicated. If there is sufficient fat present, once the submental incision is made, the neck

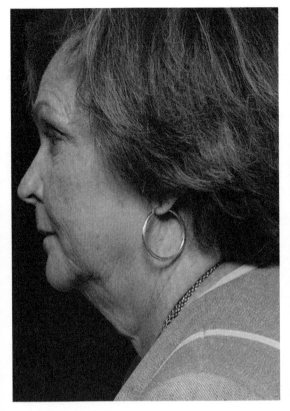

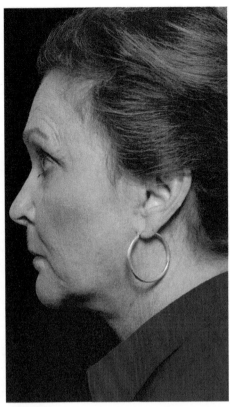

Figure 22.9 Witches chin deformity correction.

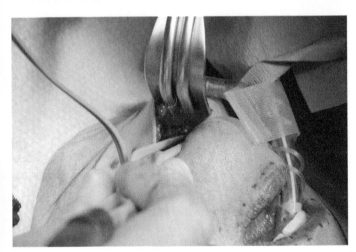

Figure 22.8 Hemostasis achieved using a lighted retractor.

skin and fat are separated in the subcutaneous plane with most of the fat left attached to the platysma. The fat is then incised transversely, approximately 3 to 4 centimeters inferior to the initial submental incision. The width of the cut is approximately 3 to 4 centimeters. Vertical incisions are then made on either side of the transverse incision back towards the submental incision. The fat is then retro-dissected off and between the platysma muscles and left pedicled just inferior to the submental incision. The soft tissues of the chin are then elevated for approximately 2 centimeters and the fat flap tucked under the elevated chin tissues and sutured into position. The submental skin incision is then closed in an interrupted vertical mattress fashion as described above. This provides vascularized soft tissue bulk and corrects the ptotic or witches chin

deformity.(Figure 22.9) If the chin has insufficient anterior projection leading to a short cervical-mental distance, an anatomic chin implant is recommended. It should be placed in the subperiostel plane at the time of rhytidectomy.(Figure 22.10)

The right face followed by the left face is then dissected. The periauricular incision is made following the preoperative markings and the proper subcutaneous plane developed sharply. A 2.7 mm liposuction cannula, without suction, is used to pretunnel the cheek flap in the developed subcutaneous plane. (Figure 22.11) The posterior skin flap is then sharply elevated in a subcutaneous plane and connected with the previous cervical dissection. (Figure 22.12) Care is taken to preserve the greater auricular and spinal accessory nerves as they emerge from the posterior border of the SCM muscle. The greater auricular nerve is the most common nerve injury during rhytidectomy and may be at increased risk with revision surgery. It emerges from Erb's point, which can be found at the posterior border of the SCM muscle, at the junction of the superior and inferior one-half of the muscle, approximately 6.5 cm below the external auditory canal. It travels under the SMAS and platysma to reach the anterior border of the SCM. Terminal branches from the main trunk travel in the groove between the SCM and the parotid fascia inferior to the ear and preauricular area. Care should be taken when dissecting as the skin can be quite thin and adherent to the muscle below the earlobe and violation of the SMAS/platysma layer can occur inadvertently, especially in revision surgery.(11) If the nerve is injured, primary repair is recommended.

In general, cheek skin elevation is then carried subcutaneously for approximately 6 cm and connected with the previously elevated cervical flap. The SMAS is then incised approximately 3 cm in front of the ear from the inferior border of the zygoma to the mandibluar border and a sub-SMAS elevation carried out

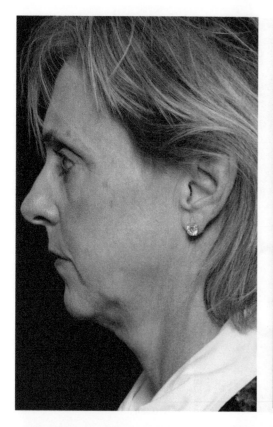

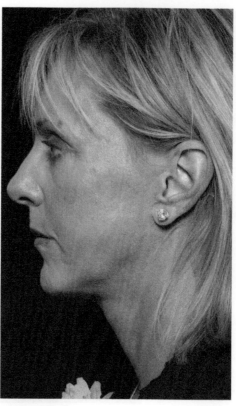

Figure 22.10 Before & after facelift with chin implant.

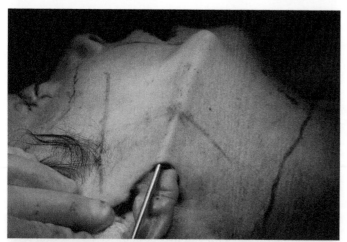

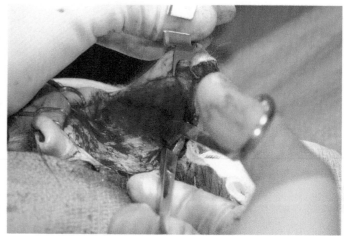

Figure 22.12 Postauricular dissection.

for 3 to 4 cm. Vertical spreading dissection is recommended in the direction of the facial nerve with care to be directly beneath the SMAS layer.(Figure 22.13) A strip of SMAS is then removed from in front of the ear and may be used for soft tissue grafting if needed. (Figure 22.14) The SMAS flap is then retro-displaced posteriorly and superiorly and secured with 3–0 PDS horizontal mattress sutures.(Figure 22.15) The first suture is placed at the point of maximum flap mobility which is determined preoperatively at the time of marking and is usually located about 3 cm inferior to the EAC at a point 3 cm anterior to the ear. It is then secured to the parotico-masseteric fascia at a point about level with the EAC just in front of the ear. Multiple sutures are then used to complete the SMAS imbrication.

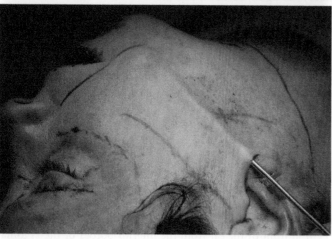

Figure 22.11 Cheek flap pretunneling with cannula.

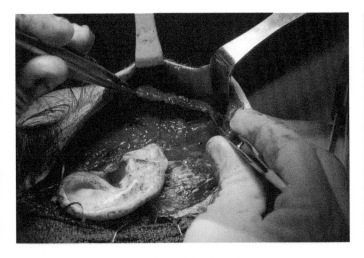

Figure 22.13 Facial dissection with SMAS flap elevated.

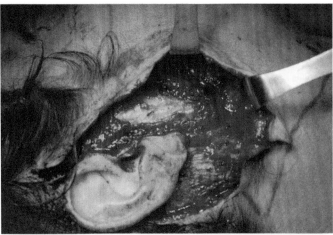

Figure 22.14 Strip of SMAS fascia removed.

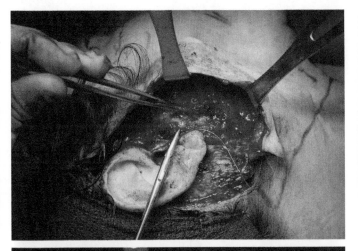

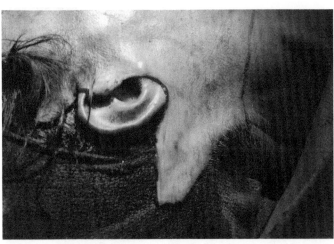

Figure 22.16 Skin flap re-draped posterior-superiorly.

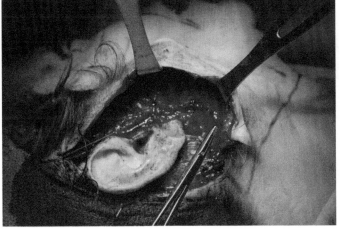

Figure 22.15 SMAS flap retro-displaced posterior-superiorly.

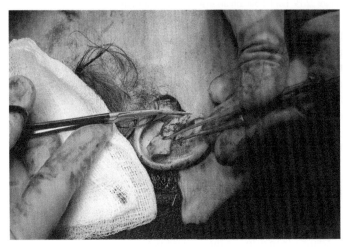

Figure 22.17 Excess skin excised.

Bi-polar cautery on a low setting is used throughout the procedure and meticulous hemostasis is confirmed prior to wound closure. The skin is then brushed with a surgical gauze sponge posteriorly and superiorly, not pulled tightly, and the flap secured with temporary staples at the helical root and at the high point of the flap posteriorly. (Figure 22.16) The excess skin is then trimmed following the contours of the ear. (Figure 22.17) The skin flap is left a bit excessive at the tragus and trimmed of all subcutaneous fat. (Figure 22.18) In a male facelift a Colorado tip cautery is used to ablate hair follicles in the area of the tragus. When trimming

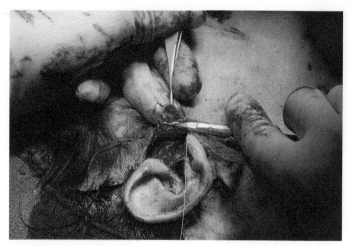

Figure 22.18 Tragal skin defatted.

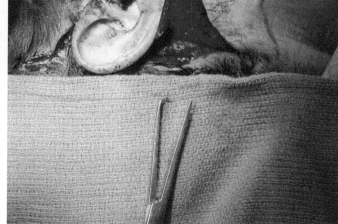

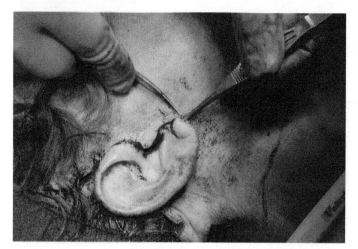

Figure 22.19 Ear lobule intentionally bunched upward.

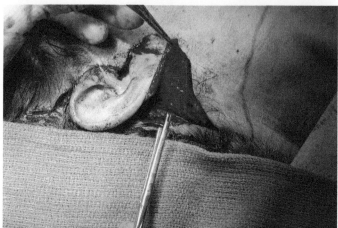

the flap, the earlobe is intentionally bunched upward a bit to avoid postoperative inferior displacement. (Figure 22.19) Posteriorly along the hairline, the skin flap excess is determined using a Pitanguy flap-marking forceps and trimmed.(Figure 22.20) The judgment of flap re-direction, tension of pull and amount of skin excision can only be gleaned from experience.

Closure begins by recreating the anatomically important pre-tragal depression. A buried 4–0 vicryl suture is placed in the SMAS just anterior to the tragal cartilage and then through the dermal undersurface of the neo-tragal skin which pulls it down in this area, thus recreating this crucial anatomic feature.(Figure 22.21) Without this maneuver, the tragus may be blunted or lost altogether, which is a tip off that a facelift has been done. The anterior ear incision is then closed with interrupted 5–0 prolene sutures supplemented by a running 6–0 prolene in front of the ear. Postauricular closure is accomplished with a running, 5–0 plain gut suture. The temple and posterior hairline incision are closed in layers using buried, interrupted 4–0 vicryl or monocryl sutures and a running 5–0 prolene suture for the skin closure. The holding staples are then removed. (Figure 22.22) No drains are used. They have never been shown to reduce hematoma formation and may leave marks on the skin, and create anxiety for

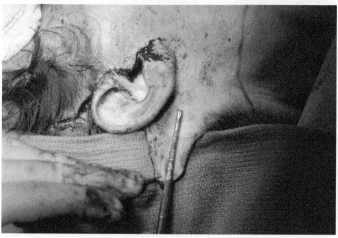

Figure 22.20 Pitanguy flap marking forceps used to contour cervical skin flap.

the patient. A nonconstricting, sterile dressing is applied consisting of antibiotic ointment, telfa, 4 × 4's, cotton fluff and a #9 surgiflex bandage. An artistic sensibility, married to skillful surgical technique and judgment are required to obtain superior, consistent results. Excellence is in the details.

Postoperatively, adequate analgesia and antiemetic medication should be provided for your patient to reduce pain and vomiting as both are known to elevate blood pressure and predispose to hematoma formation. Additionally, a course of oral antibiotics

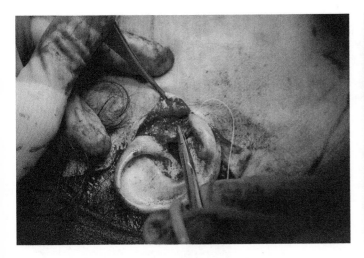

Figure 22.21 Suture placed to re-create pretragal skin depression.

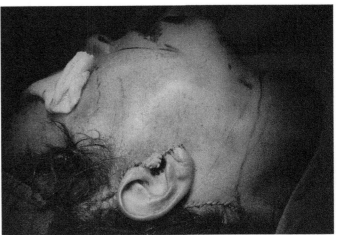

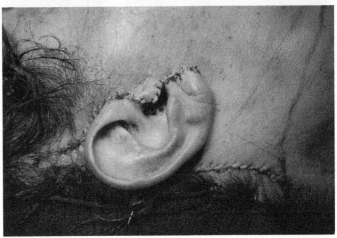

Figure 22.22 Facial incision closed.

covering gram-positive bacteria is prescribed and wound care reviewed with the patient and their care provider. This should supplement comprehensive preoperative education. On postoperative day one, the nonconstricting, sterile bandage placed at surgery is removed. An elastic facial support is then placed which is to be worn for 22 hours per day the first week and then worn only during sleep for two more weeks. The patient is encouraged to shower and wash their hair with baby shampoo daily. All incisions are cleaned with peroxide and dressed with mupirocin 2% ointment twice daily. A professional care provider is recommended for all patients recovering from cervicofacial rhytidectomy for the first 24 hours. Finally, all nonabsorbable sutures are removed at 1 week postoperatively. Routine follow-up care intervals from the day of surgery, after the first week, are as follows: 3 and 6 weeks, 3 and 6 months, 1 year and then yearly if the patient is willing to return.(Figure 22.23)

Secondary cervicofacial rhytidectomy is commonly combined with other facial cosmetic procedures to address the multiple age related changes that occur with time. These may include mid-face lifting, brow lifting, blepharoplasty, skin resurfacing, rhinoplasty, fat transfer, facial implants, ear lobule reduction, hair grafting and other ancillary procedures intended to enhance facial harmony and create youthful attractiveness. Even though you may be comfortable with the technical execution of all of these procedures, excellent aesthetic outcomes require keen aesthetic judgment. Remember to respect the patient's youthful aesthetic and resist the urge to create the "perfect" feature if it will make the patient look "different", particularly if all the patient wants is to look rested, refreshed and possibly more youthful. In fact, most patient fear looking different and if you change their "look" without agreeing to this change preoperatively, even though you may be pleased with their surgical outcome, the patient may not be happy.

As a way to make the patient and your surgical results look their best, it is often helpful to have the patient seen by both a hair stylist and cosmetics specialist to critically evaluate what hair style and make-up would best suit the patient, particularly in light of their surgical enhancement. It is quite common for older women to wear too much make-up thinking that they are hiding skin imperfections when all they are doing is highlighting their wrinkles and making their face look older. As women age they need to update their make-up and hairstyles to enhance their changing appearance and to maintain a contemporary look. Aesthetic surgical enhancement is often the perfect time to reevaluate the patients other aesthetic needs and you, as their surgeon, should feel comfortable raising these issues, making suggestions for improvement and/ or referring them to an expert of your choice. If handled well, your patient will respect your concern and appreciate your global view of their appearance.(Figure 22.24)

CORRECTABLE PROBLEMS FROM PREVIOUS CERVICOFACIAL RHYTIDECTOMY

For cases in which patients are focused on a particular problem created by a previous face-lift procedure, such as hypertrophic scar, hair loss, pigmentary changes, contour deformities or malposition of the lobule, the problem at hand will dictate the procedure recommended.

Hypertrophic Scar

Unsightly scars may result from poor incision placement, excess tension during closure or poor healing. If a scar is hypertrophic, serial steroid injections, massage and daily topical liquid silicone occlusion are appropriate initially for at least 6 months to a year postoperatively. If these interventions fail to improve the scar's appearance adequately, scar revision is appropriate.

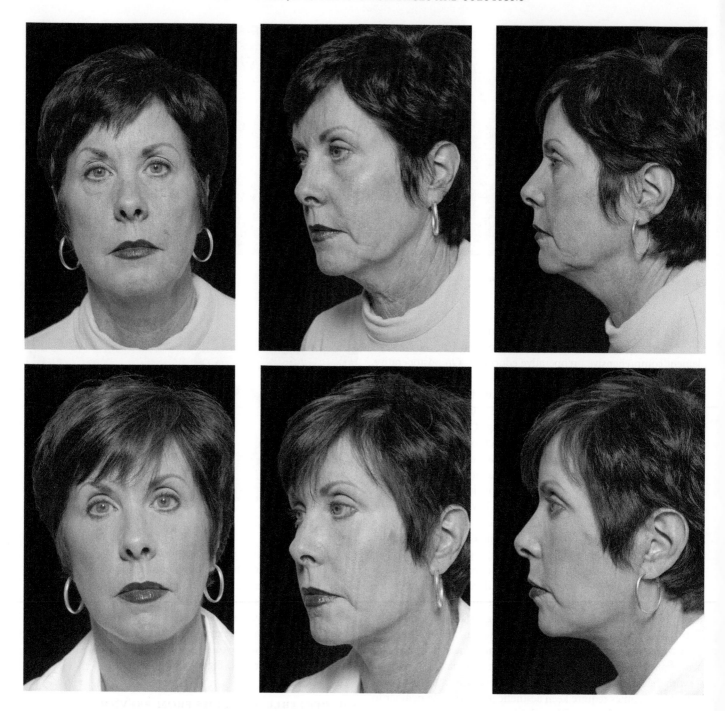

Figure 22.23 Before and after of patient shown in technique photos (take out 3 months follow-up).

Previous studies have demonstrated 50–100% efficacy of intralesional triamcinolone injections in the treatment of hypertrophic scar, with doses usually beginning in the 10 mg/ml range. Injections are typically spaced at 3–6-week intervals for several months, however, dose and frequency of injection will be dictated by the surgeon's experience.(16)

Silicone gel sheeting has been used extensively as an early, noninvasive treatment of hypertrophic scars since the 1980s. Early studies, though uncontrolled, demonstrated improvement in scar appearance in up to 81% of patients.(16) No conclusive evidence has been documented in controlled studies, however, anecdotal

evidence supports the recommendation of either silicone sheeting or topically applied liquid silicone to modify hypertrophic scars. The mechanism of action is thought to be secondary to occlusion, which results in improved local tissue hydration and the recognition that fibrogenic cytokines are reduced in scar tissue treated with topical silicone.

The 585-nm pulsed dye laser (PDL) is currently considered the laser of choice for the treatment of hypertrophic scars. The most common side effect of 585-nm PDL treatment is purpura, which is usually self-limiting over the course of 7–10 days. Hyperpigmentation may also occur, and is more common in

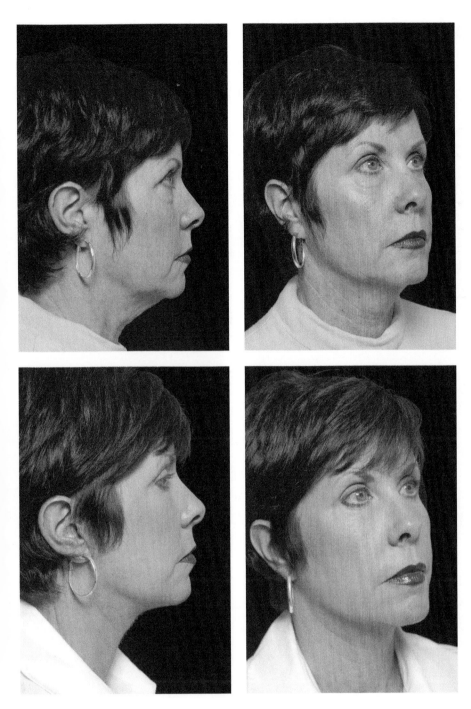

Figure 22.23 (Continued).

darker-skinned individuals.(17) Overall, PDL has been shown to be efficacious in the reduction of hypertrophic scars, especially when combined with intralesional steroid injections.

As an additional noninvasive intervention, imiquimod 5% cream, a topical immune response modifier approved for the treatment of precancerous skin lesions, has demonstrated efficacy in the reduction of keloids after surgery, and has therefore been considered as a treatment for hypertrophic scars. Therapy consists of rubbing the cream over the scar for 3–5 minutes every 3 days for a period of 8 weeks.(17) Although small studies have demonstrated efficacy of this treatment, larger studies with longer

follow-up will be necessary before this intervention can be definitively recommended.

Alopecia

Temporal hair loss after rhytidectomy can be a distressing complication, occurring temporarily in up to 8.4% (18) of patients, and permanently in 1–3%.(11)(Figure 22.25)

Unlike scars that must wait 6–12 months for revision, loss of hair can be remedied soon after its occurrence following a facelift. Once the surgeon is assured that telogen effluvium, the loss of hair due to surgical trauma leading to hair follicle shock, is not

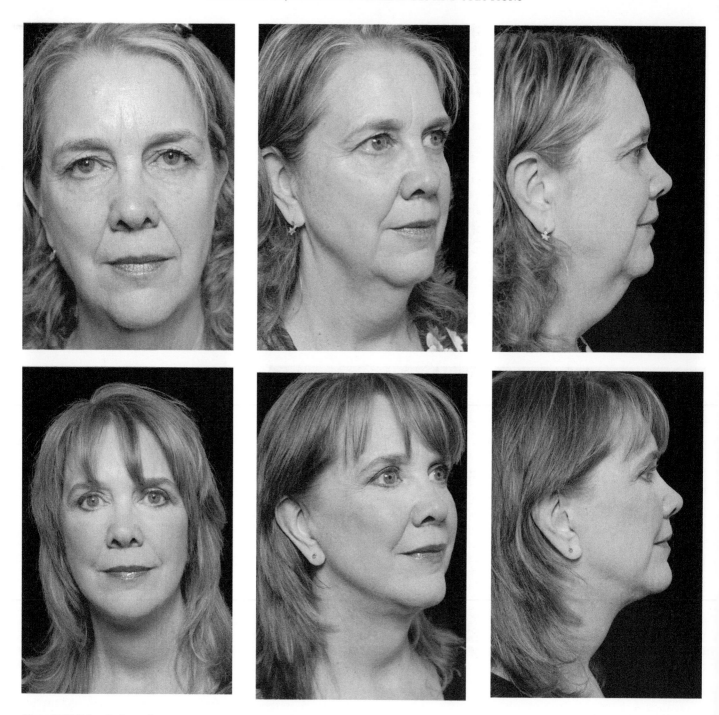

Figure 22.24 Before & after make-over.

the reason for the patient's hair loss, hair restoration can proceed. Most commonly, the temporal tuft requires restoration, which can be accomplished with several hundred micro-follicular unit transfers to achieve a natural-appearing result.

In a retrospective study by Eremia et al. 60 patients received either 2% or 5% topical minoxidil for 2 weeks before surgery and 4 weeks after surgery, with a 5-day break from the day of surgery. Patients were followed postoperatively for 3–6 months. Only 1 patient suffered temporal alopecia 6 weeks after discontinuing minoxidil, which resolved after 4 weeks of restarting minoxidil therapy. Side effects of minoxidil were not observed during this investigation. Although this was a small study, there are early indications that application of topical minoxidil pre and postoperatively in the rhytidectomy patient can prevent temporal hair loss.

Skin Pigment Changes

It is critical that patients apply sun block that covers both the UV-A and UV-B spectrum during the healing period. However, patients with Fitzpatrick IV-VI skin types may suffer from postinflammatory hyperpigmentation after rhytidectomy. This will most likely fade over a period of several months. In the interim, hydroquinone 4% is appropriate topical therapy. Patients may

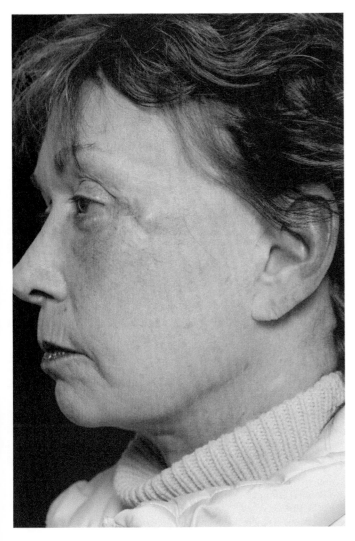

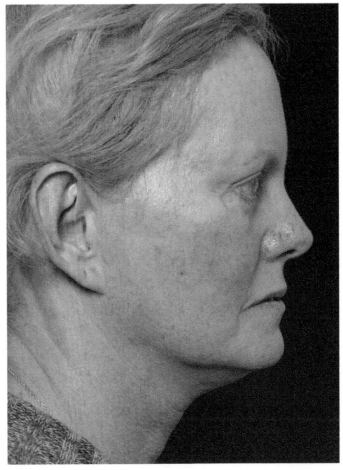

Figure 22.26 Pixie ear deformity after facelift.

Figure 22.25 Temporal alopecia after facelift.

also benefit from micro-dermabrasion to remove the deposited excess melanin and/or intense pulsed light therapy to photo-bleach the unwanted pigment. Hypopigmentation, however, may be longer-lasting, and is often found in areas of excessive skin tension or electrocautery injury of the dermis intraoperatively causing a permanent loss of melanocytes.(11)

For the past 15 years, dermatography, or medical micropig-mentation, has been applied with excellent results in a wide range of indications, including depigmentation caused by vitiligo and surgical interventions in plastic surgery. Many articles and case reports have mentioned the use and complications of medical tattooing, citing infection risks, subsequent use of MRI scans, etc. However, in those who are appropriately trained and in patients who are appropriately chosen, it appears that the use of this technique can result in effective recreation of normal pigment in depigmented areas.(19)

Less invasive methods of concealing hyper- or hypopigmented skin postoperatively can include the judicious use of concealers and make-up. It is often helpful to have the patient educated by a professional make-up artist in the proper application of these products to maximize camouflage while maintaining a natural appearance. The patient may also choose to change their hairstyle to improve coverage of the dyschromic area.

Contour Deformities

Areas most susceptible to contour deformities after rhytidectomy include the submentum and neck, which result from overzealous liposuction of the area or a lack of platysmal muscles plication in the midline. This may lead to a "cobra deformity".(11) Most of these contour deformities will resolve over a period of several months. Some, however, may require the use of massage, steroid injections, or revision with the use of autogenous fat transfer to the affected region.

To prevent prolonged edema after fat transfer, some have utilized the technique of "fat rebalancing," involving the use of multiple, smaller procedures of transfer over a 1–2 year period. Fresh fat is used the first time, but in most patients, frozen fat is injected on subsequent visits. The entire face is treated with small quantities of fat, typically 20–30 ml, reducing the downtime for patients to 1–10 days. Micro-liposuction of the jowls and other areas may also be performed during these visits for aesthetic bal-ancing.(20)

Lobule Malposition

The creation of a pixie or satyr ear deformity is, in most cases, preventable. (Figure 22.26) Causes for this deformity may include improper incision placement around the lobule, aggres-sive skin removal, or excessive tension at the time of closure. Mild traction deformities can be corrected as soon as six months after rhytidectomy. More severe deformities may require waiting up to 1 year for correction.

In order to prevent this dilemma, the preauricular segment of the incision should follow the lobule attachment to the face closely and be more curvilinear than straight. When contouring the cheek and neck skin flap it is important to leave the lobule slightly bunched upward, which will reduce the tension of the closure and avoid this complication. The lobule will assume a normal position during the healing process. However, if you do not anticipate skin flap contracture in this the most dependent portion of the incision, the lobule may be pulled down undesirably.

Correction of the pixie-ear deformity can often be accomplished with a simple V-Y advancement flap technique. In the case of a pixie-ear deformity in combination with an excessively small lobule, where the resultant V-Y advancement would decrease the size of the already-small earlobe, the use of cartilage to increase the size of the earlobe may be appropriate.

A V-shaped skin incision is made along the line of the lobule-cheek attachment. A subcutaneous tunnel is then made in the lobule through the skin incision. A piece of conchal cartilage is harvested and then inserted to enlarge the size of the lobule. According to Park (21), a dermal-fat graft from the sacrococcygeal region may then be harvested and placed inside the lobule pocket to add further soft tissue bulk. The tip of the V-shaped flap is then loosely attached to the infra-tragal cartilage and the skin closed.

SUMMARY

Any time a patient presents for secondary facial aesthetic enhancement, it is important to keep in mind that as cosmetic surgeons, our primary goal is to make that individual feel good about themselves. It does not mean that we need to create an idealized facial feature or the perfect face. In fact, most patients are quite satisfied with looking rested, refreshed, healthy and natural. The patient may have been quite pleased with their initial cosmetic surgery experience or may have been left feeling dissatisfied or in some cases frustrated or angry as a result of legitimate aesthetic complaints following their previous procedure. In any event, the patient is now entrusting their face to you. If you deem it appropriate to treat the patient, assume that they are hearing everything for the first time. Never think that just because a patient has had a procedure done before, they understand the surgical concepts adequately and that their expectations are realistic. Realize that you cannot be an expert in every technique. In order to minimize risk to the patient, choose procedures that work best in your hands. This is not meant to stifle professional growth, but does stress the point that cosmetic surgery should

entail minimal risk while delivering consistent and reproducibly excellent aesthetic results. If you deliver complication-free facial aesthetic enhancement, which appears natural and respects both the patient's desires and youthful anatomy, you will have a satisfied and happy patient.

REFERENCES

1. Tobin H. What makes a patient unhappy. Facial Plas Surg Clin N Am 2008; 16: 157–63.
2. Becker F, Castellano R. Safety of face-lifts in the older patient. Arch Facial Plastic Surg 2004; 6: 311–4.
3. Baker TJ, Gordon HL, Mosienko P. Rhytidectomy: a statistical analysis. Plast Reconstr Surg 1977; 59(1): 24–30.
4. Baker DC. Complications of cervicofacial rhytidectomy. Clin Plas Surg 1983; 10(3): 543–62.
5. Grover R, Jones M, Waterhouse N. The prevention of hematoma following rhytidectomy: a review of 1078 facelifts. Br J Plas Surg 2001; 54: 481–6.
6. Rees T, Barone CM, Valauri FA et al. Hematomas requiring surgical evacuation following face lift surgery. Plast Reconstr Surg 1994; 93(6): 1185–90.
7. Perkins SW, Williams JD, Macdonald K et al. Prevention of seromas and hematoma after face lift surgery with the use of postoperative vacuum drains. Arch Otolaryngol Head Neck Surg 1997; 123(7): 743–5.
8. Kamer FM, Song AU. Hematoma formation in deep plane rhytidectomy. Arch Facial Plast Surg 2000; 2(4): 240–2.
9. Jones BM, Grover R. Avoiding hematoma in cervicofacial rhytidectomy: a personal 8 year quest. Reviewing 910 patients. Plast Reconstr Surg 2004; 13(1): 381–7.
10. Straith RE, Raju DR, Hipps CJ. The study of hematomas in 500 consecutive face lifts. Plas Reconstr Surg 1977; 59: 694–8.
11. Moyer J, Baker S. Complications of Rhytidectomy. Facial Plast Surg Clin N Am 2008; 13: 469–78.
12. Rees TD, Liverett DM, Guy CL. The effect of cigarettes smoking on skin flap survival in the face lift patient. Plast Reconstr Surg 1984; 73: 911–6.
13. Rees TD, Aston SJ. Complications of rhytidectomy. Clin Plast Surg 1978; 5(1): 109–19.
14. Vecchione TR. Rhytidectomy flap necrosis in Reynaud's disease. Plast Reconstr Surg 1983; 72(5): 713–9.
15. Daane SP, Owsley JQ. Incidence of cervical branch injury with "marginal mandibular nerve pseudo-paralysis' in patient's undergoing face lift. Plast Reconstr Surg 2003; 111(7): 2414–8.
16. Reish R, Eriksson E. Scar treatments: preclinical and clinical studies. J Am Co of Surgeons 2008; 206(4): 719–30.
17. Zurada J, Kriegel D, Davis I. Topical treatment for hypertrophic scars. J Am Acad Dermatol 2006; 55(6): 1024–31.
18. Knuttel R, Torabian SZ, Fung M. Hair loss after rhytidectomy. Dermatol Surg 2004; 30: 1041–2.
19. van der Velden E, Baruchin A, Jairath Oostrom CAM et al. Dermatography: a method for permanent repigmentation of achromic burn scars. Curr Opin Otolaryngol Head Neck Surg 2005; 13: 349–53.
20. Butterwick KJ, Nootheti PK, Hsub JW, Goldman MP. Autologous fat transfer: an in-depth look at varying concepts and techniques. Facial Plast Surg Clin North AM 2007; 15(1): 99–111.
21. Park C. A new method for the correction of small pixie earlobe deformities. Ann Plast Surg 2007; 59(3): 273–6.

23 Dealing with the dissatisfied patient
Sigmund L Sattenspiel

INTRODUCTION

Caring for the dissatisfied patient presents one of the greatest challenges to the cosmetic surgeon. There are numerous articles suggesting both diagnostic ideologies and management regimes. The ultimate strategy for handling the difficult patient will periodically elude even the most experienced surgeon with the best interpersonal skills.

While I may not have all the answers, I have some thought provoking concepts regarding this most stressful and perplexing problem in our emotionally charged specialty involving surgery of appearance. My thoughts are based on 35 years of observations and experience in the private practice of facial plastic and cosmetic surgery. I have had the opportunity to closely scrutinize, assess and evaluate unhappy and dissatisfied patients as well as the majority of patients who are happy with their results. Powers of observation and the awareness of patient emotional nuances have contributed to my development of valuable management techniques. The purpose of this discussion is to share my experience and views with my colleagues who, hopefully, will benefit from my successes as well as my misadventures.

The mercurial kaleidoscopic uncertainties and current comfort levels of peoples' lives significantly impact the degree of acceptance of their surgical results. Through the years, I have often seen patients whose satisfaction levels fluctuate. When they are content and socially stable, they enjoy the benefits of their surgical results. When their lives are in disarray, they express unhappiness with their results. In general, people who are happy and content are pleased with their results, whether or not these results are objectively great. To put it in the vernacular, if they have their act together, they enjoy their surgical outcome. Conversely, unhappy, maladjusted people rarely express pleasure at their results. McCollough (1) states that you cannot turn an unhappy person into a happy person by performing an operation. The surgical knife does not convert unhappiness. Many of these unhappy patients present some very difficult management problems for the surgeon.

OBSERVATIONS

There are at least three terms, not necessarily mutually exclusive, that are used to describe troublesome patients: difficult, unhappy, dissatisfied. The difficult patient is one who is a complainer and may give the surgeon a hard time. This patient may or may not be truly dissatisfied. The unhappy patient may be unhappy in life of which the surgical result is a part of that process. This patient may be compliant and may not always be truly dissatisfied. The dissatisfied patient may or may not be difficult or truly unhappy with life; but, more often than not, this patient is also unhappy and difficult.

The determinants creating patients who are dissatisfied with their results fall into two basic categories, objective results and subjective results. Objective dissatisfaction with results is usually real, easy to identify and understand. The physical findings are usually seen by both the patient and the surgeon. Whether or not the patient would derive benefit from correction or if surgical correction is even feasible is another matter. Objective dissatisfaction is not necessarily associated with patient psychopathology.

Subjective dissatisfaction refers to patients who complain of resultant deformities or sensations that represent patient perceptions. These findings are not physically identifiable to the surgeon. Internal psychopathology presenting as personality disorders, emotional instability influenced by social forces, marital instability, conscious or subconscious unrealistic expectations, and failure to establish a positive physician–patient rapport are some of the important factors contributing to subjective dissatisfaction. Based on one or two consultation sessions, it is often very difficult to adequately assess the patient and determine who is likely to be irrationally dissatisfied postoperatively. There are patients with obvious psychotic or neurotic symptoms that manifest extremely bizarre behavior. Despite these red flags, I have performed surgery on some very eccentric personalities who have become model patients that are very accepting of their results. On the other hand, a seemingly well-adjusted and overtly compensated paranoid schizophrenic may be very hard to spot preoperatively. I missed one such patient and the postoperative experience was not fun.

There are various types and degrees of neurotic and personality disorders, often influenced by social and environmental factors. Emotional symptomatology may be hard to discern. Although often not readily apparent, it is my experience that psychosocial sexual factors offer the best predictable indicators of a patient's ultimate response to and acceptance of surgical results. Underlying psychiatric disorders notwithstanding, I have seen that patients who are well-adjusted in their social milieu, referring to family, work and personal relationships, are usually accepting of their cosmetic outcome. Within the patient's social environment, it is my opinion that the most important element pertaining to postoperative satisfaction is personal intimacy. Time and time again, I have seen that the most satisfied patients are those who are the most secure with their spouse, companion, partner, boyfriend or girlfriend. Marital disharmony should be a clue for potential postoperative dissatisfaction. A depressed woman with a cheating husband who obsessively fixates on her appearance will most likely be unhappy with her postoperative results, as well as everything else. Therefore, it is imperative that the surgeon obtain a good social history of the patient during consultation. The importance of psychosocial sexual factors cannot be overemphasized.

Every experienced surgeon has encountered problem patients who are irrationally dissatisfied with their results, complaining of problems and deformities that are minimal or do not objectively exist. Often, surgeons will regret having operated on these people. Well-respected surgeons performing cosmetic surgery have defined personality types of patients who are most likely to be unreasonably dissatisfied.

Adamson (2) describes 12 dangerous personality types in whom caution should prevail and avoiding surgery should be a consideration. He indicates, and I agree, that patients with depressive disorders tend to present the greatest overall problem. These are unhappy people. Interestingly, he states that ten percent of the population is depressed (2 times greater in females). Furthermore, he mentions that the majority of people in society are somewhat unhappy, exhibiting a pessimistic tendency. Tardy (3) lists fifteen categories of patients with a high predictability of being unhappy with their results. Chatham (4) describes thirteen potentially problematic patient types. He describes the demeanor and behavior of each type indicating the degree of difficulty of identification by the surgeon and the degree of risk to the surgeon if surgery is performed.

Experienced cosmetic surgeons have seen most or all of these types of patients depicted by these and many other authors. Goin and Goin (5) in a classical text on the subject of the psychological effects of plastic surgery, describe these same stereotypical personality types that predispose to resultant dissatisfaction. A large number of patients present to our offices with these disconcerting personality types as well as many others with eccentric effects. Unfortunately, if we only operated on those whom we believed to be obviously normal, rational, well-adjusted, intelligent, comprehending, compliant, warm, pleasant individuals, we would most likely perform little surgery. It is very hard to accurately predict who will be happy. So many people who appeared to have somewhat unstable personalities, presumably considered to be unsuitable candidates for surgery, become excellent patients who are thrilled with their results and their surgeon. On the other hand, we have all seen patients preoperatively behaving in a very benign manner displaying a pleasant, compliant and seemingly stable manner who become extremely dissatisfied postoperatively. Some even become nasty and hostile. Chatham (6) cautions the surgeon to watch out for this individual to whom he refers as a "patient from hell."

In reality, there are so many complexities that make up an individual's personality, it is often difficult to adequately predict a patient's acceptance of surgical results. Authors, including Terino (7), have recommended the use of preoperative patient questionnaires. Some have extolled the virtues of psychological evaluations. I disagree with these concepts. I feel that these steps are cumbersome, time consuming and are of questionable value as true predictors of postoperative satisfaction. Furthermore, a number of patients will be turned off by these questionnaires and psychological evaluations. I do agree, however, that there are occasional patients for whom psychiatric consultation may be beneficial. These patients include those who are obviously troubled, on multiple psychiatric medications or currently undergoing psychotherapy.

Based on long-term experience and intense introspection, I have come to the conclusion that the most important preoperative determinant of patient satisfaction is the "sixth sense" of the surgeon. The surgeon should be cognizant of all the various personality aberrations that patients may display and weigh the relative value of these traits in developing a feeling for predictability of a successful outcome. Placing a patient into a category is not as important as the internal gut feelings of the surgeon. Adding careful thought and consideration to the powers of observation, that we are taught to develop in medical training, to the background knowledge elaborated so eloquently by many authors, often will enable the surgeon to determine when to operate and when to reject surgery. Intelligent discretion is wise patient management.

When patients present to my office for a consultation, I pay as much attention to their social history, demeanor, desires and responses to questions and recommended corrective options, as I pay to their physical findings. My careful assessment offers me a degree of predictability for a potentially successful outcome. It is often stated by my colleagues that they rely heavily on the input of their staff. I respectfully disagree. While I do listen to the opinions of my staff, I prefer to carefully assess each patient and discuss my findings and perceptions with my clinical coordinator of over 30 years. Finally, I formulate my opinions based on my own judgment. This is the sixth sense to which I have referred. Thereupon, I decide whether or not to schedule surgery.

Surgery is most often scheduled for at least a couple of months following the initial consultation in our office. A second visit is routinely scheduled preoperatively several weeks prior to the surgical date to finalize surgical details that includes reiteration of the proposed surgical plan, obtaining of informed consents, providing instructions and taking of photographs. The interim lag time and the second visit offer me further opportunity to assess the patient as to suitability for surgery, medically and psychologically. On occasion, there are additional office visits and/or phone conversations with these patients. I continually assess each patient with the concept of predictability of patient satisfaction in mind. Despite comprehensive evaluation, with thoughtful and careful scrutiny of the patient in an attempt to avoid undesirable problems, I am not always right. At times, I have missed the boat!

MANAGEMENT

When the surgery is completed, postoperative patient management commences. Chatham (8) suggests that the emotions of dissatisfaction may follow similar paths to those of grief following loss. He makes reference to Gorney (9) in presenting five stages of patient dissatisfaction: 1. surprise 2. disappointment 3. resentment 4. focused anger 5. retribution. I have observed these stages in dissatisfied patients of mine and of others. Focusing attention to these stages in dealing with the dissatisfied patient should allow the surgeon to provide better management skills and preparation in attempting to assuage emotionally symptomatic patients.

I begin careful and close management of patients immediately following surgery. Rapport is established with the accompanying caretaking family, companions or friends beginning in our Recovery Room. Two personal phone calls are made to each postoperative patient at home, one call in the afternoon by our nursing staff and one call made personally by me that night. Every postoperative patient is seen by me on the day after surgery. Communication is both verbal and sensate. Eye contact and touching are important. Compassionate reassurance is offered with conspicuous care and concern. At each visit, I am constantly assessing the affect of each patient. I check for signs and symptoms of unusual or unexpected behavior. Careful scrutiny of physical findings of the operative sites combined with behavioral observation is the hallmark of postoperative vigilance.

Except for expected bruising, swelling and discomfort, obvious surgical complications or very conspicuous physical irregularities, it is unusual for patients to complain of dissatisfaction in the immediate postoperative period. There is a transient postoperative depression that occasionally occurs in susceptible individuals. This situation is usually short-lived and should not be confused with true dissatisfaction. In general, it usually takes at least a few weeks for the problem patient to emerge. Assuming that there are no obvious objective physical abnormalities, the subconscious emotional agendas generally begin to surface when the initial impact or shock of surgery and the preoccupation with the early postoperative phase has worn off. At this time, perhaps a few weeks to several months after surgery, patients will closely observe and even microdissect their results. Minor concerns are readily resolved. Patients who are pleased will often state so and get on with their lives.

Those patients who are dissatisfied with subjective results will progressively obsess over their findings and express their sentiments of dissatisfaction to the surgeon. In some cases, these sentiments, if not addressed suitably to the patient, will continue and may progress to anger and hostility. Accordingly, these first several months are critical in the doctor-patient relationship. Whereas the doctor must cultivate a rapport preoperatively and hand-hold the patient after surgery, the doctor must actively maintain rapport with the patient in this crucial several month postoperative phase. This is easier said than done.

The maladjusted, emotionally labile, depressed, unhappy individual who may be socially discontent or involved in an unfulfilling marital relationship will usually be difficult to manage. Patient expectations, realistic or unrealistic, may present on a conscious level but are often subconscious. Patients may expect their occupational, social or marital situation to improve. They may anticipate greater recognition and approval from others. They may expect a rekindling of their spouse's affections and desire for them. Some of these difficult patients may complain of undue pain and suffering in an attempt to gain the sympathies of spouses, companions, family members. These complaints provide secondary gain and motivation to attract attention to their unfulfilled emotional needs, real or perceived. There is an entity, chronic pain syndrome, described by Bunden and referenced by Adamson, (10) whereby the patient's pain is emotional rather than physical. Goldwyn (11) mentions that some patients complain of pain well beyond an appropriate period of time signifying displeasure and often symbolizing depression. True physical pain should be minimal following facial cosmetic surgery since cutaneous nerve twigs are temporarily separated from underlying attachments when making incisions and developing flaps. Barring infection or other unusual postoperative consequences, significant pain is rarely experienced and should not be expected, especially after the first several postoperative days. In some patients, emotional pain is confused with, substituted for and experienced as physical pain. These complaints of pain, unhappiness and dissatisfaction are usually based on emotional or psychological dysfunction at the subconscious level.

In addition to those who express subjective complaints of dissatisfaction relatively early, there are patients who will be seemingly content with their results until much later. We have seen patients who have expressed pleasure at their findings during each postoperative and follow-up visit only to reveal their displeasure for the first time at 1 year or later. At this time, they may state that they were never truly pleased. Furthermore, I have experienced patients who display a capricious attitude toward their results. They manifest cyclical periods of satisfaction and dissatisfaction. When patients are dissatisfied with their results, they will express their reasons and point out their physical areas of discontent. Some patients will indicate an overall unhappiness with their results, being unable to give specific reasons. In most of these cases of subjective dissatisfaction, I will tactfully delve into their current social situation. Invariably, there are some highly charged psychosocial, and perhaps sexual, factors that are contributing to their dissatisfaction. The patient may develop hostility and blame the surgeon. This attitude toward the surgeon may represent a transferred subconscious anger towards a spouse. This Freudian transference is consciously more socially acceptable to a patient who is not able to confront his or her spouse.

Dealing with the dissatisfied patient is usually extremely disconcerting to the caring and compassionate surgeon. So how do we or should we manage patients who complain?

A. Objective management

There are complaints that involve objective physical findings identified by the patient and conspicuously recognized by the surgeon. These findings should be addressed in the most medically appropriate, efficacious and expeditious manner. The doctor must be honest and realistic internally as well as with the patient. If there are early postoperative findings that have a reasonable chance of resolution or improvement with time, such as edema, bruising, hyperpigmentation and chemosis, then observation and reassurance may be appropriate. On the other hand, when postoperative results reveal early adverse physical features that obviously will neither change nor improve with time, these findings should be addressed without unnecessary delay. Too often, there are surgeons who deny to themselves or falsely tell their patients that these aberrations will change and improve with time and patience. This attitude usually emanates from either the lack of desire to attend to the problem or the hope that the patient will get use to or forget about the undesirable feature. The obvious deformities will not disappear and neither will the patients. Not only will they annoy the patient and haunt the surgeon but they create poor public relations. Family, friends, co-workers will all see these results and listen to the complaints about the results and the surgeon. Future business will be lost.

Obvious objective postoperative irregularities should be remedied as soon as physically appropriate. Understandably, even minor revisions should not be attempted until a desirable degree of surgical healing has taken place. Imperfections should not be treated early if intervention at this time would be detrimental to the outcome. However, potentially beneficial corrections should be made as soon as possible. For example, an obviously high residual cartilaginous septal supratip elevation post rhinoplasty can easily be trimmed without extraordinary delay. Also, after a couple of months, a soft tissue supratip elevation may be conservatively injected with a dilute corticosteroid. The same is true for periauricular hypertrophic scars following a facelift. Submental bilateral dog ear deformities appearing after the correction of a large anterior cervical wattle can be revised without undue delay. Excess residual skin following an upper lid blepharoplasty and residual fat following a lower lid blepharoplasty can easily be addressed at least a few months after surgery. Some findings may appear later, such as a nasal bossae. As soon as these become conspicuous and bothersome to the patient they should be corrected. The list goes on but the principle remains that the nature of the patient's complaints should be appreciated and corrections should be made as soon as physically feasible. Do not wait! The prudent surgeon deals with the objectively displeasing feature sooner rather than later. The benefits are multiple. Patients will usually appreciate the surgeon's concern and willingness to attend to the problem and enjoy the more pleasing refinements before they have a chance to dwell on their displeasure. At first, they will point out a feature. With time, they will develop a growing and pervasive dissatisfaction with their results and with their surgeon for not addressing their concerns. If possible, it is best to avoid this prolonged patient dissatisfaction and the acrimony that may develop. When I have made necessary corrections early on, I have noticed that, with time, these satisfied patients often have truly forgotten that they had, what they perceived to be, a minor adjustment. Interestingly, in a couple of years, patients will rarely recall even more extensive revisions when they are conducted early. The entire long-term follow-up scenario becomes as comforting to the surgeon as it does to the patient. The surgeon and patient will actually enjoy seeing each other during their office visits, often trading niceties on subjects unrelated to medicine.

What if the surgeon sees an objective irregularity that is not seen, not appreciated or not a concern of the patient? In general, unless the deformity is so conspicuous and unsightly that the patient will most likely eventually complain or have it pointed out to them by others, it is best to avoid any related conversation. In most cases, it is best that the surgeon accept less than his or her perceived ideal perfection and avoid opening a can of worms. I agree with Adamson (12) who advises acceptance of patient contentment.

Another situation may present where there is an obvious physical abnormality requiring revision that the surgeon does not feel comfortable managing, be it lack of experience, knowledge or technical skill. This patient should be referred to another surgeon who is skilled and experienced in revising the specific surgical irregularies.

B. Subjective management

Dealing with the subjectively dissatisfied patient is another story. This management is much more difficult than recognizing and surgically revising correctable physical features objectively displeasing to the patient. In caring for these unhappy patients, the physician's skills and maneuvers transcend surgical expertise. Therapeutic considerations are much less exacting. Appreciating patient nonverbal motivations, assessing patient hidden agendas, understanding unexpressed concerns and diagnosing contributing psychopathological entities present complexities that even the most experienced erudite surgeon will often have trouble resolving. The competent surgeon well-trained in diagnosing and correcting physical features will usually have significant difficulty handling unrealistic and emotionally distraught patients. Unfortunately,

there is no way around it; these patients must be managed. No one has all the answers and certainly not I. There are controversies and gray areas concerning methodology and management. Nevertheless, there are some therapeutic principles that may be applied in seeking to effectively handle the dissatisfied patient. More often then not, these principles have served me well in caring for the surgically unfulfilled, dissatisfied and often irrational patient.

First and foremost, never ignore the patient. Listen attentively to all complaints. Keep eye contact with the patient and display a demeanor of comprehension, compassion and caring. The affect of the surgeon should be noncommittal, warm and compassionate at all times. The more irrational or bizarre the complaints or the more defiant the patient behavior, the greater should be the composure of the doctor. The surgeon must never give any indication of an emotional reaction. It is critical to maintain an affect of understanding that is devoid of any signs or facial intonations of negativity. Listen to the patient and keep listening. Let the patient speak and keep speaking. Delay any response. Occasionally, the patients will experience a beneficial catharsis. Sometimes they will just wear themselves out. The surgeon should wait as long as possible before attempting any response. When it is inevitably appropriate, the response should be delivered in a pleasant, soft-spoken manner to assure the patients that their sentiments are appreciated. During these follow-up sessions, I recommend that the surgeon be seated near to and directly facing the patient while maintaining direct eye contact. There should be a hint of a subtle understanding smile. The surgeon's seat should be slightly higher then that of the patient. This is an important nonverbal communication. If the patient is seated higher then the doctor, it gives the patient a sense of control, empowerment and entitlement. The doctor being slightly higher lends a degree of authority. The surgeon sitting much higher then the patient may be construed as exerting overpowering superiority as well as a demeaning gesture interpreted by the patient as a sign of admonishment as well as a literal and figurative put-down.

The best initial response from the surgeon is to pause. Let the dust settle and allow the patient, as well as the surgeon, to be somewhat composed. Next, and very important, repeat the patient's main complaints in a question form. As an example, the surgeon might state, "If I understand you correctly, you are dissatisfied or unhappy because . . . ." The last part of this sentence includes the patient's stated complaints. Next, listen again. To continue listening cannot be over emphasized. The conversation can go back and forth this way for awhile. This represents an effective psychotherapeutic modality called reflective listening. This technique is discussed and employed by Sykes.(13) It is important to avoid direct responses to these patients. Thank them for sharing their concerns and expressing their feelings with you. Indicate that you appreciate these concerns and reassure them that you will work with them. At this time, do not offer reassurance that everything is or will be "just fine". Do not tell them that their results are or will be terrific. These patients do not want to hear these statements as they threaten the true underlying reasons for their dissatisfaction. Responses are often best put in the form of questions that do not potentially threaten their subconscious emotional inadequacies. A logical discourse presenting reasons for or even refuting the findings should not be held. It is hard, and often impossible to have rational explanations accepted by irrational patients. This concept is so hard for most surgeons to fathom. Time and time again, we all get caught in this trap. It is best for the surgeon to pause and take hold in order to avoid inappropriate responses at an inopportune time creating an unmanageable situation. Explanations are not what these patients want to hear because their true disorders are not surface issues. Furthermore, the surgeon must never be judgmental and must never challenge the patient. The surgeon should not attempt to justify and offer lengthy dissertations defining the benefits the patients have derived from their services. Strange as it seems, trying to justify good objective results to a subjectively dissatisfied patient by showing them their before and after photos rarely mollifies their displeasure. In fact, it may even escalate the emotional conflicts of the patient. It must be remembered that what they see is not what the doctor sees. What they see is what they are looking for. They are viewing their inner disorders, not the physical differences displayed on before and after images. When unhappy patients are shown these photos, they do not see themselves. These images are foreign to them. Sometimes, the better the results, the more they feel challenged and personally threatened. These patients are emotional and not rational. The photos they are viewing are subject to personal interpretation, similar to Rorschach, Thematic Apperception (TAT) and other similar psychological personal interpretive tests.(14)

Considerable hand holding is essential in all patients from the first postoperative day. Continual close contact with the complaining, difficult and dissatisfied patient cannot be overstated. In general, it is my management style to see postoperative patients at frequent intervals in order to assess their results and progress. In fact, I virtually never truly discharge a patient. This principle has served me well. In addition, from an unrelated but beneficial practice standpoint, long-term returning patients will often seek additional major as well as adjunctive procedures.

Problem patients are intentionally seen by me more often than satisfied patients. I listen and listen again to their complaints and I express my concern for their well-being. I try to get to know them as individuals, not just surgical patients. At times, I will try to tactfully shift gears by altering the dialogue to more pleasant and subjective matters. Seeing these patients frequently, getting to know them and attempting to establish a positive bond is often a very beneficial tact. In addition, whenever possible, I try to do a little physical something to the patient or at least make a recommendation for the patient during each visit. Encouragement and hope for a favorable outcome should be the message but care should be taken to avoid making overt statements in this regard. And, of course, never tell a patient that "there is nothing wrong" when there is plenty wrong with them internally. The surgeon must use discretion and be careful to avoid patronizing these patients. Careful thought must be given to the specific management of each patient prior to and during the follow-up visit. When I am about to see a known dissatisfied patient, I carefully review the case in advance, plan my responses to potential expected complaints, take a breath and

enter the examination room with a composed manner and a friendly smile.

Often, with good technique, time heals. Sometimes it does not. Despite best intentions, sometimes rapport is never established or maintained, communication disintegrates, the patients remain dissatisfied and, perhaps, antagonistic. At this point, recommendation may be made to the patient to obtain consultations with other well-respected surgeons who can be trusted to render fair and nonprejudicial opinions. If this option is unsuccessful, suggestion can then be made to the patient to seek the advice from an experienced professional therapist who might help them to understand and deal with issues contributing to their surgical dissatisfaction. However, one must be careful in making this recommendation. An unreceptive patient who refuses to accept that they may have underlying emotional issues may react very negatively and accuse the surgeon of indicating that their complaints are totally unrealistic.

With time, some of these patients' emotional conflicts will resolve and their perceived surgical dissatisfaction will abate. With some patients, another and greater incident will impact their lives. In this case, they will redirect their outward dissatisfaction towards this subsequent episode and transfer their aggression to other individuals.

There are patients whose emotional disorders and social and marital problems never improve and they remain unhappy and resentful of the surgeon. Despite the best intentions and efforts, the surgeon fails to adequately alleviate patient dissatisfaction. After a lengthy and literally exhaustive attempt, the time has finally come to be frank with the patient. The surgeon should be pleasant, look the patient in the eye and state that there is no further treatment recommended. The surgeon should further explain that procedures were performed to the best of his or her ability and that any additional procedures would not yield any improvement and may be associated with potentially harmful risks. Therefore, further surgery is not in the best interests of the patient. This discussion must be conducted with care since resultant patient frustration could lead to potential litigation or, very rarely, to threats of violence. An alternative approach could be to continue to offer to see the patient at frequent intervals and drag out the situation in the hope that the patient will eventually develop other agendas, focus on other nonrelated issues, or resolve some of the underlying psychosocial elements contributing to the dissatisfaction. This patient may go to another surgeon or just tire of the entire process and move on.

Another important point should be made. As Goldwyn (15) elucidates, when a patient comes for a consultation presenting with complaints and dissatisfaction with previous surgery performed elsewhere, the consulting surgeon should never make any negative or condescending remarks regarding the initial surgeon, surgery or results. Negative facial expressions, such as frowns or grimaces by the surgeon, are just as bad. When patients consult with me regarding an objective postoperative deformity, I often tell these patients that the original surgeon was most likely well-intended, the physical findings are evident and we should proceed with discussing potential corrective options. When I do not observe any objective physical abnormalities, I tell the patient that I do not see any significant physical deformities and I reassure the patient that the surgery appears to have been performed well by the original surgeon.

PERSONAL PATIENT CASE EXAMPLES

A few brief examples of dissatisfied patients experienced in my practice can highlight some of the concepts to which I have eluded in my discussion.

1. An Irish woman with a hook nose wanted to look Irish. She desired a turned-up nose emphatically stating that she did not want my recommended "natural" nose. Rhinoplasty resulted in a beautiful, surgically undetectable natural nose. This was exactly what she did not want. She was extremely unhappy with me for 6 months until she became serious with a Jewish man. Now, she loved her new nose. When he left her the following year, once again she hated her nose. Her next boyfriend was Italian. While she dated him she was happy with her nose. This scenario went back and forth with her nasal satisfaction depending on the ethnicity and success of her relationship at the time. When I saw her a few years later, her nose was no longer an overriding concern in her life. She was pleased with the contour of her nose. Despite an objectively superb nose by surgical aesthetic standards, this patient's satisfaction was significantly influenced by psychosocial sexual factors.

2. A pleasant 64 year old woman had a facelift and blepharoplasty performed by me. She did not inform her husband who was at their winter home in Florida. I did wonder about this situation but I did not openly question their relationship. The objective results of surgery were excellent as readily confirmed photographically. However, when this patient returned from Florida 6 months later, she indicated displeasure with her results. She obsessed with virtually unapparent physical features including a palpable Adams apple, minimally noticeable submaxillary glands and so forth. Interestingly, she came to the office with a friend who could not understand her complaints. Her husband remained in Florida. He was never told about the surgery and he never noticed her substantially improved appearance. Most likely, he did not notice his wife at all. Obviously, the surgery did not re-attract the attention or affection of her husband and did not re-establish a more positive relationship with him. This case also illustrates the psychosocial sexual dynamic.

3. A 57 year old female, who could pass for much older, had an uneventful, uncomplicated, successful facelift and blepharoplasty. She was quiet, benign and compliant with little affect both pre and postoperatively. She never complained of anything until her 6 week postoperative visit during which time she not only complained of severe uncontrollable "pain all over," but she was outwardly screaming with pain and obvious rage. She said that it was too painful for her to wear the jewelry given to her by her husband. Furthermore, she could no longer enjoy hugs and kisses from her grandchildren because of the pain that it caused. There were no detectable physical abnormalities. This patient was completely out of control. Her husband, who was in the office waiting room, heard her scream and the commotion and came in to rescue her and take her home. Interestingly, her husband had never

been present in the office before. I had never met him. He did not come with his wife on either the initial consultation or the preoperative visit. He did not appear during or after the surgery and he did not accompany his wife to any of the postoperative visits during the previous 6 weeks. This patient did not even put her husband's name as the next of kin or closest relative on the original information form. In fact, there was no written or verbal mention of her husband at all. Indeed, this patient was in pain, not physical but emotional pain. Obviously, the surgery failed to resolve or ameliorate her marital issues. She had to resort to extreme measures to try to regain the attention and, hopefully, physical affection of her husband. This case represents another example of the influence of the psychosocial sexual dynamic.

4. A heavy, relatively unattractive, pleasant 67 year old woman with a short neck and thick facial features had a facelift and blepharoplasty performed by me. I felt that I had performed a good procedure and I expected to have a nice improvement. This woman was always accompanied by her husband who was obviously caring and who expressed his desire for her happiness. He would hold her purse and often hold her hand during visits. On a follow-up visit to the office 6 months postoperatively, I looked at this patient's preoperative photos. I was dismayed to see that, in my clinical judgment, there was little overall improvement in her appearance despite my best surgical efforts. The patient and her husband asked if they may see the preoperative photos. I was somewhat hesitant to show these photos to them for fear of a negative reaction. Nevertheless, they looked at the photos and they were overwhelmed with joy. They liked what they saw indicating to me that the improvement was dramatic. The husband stated, "My wife is so beautiful!" The patient agreed and she beamed. She was thrilled with results that I had seen as minimal at best. This case represents a positive psychosocial sexual marital dynamic.

5. Many years ago, I performed several rejuvenation procedures on a 69 year old woman who had experienced a hard life contributed to by alcohol and substance abuse. She could have easily passed for being in her late 80s. She had what I had called a "hound dog" look. She appeared sad but she was not clinically depressed and she was in a good marriage with a caring, devoted husband. Several rejuvenation procedures were performed at the same sitting. Her surgical results were outstanding. Postoperatively, we treated her to a makeover including hair styling. Her husband treated her to new outfits. This transformation made her stunning. Ultimately, she was lost to follow-up. A number of years later, while attending a local event, an elderly man came up to me and introduced himself as the husband of this patient. He informed me that she had passed away a couple of years ago. Tears came to his eyes as he thanked me for what I had done for his wife. It may sound morbid, but he said that his wife looked so beautiful as she lay in her casket at the funeral. Although she only lived for a few years after her surgery, he stated that these were her happiest years. He attributed this happiness to my surgical efforts and kindness. I have no illusions that I was truly responsible for transforming this patient into a happy individual. Perhaps, I just tweaked a psychosocial dynamic that sparked her own transformation ultimately giving her a few years of bliss.

6. A slender 29 year old female requested a fat transfer to fill up her cheeks. I transferred 3cc of fat from the inferior aspect of each buttock (the only place where she had any subcutaneous fat). She loved her cheeks but she complained that her buttocks virtually disappeared and that her underwear kept falling down. Physically, her buttocks appeared exactly the same as they did preoperatively and her complaints of her underwear falling down made no rational sense since underwear is supported at the hips. Despite her irrational complaints, I saw this patient at frequent intervals for 12 months. To my surprise, at the 1 year postoperative visit, she made no mention of her buttocks. She expressed complete happiness with the prominent appearance of her cheeks. Interestingly, it appeared to me that most of the transferred fat in her cheeks had absorbed. She was accompanied by her husband at that visit. He was holding her hand. Apparently, he was paying more attention to her. The scenario in this case illustrates the psychosocial sexual dynamic.

7. A 69 year old divorced woman desired to look more youthful. Facelift and blepharoplasty was scheduled. As the time for her proposed surgery neared, her behavior became somewhat irrational. In addition, she was poorly compliant regarding her preoperative medical evaluations and instructions. I developed a feeling that she would not react favorably to her ultimate surgical results. Accordingly, my sixth sense led me to cancel the surgery. I refunded her fees. Was preventive discretion the better part of valor? Most likely.

There have been a number of happy and not so happy endings in my long-term experience. Some situations have worked out well, others have not been so fortunate. There have been patients who turned out to be diagnosed with significant obsessive-compulsive disorder, profound clinical depression, body dysmorphic syndrome, paranoid schizophrenia. In some of these cases, the psychopathology was detected by me and I was able to avoid surgery. Some cases I discovered early, referred for treatment and obviated significant problems. Occasionally, I missed the diagnosis. I recall one male rhinoplasty patient who committed suicide many years later. Fortunately for me, this incident was far removed from and completely unrelated to the surgery. Also, many years ago, I had a male patient who I felt presented a potential physical threat to me. Fortunately, this situation defused and faded.

CONCLUSION

There is a tendency in medicine, as in society, to assume that all people are normal, rational, stable, understanding and somewhat intelligent, as long as they do not act bizarre. A further assumption in cosmetic surgery is that patients know what they want. So often at medical meetings, I hear my colleagues say, "my patients want" this or that, as if each surgeon has patients whose desires are set apart and different from other surgeons. Do patients know what they want? When adding internal and external psychosocial factors to patient uncertainty and ambivalence, it is no wonder that there are subjectively dissatisfied patients. They are unsatisfied people who have become dissatisfied patients. The surgery did not help them.

The exigencies and vicissitudes of peoples' lives significantly influence the degree of acceptance and satisfaction with their results. In essence, if they have their act together, they usually enjoy their surgical outcome. At least they do not dwell on it. Happy people are happy people. Happy people are usually happy patients. Unhappiness pervades everything that touches people's lives, especially cosmetic surgery since it is so emotionally charged. As previously stated, happiness cannot be created with cosmetic surgery.

Patients presenting for consultation regarding cosmetic surgery are looking to improve their physical appearance. In reality, they are seeking to improve their self-image as well as their projected image. Their motivation may be based on apparently logical objective criteria considered to be rational and understandable. These people tend to be accepting of their results, even if they are less than ideal. On the other hand, some people present with hidden agendas that may include overt and subconscious issues that they are attempting to resolve by enhancing their physical features. Sometimes this works out; often times, it does not. Environmental factors and situational conditions impact how patients feel about their surgical results. Patients who present with emotional disharmony, functional instability, personality disorders or other psychosocial pathology may become potential postoperative nightmares. For centuries, many pundits have described these people and placed them neatly into categories, warning the surgeon to stay away from these obviously troubled people and refuse surgery. However, despite the many advocated methods of evaluation, Wright (16) indicates that research has shown that no single method has proven to be a reliable means of preventing postoperative dissatisfaction. Furthermore, there have been clinical observations and studies, eluded to by Gifford, (17), suggesting that psychological symptoms per se do not necessarily carry a poor psychological prognosis for cosmetic surgical satisfaction.

All of the theories and erudite treatises on this subject notwithstanding, in reality it is often very difficult to determine who will be an unfulfilled or dissatisfied patient after surgery. In my opinion, in addition to the evaluation of physical features, a comprehensive social history should be obtained and scrutinized as part of an integrated patient assessment during the consultation and prior to performing any procedures. Psychosocial sexual prognostic indicators are the best determinants of ultimate patient satisfaction or dissatisfaction to which the surgeon should become cognizant before conducting feature altering surgery. In addition to all the formulated diagnostic criteria, the most important consideration in preventing potential patient difficulty is the sixth sense of the surgeon.

While diagnosing the potentially dissatisfied patient is difficult, management is much more difficult. When surgery is not rejected by the surgeon and a potentially distraught patient is missed, the postoperative management must be orchestrated thoughtfully, conducted skillfully and performed with exceptional care. In experienced hands, the surgery is easy. Dealing with the difficult patient can be an overwhelming arduous task.

Through the many years I have been treating cosmetic patients, principles of care have evolved. It gives me pleasure to share my experienced based observations, conceptual opinions and management methodology with my colleagues.

REFERENCES

1. McCollough EG. The act of building a successful facial plastic surgery practice. Facial Plast Surg Clin N Am 2008; 16(2): 187–90.
2. Adamson PA, Chen T. The dangerous dozen–avoiding potential problem patients in cosmetic surgery. Facial Plast Surg Clin N Am 2008; 16(2): 195–202.
3. Tardy E, In Connell BF, Gunter J et al. Roundtable: discussion of "the difficult patient". Facial Plast Surg Clin N Am 2008; 16(2): 250–3.
4. Chatham DR. It's a jungle out there: survival guide for the facial plastic surgeon. Facial Plast Surg Clin N Am 2008; 16(2): 207–16.
5. Goin J, Goin MK. Changing the body: Psychological Effects of Plastic Surgery. Baltimore: Williams and Wilkens, 1981: 39–60, 137–162.
6. Chatham DR. Essays on patient management and elective surgery. Facial Plast Surg Chin N Am 2008; 16(2): 260–1.
7. Terino E. Psychology of the aesthetic patient: the value of personality profile testing. Facial Plast Surg Clin N Am 2008; 16(2): 165–71.
8. Chatham DR. Essays on patient management and elective surgery. Facial Plast Sur Clin N Am 2008; 16(2): 259–65. Ref from: Kubler – Ross E. and Kessler D. On grief and grieving: finding the meaning of grief through five stages of loss, New York, Scribner, 2005.
9. Chatham DR. Essays on patient management and elective surgery. Facial Plast Sur Clin N Am 2008; 16(2): 259–60. Ref from: Gorney M. Lecture at AAFPRS Fall Meeting. New Orleans, (LA) September 23–5, 1999.
10. Adamson PA, Kraus WM. Management of patient dissatisfaction with cosmetic surgery. Facial Plast Surg II 1995; 11: 103. Ref from: Burden G. Chronic pain syndrome, a behavioral abnormality. In: Medical Post, Toronto. Maclean, Hunter, February 22, 1994: 37.
11. Goldwyn RM. The dissatisfied patient. In: Goldwyn RM, ed. The Unfavorable Result in Plastic Surgery: Avoidance and Treatment, Boston: Little, Brown, 1972: 14.
12. Adamson PA, Kraus WM. Management of patient dissatisfaction with cosmetic surgery. Facial Plast Surg 1995; 11: 99–104.
13. Sykes JM. Patient selection in facial plastic surgery. Facial Plast Surg Clin N Am 2009; 16(2): 173–6.
14. Diamond S. Personality and Temperament. New York: Harper & Brothers; 1957.
15. Goldwyn RM. The consultant and the unfavorable result. In: Goldwyn RM, ed. The Unfavorable Result in Plastic Surgery: Avoidance and Treatment, 2nd edn Boston: Little, Brown, 1972: 15–7.
16. Wright MR. Management of patient dissatisfaction with results of cosmetic procedures. Arch Otolaryngol 1980; 106: 466–71.
17. Gifford S. Cosmetic surgery and personality change: a review and some clinical observations. In: Goldwyn RM, ed. The Unfavorable Result in Plastic Surgery: Avoidance and Treatment, 2nd edn Boston: Little, Brown, 1972.

24 Psychiatric considerations for aesthetic procedures face to face: Straight talk

Harish Kumar Malhotra

INTRODUCTION

Before writing, I asked my aesthetic surgeon colleagues as to what they would like to know from this chapter. The need was unequivocal. They felt lack of confidence in communicating about emotional issues. They wanted to know how to communicate about emotions with a patient for the aesthetic surgery so that they could minimize psychiatric complications and malpractice suits.

Some of them showed out right abhorrence, "I don't have two hours to hold hands".

I am going to stress on the communication so that you can get to know your patient, recognize psychiatric aspects of her problems, treat or refer her to a mental health professional for help. Addressing a female patient has been done for ease of writing. It includes male patients.

HOW TO RECOGNIZE PROBLEM PATIENTS

Some patients make you uncomfortable. Tune in to your inner self and do not deny the discomfort. Recognize it as a red flag. It helps you to investigate further and get timely psychiatric help for your patient. However, there is a wide variation in normal behaviors. Remember, apples are red but not all red things are apples.

Rees (1) pointed out such common observations. Watch out for

- Patients who are hyper critical of their defects
- Patients who have an unrealistic image of themselves
- Flat and monotonous voice
- Woman 40 years or older for rhytidectomy
- Patients who are pushy, obnoxious, over demanding, uncooperative and difficult to communicate with
- Patients who apply undue pressure to obtain an early appointment
- Patients who expect appointments at times other than normal allotted time
- Patients who interfere with the normal office structure
- Patients who show extreme irritation and intolerance to the office staff for minor delays in appointments
- Patients who go through your bookshelves, drawers or your personal effects
- Visible differences between the patient and the family members regarding the need for surgery or its payment

In addition, extreme deviations in the manner of speech, behavior, personal hygiene, dress and seductiveness should raise doubts in you. Extreme anger, criticism of previous surgeons, undue praise and attempts to develop extraprofessional relationship with you may indicate the need to explore further. Watch the patient when they are alone and when they think they are unobserved in the waiting room and examination room. If they talk or gesture to themselves, it may indicate psychosis.

THE INITIAL SESSION

Edgerton and colleagues (2), stated that it is "the patient's evaluation of the surgical result, not the surgeon's, that will determine any change in her sense of the deformity, and hence produce, or fail to produce, the desired psychological response."

The goal in the initial session is to reframe your patient's visit as an attempt to solve a problem in her life. She has considered many solutions for the problems of her appearance. She has thought, researched and come to you to solve a crisis in her life. In an average person, one would use the word "issue" instead of a "crisis". She, finally, decided that the best way is to alter her appearance with your help. You want to find out whether realistic reasons or a psychiatric disorder is guiding her decision for aesthetic surgery.

Use an open-ended style interview to find out the strengths and weaknesses of your patient and decide whether to operate or not. Please document your findings and your rationale in either case. It is your findings and documented reasons, which will be your best witness in a malpractice suit.

Investigating your patient's set of mind will require empathy and a good rapport with her. Your first interview with her is not only investigative but also serves to develop a therapeutic alliance with her. Only then, would she agree to your suggestions for surgery or alternatively a medical intervention. She must believe that you are in her camp and understand her needs.

In the end whatever you do, you cannot predict an individual out come. The good and bad prognostic factors only recognize good and bad prognosis groups and not individuals. However, a good history may reduce your risk of making mistakes.

Reframe the visit to you as a step to solve her life's problem. The following is based on rules of crisis intervention (3)

1. Validate the patient's sense of discomfort with her appearance and wanting relief by altering it
2. Reframe aesthetic surgery as a problem solving behavior.
3. Commend your patient for coming to you for solving her problems
4. Reduce your patient's anxiety about her desire to come for aesthetic surgery.
5. Develop the idea of studying her desire for surgery in the context of problem solving.
6. Now you are ready to explore the patient's perceived problems and analyze how the aesthetic surgery fits as a solution in the larger picture of her life.

THE CHECKING OUT PROCESS

Your patient has been thinking of how you would react to her request for surgery. She started evaluating you on the internet. She continued to evaluate you as she entered your parking lot, saw your name in the directory and walked in your office. She thought about you as she waited in your waiting room and observed how your staff and you greeted her. You are revealing your attitudes to her each time you ask a question. The extent of her self-revelation will depend on her perception of you as an empathic doctor. Your interview of your patient is a two way street. You think that you are evaluating the patient; however, patient is evaluating you too.

OPEN-ENDED INTERVIEW TECHNIQUE (4)

If a significant family member is accompanying the patient it may be a good practice to see the patient alone first. Later the family member can be invited in to participate in the final decision making if your patient so desires

Surgeon looks at the family member and says," Would it be okay if I interviewed Jenna alone first and than if needed I can invite you to get your input?" Usually the family member agrees to that request. This way you can get to know what your patient wants. Later if the family member comes with a different agenda, that will give you a red signal.

An open-ended interview in a comfortable environment, preferably sitting down face to face in your office, will give you the best harvest. Sit with a pleasant eye contact, and a non-rushed demeanor. Give a sense of timelessness i.e. uninterrupted time to the patient. After your interview, you may call a nurse in while you examine the patient. (Wrong scenario: An anxious patient sits on the edge of an examination table in a paper gown; the nurse stands there as your chaperone. You are talking to the patient while looking at the forms she filled in your waiting room.)

Few examples of closed ended and open-ended questions are as follows.

You put the chart down. You look at her and sit close enough where patient can touch you if she wants to.

Surgeon:	Tell me what brings you to me today. (Open ended question)
Surgeon:	I understand you are here for a face-lift operation (Avoid closed ended question)
Patient:	I have been thinking about getting some lines on my face taken care of. I want my chin to be tightened. I want my forehead to look less worried. I have felt that I look tired lately. I have been hesitating. Finally, I faced the situation and called you.
Surgeon:	How do you feel about being here? (Open ended question).
Patient:	I feel anxious because I have never been to a plastic surgeon before
Surgeon:	Please tell me what makes you anxious.
Wrong response:	Don't worry; I will take care of you.
Patient:	I wonder how I will look after the surgery. Some times, I feel that I can't hide my age and I feel I am losing the grip on my life. I used to be a model. I was considered very beautiful.

You let her tell you her conflicts about her concerns and fears about any procedures. She also tells you what she heard from her friends. While you listen to her, you make affirmative responses including Hum…um…..um sounds, head nods and blink your

eyes. She sees and hears that you are listening with interest. Let your facial expressions mirror the patient's feelings. Smile if she expresses a sense of humor and express concern if she shows emotional pain.

Do not interrupt while the patient is talking so that she can formulate her ideas and her story. You can make mental and written notes so that you can respond to later. Her anxiety level is very high. Doctors become bigger than life in the patient's perceptions. Therefore, she can easily misinterpret any hurry or poor eye contact as lack of interest.

If the patient hesitates and stops, do not jump in. Summarize what she said and ask her to go on.

| Surgeon: | You were saying that you were a beautiful woman and lately you feel that you have been losing a grip on life! Please tell me about that. |

A small investment of time at this moment will go a long way to save a lot of wasted time later on.

Alternately, the patient tells you that she has been to plastic surgeons before.

Surgeon:	Who was the surgeon? (Closed-ended question)
Patient:	Dr. Smith
Surgeon:	Tell me about your previous experience with aesthetic surgery. (Open-ended question)

The patient will tell you the reasons, the doctors, the experiences and the positive and negative consequences of surgeries. She will tell you how she felt about the previous doctors.

| Surgeon: | How did he treat you? |

Her feelings about what he said, what he did and her reactions to the surgeon may give you clues about how she will react to you and treat you. It will make you aware of her expectations from the surgeon, the surgery and the surgical experience.

The above is only possible if you keep sufficient time for your new patient. If you don't have time, ask the patient to come again when you have the time for her. You have to decide where you would like to spend your time, now in your office or later in the courtroom.

VALIDATION OF PATIENT'S NEEDS TO SOLVE THE CRISIS:

You want to find out what broke the camel's back. What made her come to your office today?

Surgeon:	Tell me how you feel about the shape of your nose. (Correct, open-ended question)
Patient:	I never liked my nose.
Surgeon:	Tell me about it (Facilitation)
Patient:	I don't like the shape. It is unattractive
Surgeon:	Unattractive! (Correct Reflective response)
Patient:	Yes, my husband says it is unattractive
Surgeon:	Your husband says it is unattractive! (Correct repetition to find more information)

Patient starts crying.

Surgeon: Please don't cry (Wrong response)

Surgeon: I see tears in your eyes. What brought the tears? (Correct: You observe and verbalize her behavior)

Patient: My husband used to like me all these years. He criticizes my appearance and my nose since he started cheating on me with his secretary. I will show him, who has a better nose

Surgeon: Operation on your nose will not take care of your marriage (Wrong response)

Surgeon: Please tell me more about your relationship with your husband (Correct open-ended exploration response)

Patient: He has been having problems with his mom and his business and he is taking it all out on me...............

She tells you about her problems openly.

METAPHORS AND STORIES HAVE BEEN USED SUCCESSFULLY IN PSYCHOTHERAPY (5)

You tell her a story of a patient who has magical and unrealistic expectations from aesthetic surgery.

Surgeon: Mrs. Smith! Make-believe that you are an owner of an auto body shop. Make believe that I am a customer who brings my car to you. I am upset about a minor scratch on my car. You want to find out why I want to spend so much money to fix that small scratch. I tell you that I tried to sell my car; I was offered only $5,000. I am wishing that by making my car perfect looking, I might be able to get $25,000 for my car.

Would you start fixing that minor scratch on my car or would you sit down to explain that the minor repair will not bring that kind of a price. When a Honda goes in for a repair, a Honda comes out of the workshop. It does not turn in to a Mercedes Benz.

Some time, people over estimate the results from aesthetic surgery. A woman who is having marriage problems, a man who cannot find a mate, and a worker who cannot rise in his job may turn to aesthetic surgery to solve their problems. The woman needs to work on her marriage problems with the help of a marriage counselor. The man who cannot find a mate needs to work on his interpersonal and social skills. The worker who cannot rise in his job needs to go for managerial training. He needs to work on the inside of his head rather than to grow hair on the outside of his head. If only growing hair on the head would bring managerial jobs then all his coworkers with hair would be managers. A woman with small breasts and marriage problems becomes a woman with large breasts and marriage problems after the surgery.

Your desire to get surgery in an attempt to get your husband back does make sense to me. However, I feel that problems of his business and his mother will still be there after your operation. My recommendation is to get help to settle those problems in your marriage first. Once you both have taken care of those then we can reevaluate your needs for aesthetic surgery. I do have the names of very competent marriage counselors who could take care of the other problems first.

Patient: OK, I am open to that. I was thinking about it too but I was not sure.

BODY DYSMORPHIC DISORDER (6)

If the patient were dissatisfied with her **normal** face and body parts, the chances are that even after surgery, she would remain dissatisfied. A patient who remains dissatisfied with normal body may have Body Dysmorphic Disorder.

Surgeon: What brings you to me today? (Open ended)

Surgeon: So I see that you have come to me for your nose problem (Closed ended)

Patient: I would like to have some changes done to my nose

Surgeon: Please tell me about it (Open ended)

Surgeon: I see here that you want to have the bridge of your nose made less prominent(Closed ended)

Patient: I think my nose is ugly.

Surgeon: Yes, please go on? (Encourages talking more)

Surgeon: I don't see any problem with your nose (Stops communication)

Patient decides that you don't have the ability to see her defect, may become hostile towards you and move to the next doctor.

Patient: I would really appreciate if you could help me because my life has come to a stand still with this ugly nose.

Surgeon: It must be so difficult to feel that way. Would you please tell me how it has brought your life to a stand still? (Correct empathic response)

Surgeon: Look, I am a plastic surgeon and I do this all day for the last 15 years. I don't see a problem there. (Non-empathic response)

Patient: When I go out, people look at it. It is so uncomfortable. I have stopped going out to the market until it is late at night when there are only a few people.

Surgeon: This must be so difficult to have to stay home to avoid that humiliation. How else does it hinder your life? (Correct Affirmation and more exploration)

Surgeon: How could people be looking at you? I am telling you that you have a normal nose. (Non-empathic response)

Patient: I am always worrying about it. It is such a relief to come to you to get this hideous ugliness taken care of. I am sick of watching my face. I keep looking at it in the mirror. I have lost a job because I was always late taking care of my nose. No one understands. I had a girl friend. She was very insensitive to my problems and forced me to go out to places with her. Finally, we broke up.

Surgeon: That must have been so painful. (Correct empathic response. By this response, the surgeon is not agreeing with patient's request for surgery. He is agreeing with the patient's distress. This helps to establish rapport. Later the surgeon will talk about why the surgery is not a good idea)

Surgeon: She was right. You should have tried to go out. You seem to have Body Dysmorphic Disorder (Non-empathic response)

Patient: Yes it was! I have become so depressed after that.

Surgeon: I understand your distress. I would feel similar pain if I were in your shoes. (Empathic response. Surgeon is not saying that her nose has problems. He is saying that it must be distressing to have the pain of Body Dysmorphic Disorder)

Surgeon: You are unnecessarily making yourself miserable. Believe me your nose is all right. Actually, it is a pretty nose (Wrong response)

Patient: Would you help me?

Surgeon: Yes, I would help you. (Helping to solve her problem of distress)

Surgeon: No, I am not going to operate on you. (Wrong. Patient has discovered that you don't understand and she is thinking about the second surgeon on her list)

Patient: would you correct my nose?

Surgeon: I can feel your distress about your perceived defect in your nose. Any one in your situation will feel the pain you feel. The surgery and its after math can be very stressful. Yet you may not like the results after surgery. Let me explain to you how I will help you. There are many ways to solve this problem. Operation is the last resort. There are many treatments available for your problem. Let me tell you a story to make a point.

THE STORY FOR A BODY DYSMORPHIC DISORDER PATIENT

A woman took her car to a glass shop. She told the young shopkeeper that her windshield was cloudy. She told him to replace it. The shopkeeper asked her to leave the car, in his shop and come the next day. He diligently found one of the best windshields and replaced it. He was very happy with his work. The next day, the customer came, saw the windshield and was very unhappy with it. She said that the windshield he replaced was cloudy too. The shopkeeper put in a second windshield. The woman said this was cloudy too. The shopkeeper was very frustrated and they had an argument. She complained to the better business bureau that he was a dishonest shopkeeper because he used cloudy windshields twice and charged her money for new ones.

The woman went to another glass shop. The elderly shopkeeper wanted to know her story. He saw a new windshield professionally installed and yet a dissatisfied customer. He asked her, how were the other window glasses in her car. The customer said that they were cloudy too. She said that once she had more money she would come and get them fixed too.

The shopkeeper shared his own life experience with her. Two years back, he felt that his windshield was becoming cloudy however; his wife told him that the windshield was clear. Finally, he discovered that he was developing cataract in his eyes. He had to undergo a cataract operation. After that, the cloudy appearing windshield started looking clear again. The problem was not his cloudy windshield. It was his vision due to cloudy lens in his eyes.

Because, she was seeing fog on the glasses even though they were clear to him, she may be developing a cataract too. Her solution did not lie in his glass shop. Her solution lay in an eye doctor's office. The woman listened to the old man and went to her eye doctor. He operated her cataract and she could see every thing clear. She came, thanked the old man, and decided not to change the windshield in her car.

Aesthetic surgeon looks at the patient and says:

I am telling this story to you because there is a brain condition called Body Dysmorphic Disorder. The person who is suffering from it sees problems in different parts of the body even though others do not see the problem. When the woman in the story saw the cloudy windshield, she was right in her own way. She did see the cloudy windshield, except that the cloudy perception was due to a cataract in her eyes. If the cloudiness were in the windshield, the glass man would have seen it too.

I am a plastic surgeon, and I have been seeing body parts for years. If there were a defect in your body, I would have agreed with you and started planning the operation right away. However, I feel that you must take care of the disease of perception called Body Dysmorphic Disorder. There are treatments available for this condition. There are medicines, and cognitive behavior therapy, which helps to correct this condition. After you have gone through the psychiatric treatment, we may sit down and discuss it again.

If you have Body Dysmorphic Disorder, and I operate, you will return dissatisfied repeatedly like the woman in the first glass shop. Repeated surgeries have bad consequences too. You may have seen the face of a well-known celebrity who has had multiple surgeries and disfigured his face. I want to save you from that fate. If the psychiatrist says that you do not have Body Dysmorphic Disorder, I would be reassured and will go ahead with planning the surgery. I have the names of few good psychiatrists. Let us try some simple treatments first.

Patient: I am sure that I have a problem that you should correct with surgery but I will listen to you and go for help. Would you operate on me after I see the psychiatrist?

Surgeon: We will cross the bridge if there is a bridge. We will cross the bridge when we come to the bridge. I am glad you are going to a psychiatrist.

A DEPRESSED PATIENT

The goal of the aesthetic surgery is to make the patient happy.(1) If a patient has any psychiatric condition, which blocks the patient's ability to become happy, then the best results will not make a difference. That is why it is important to screen the patient for any significant depression. You may note that the patient looks colorless, expression less, moves slowly, and talks in a flat voice. You may feel a sense of sadness inside you as you relate to the patient. You suspect depression.(6)

An open-ended interview for depression:

Surgeon: How are you feeling right now?

Patient: OK I guess. (She has poor eye contact with you and talks in a low flat voice)

Surgeon: OK, I Guess? (He repeats her statement to get more information)

Patient: I don't know

Surgeon: The only person who knows about your feelings is you. So tell me how you feel

Patient: I feel very discouraged

Surgeon: When you were talking to me, I saw tears in your eyes. What brought them?

Patient: I just feel down. Depressed you know.

Surgeon: I can feel the sadness in you. How long have you felt this way? (Empathic response with exploration)

Surgeon: Cheer up! A young girl like you should be enjoying life (Non-empathetic response)

Patient: It is going on for the last 4 months.

Surgeon: Could you please tell me about it. (Exploration for more information)

Patient: About 4 months back, my brother died in an auto accident. It was a painful loss. He was my friend. It has been difficult. (Patient starts crying)

Surgeon: (He hands over some tissues to the patient) I can see the sadness and depression. Please tell me about it.

Surgeon: Please do not cry. (wrong response because crying is a nonverbal communication of the internal state of her psyche)

Patient: Little things have overwhelmed me.

Surgeon: hum... um …

Patient: I cry all the time.

Surgeon: yes

Patient: I cannot sleep well.

Surgeon: Tell me about your sleep problems.

Patient: I get exhausted easily so I fall asleep early. However, my sleep remains interrupted all night and I stay awake in my bed at 4 AM.

Surgeon: I see. Please tell me more.

Patient: My mind keeps racing.

Surgeon: How is it affecting your day?

Patient: I cannot focus my mind on any thing.

Surgeon: yes

Patient: I read a page of a book and do not know what I read. I am having difficulty making decisions.

Surgeon: It must be so difficult to feel that way. Has it affected your ability to get joy out of things?

Patient: I was so fond of movies. Now I don't feel like seeing one. Even if I do go to one on the insistence of my family I can't concentrate on it and really do not get any enjoyment.

Surgeon: How has if affected your physical health.

Patient: I feel very weak. I have no energy in my body and soul. I have lost my appetite and have lost five pounds of weight in the last 2 weeks without dieting.

Surgeon: How has it affected your self-confidence and self-worth?

Patient: I feel inferior and ugly that is why I came to get your help. I have never felt so unattractive. I would not mind if I did not wake up ever. I need a lift. I need some facelift.

Surgeon: I can hear how unattractive you feel. I can feel your depression as I listen to you.

Patient: Would you give me a face-lift? May be it will lift my spirits.

Surgeon: I would definitely like to help you. In your case, we have to take care of your depression first. In my experience, the depression can make the person feel inferior and unattractive. Once the depression is treated the patient finds that they feel good about themselves and their looks. Once the depression lifts the patient does not want to correct any thing surgically. There are effective medicines and counseling available. After you have gone through the treatment and the psychiatrist gives a green light, I can meet you again. We will discuss your surgery if you want. It is a well-known saying that the best kind of face-lift surgery for a depressed face is a smile. Let me refer you to my colleague Dr. Smith. He has helped many of my patients in the past. How do you feel about my suggested plan?

Patient: I want to feel better. I will try it. Thank you.

HIGH EXPECTATION PATIENT

A patient came to the surgeon for a rhinoplasty.

Surgeon: I want to show you what the aesthetic surgery can do.

(He made her sit in his office. He set up his new equipment and favorite toy, the camera with a software program. He showed her how her face would look when rhinoplasty was finished.)

Surgeon: This is your face and watch how the new nose will look like.

Patient: It is amazing! Science can do wonders

(She stared at her computer-generated picture with amazement)

Patient: I love it.

(Surgeon did a good job. Every thing went well. After the surgery was over, she looked at her face in the mirror.)

Patient: This is hideous. I do not like it. (She was thinking that she wanted to look like her computer-generated picture. She returned to the surgeon repeatedly, and complained to him about his botched up job.)

An alternate open Ended Interview:

Surgeon: What made you decide to have the rhinoplasty?

Patient: I have always wanted to get it done.

Surgeon: Always! (A reflective response to get more details)

Patient: Yes, always. Since I was in the middle school, the kids used to call me Tunnel Head because I had wide nostrils.

Surgeon: What made you wait until your 35th year to come here?

Patient: I have had many broken relationships. Recently, I fell in love with Jack. He is very cute. We were going strong. One day, I saw him with another girl. She has a pretty nose. I know why he left me; I felt so broken hearted. I can do any thing to get Jack back. I will use my savings to get the surgery done.

(Now the surgeon knew that she had multiple broken relationships. If her nose were the problem, she would have had difficulty <u>starting</u> relationships not <u>keeping</u> them. He knew that the new nose is not going to bring back Jack, the boy friend. Her high expectations from her repaired nose and the surgeon were unrealistic.)

Surgeon: You must have really cared about Jack. The shock of seeing him with another girl brought back the hurtful memories of your schooldays. It is natural that you tried to find a reason for the breakup. Your nose has been your life's Achilles heals. It made you suffer during your childhood. I can fully understand that you thought that if you get the nose fixed all the problems would disappear and Jack will come back. This may look like an obvious solution for a relationship problem.

Patient: That is right. I think that nose repair is the solution

Surgeon: Let me give you a new way to look at the breakup. If your nose were the problem, you could not attract so many men. They found you attractive enough with your nose. There is some problem in your relationship maintaining skills. I would suggest that you go for some counseling to work on your relationship skills. Men do get attracted to you with this nose. At this time we don't know what is the problem that makes you breakup with men? If we do not do that, you will have an expensive nose but breakups will continue. Now you blame your nose. Whom will you blame then? You will be a girl with a good-looking nose who breaks up with people just the way Elizabeth Taylor did. Once you have gone through the counseling, come back and we can discuss working on your nose again.

Initially, the patient resists.

Because of the surgeon's warmth and sincere advice, she thanks him and decides to go for psychiatric help, sparing mutual disappointment.

If you don't explore the patient's needs and operate because of your need to do the operation, you will get the anger of the patient.

After the surgery, the anger at you will be directly proportional to the high expectation that the patient came with. The patient read magazines, saw movies about plastic surgery and brought in the high expectations. Your advertisement with a perfect face may have fanned her expectations from you. The patient do not know that the results depend on not only your surgical skills but also on their body. Their skin, tissues, shape of their skull and healing physiology all affect the result. It is very important that you do not lose the sight of bad consequences of her high expectations. The enthusiastic surgeon who has good bedside manners, but gives all the information about what can go wrong may avoid problems later. Patients use denial of bad results and complications. In case of dissatisfaction, the patient's denial will work against you. The patient will say you never told them about what could go wrong.

It is important to break the shield of denial the patient comes with. The surgeon sends in a form letter before the patient comes in for consultation. You can see the example of preconsultation letter for patient elsewhere.(1) The Surgeon should not take it for granted that the patient read the letter. It is important to ask leading questions to find out the grasp of the patient of the contents of the letter. The expedience of the surgeon will determine the right dose of encouragement and caution.(1)

If you find a psychiatric problem, you may refer your patient to someone with whom you have a good relationship. If you verbalize confidence in the psychiatrist/psychologist, the patient will accept him well. If you have a negative feeling about mental health providers, it will show in your talk and will negatively affect your patient.

TREATMENT OF BDD

Experienced physicians and therapists should perform treatment of Body Dysmorphic Disorder. The patient may ask you questions as to how the mental health professional will treat her illness. She may also call you while undergoing psychiatric treatment to use you as a sounding board. If you are knowledgeable, it will help your patient to see the psychiatrist. Please use the limited therapeutic guidelines below only as basic background reference material.

1. Pharmacotherapy

Patients consistently respond to Serotonin reuptake inhibitors (SSRI) e.g. fluoxetine and clomipramine. Patients may show a complete or partial reduction in BDD symptoms. The effective treatment of BDD with SSRIs requires a relatively long duration of treatment and often needs doses, which are higher than those used for depression. An average time to respond is at least 7–8 weeks, but sometimes as long as 12 weeks. Try sequential SSRI's one after another, if the first or second one in highest doses for required time does not work. If it works, continue the treatment for 1 year because relapse is likely with early discontinuation. Combination and augmentation strategies with benzodiazepines and antipsychotics may be useful if one SSRI alone does not work. Monitor Clomipramine levels if it is used in combination with SSRI.(7)

2. Cognitive Behavior Therapy (CBT)

The therapist has his subjects list a hierarchy of distressing aspects of their appearance. He then uses exposure therapy and thought stopping to prevent distress at the sight of these features. In addition, response prevention (i.e. not letting them check their face in the mirror each time they feel doubt about their face) is used to decrease checking behavior. Each patient is taught relapse preventions in order to prepare them selves for high-risk situations.

THE TECHNIQUE OF RESPONSE PREVENTION

When the thought (inner stimulus) or a reflection of self in the mirror (outer stimulus) creates anxiety, the patient responds by repeated checking and rectifying the defect. The checking and rectifying behavior rewards the patient by temporarily decreasing the anxiety. This vicious cycle of obsessive compulsive checking and rectifying behavior becomes a self perpetuating reward system. The treatment involves breaking this reward cycle to extinguish the obsessive-compulsive behavior. Here is a simple way of doing it.

The popular story among CBT therapists is as follows.

Therapist relates the following story to the patient suffering from BDD.

There was and old woman who lived happily in a house. One day she heard a little cat meow in her back yard. She came out and saw a little kitten meowing. To make the kitten quiet she threw some scraps of food. The kitten became quiet. Next morning the kitten was sitting next to the door meowing loudly. The old woman started feeding the cat each time it meowed. Slowly the cat became bigger as she ate the food given by the old woman. The more she ate the more she grew stronger and hungrier. The scraps of food did not satisfy the cat anymore. The old woman started to bring cat food. The cat ate all the cat food and turned in to a big bobcat. She started snarling at the old lady for food. The old woman started remaining hungry so that she could bring large chunks of meet for the bobcat. One day the bobcat remained hungry after being fed. She broke the house door down. It attacked and ate the old woman.

After relating this story the surgeon asks the patient," what was the mistake the old lady made, which lead to her being killed by the cat."

The patient answers, "she fed the cat. If she had not fed the cat, it would have gone away."

Surgeon says to the patient, "in your case the cat (your BDD anxiety) is your doubt about your nose. Its mew is the need to check your face. The doubt bothers you as the mewing of the cat bothered the old woman. You feed the cat of the BDD anxiety, by examining your face in the mirror repeatedly. The cat (of BDD anxiety) becomes quiet after the feed of checking for few minutes. However, the cat of BDD becomes stronger and comes back with vengeance. It comes back with a stronger urge to check your face again. The more you check the face the stronger the cat of BDD becomes. If you starve the cat of BDD by not feeding it (by not checking it), it will become weak and you will be less uncomfortable with your face.(8)

Surgery: It is important to arrange a joint surgical/psychiatric assessment before proceeding

There are related resourced for your patients. There are also support groups for BDD patients where they meet other people who understand them and support them. There are many ways of helping your patients. Surgery is one of them.(9–11)

REFERENCES

1. Rees TD. Selection of Patients. In: Rees TD, ed. Aesthetic Plastic Surgery. WB. Suanders Company, 1994: 4–13.
2. Edgerton MT, Meyer E, Jacobson WE. Augmentation mammaplasty. II. Further surgical and psychiatric evaluation. Plast Reconstr Surg Transplant Bull 1961; 27: 279–302.
3. Chiles JA, StrosahlKD. Clinical Manual for Assessment and Treatment of Suicidal Patients. First ed. Arlington, VA, USA: American Psychiatric Publishing, 2005: 78–82.
4. Shea SC. Psychiatric Interviewing: The Art of Understanding. 2nd ed. Philadelphia: WB Saunders Company.
5. Barker BA. Using metaphors in psychotherapy. Brunner/Mazel, 1985.
6. American Psychiatric Association: Diagnostic and Statistical Manual of Mental Diorders. 4th Edition, Text Revision ed. American Psychiatric Association, 2000: 369–376.
7. Phillips KA, Hollander E. Treating body dysmorphic disorder with medication: evidence, misconceptions, and a suggested approach. Body Image 2008; 5(1): 13–27.
8. Neziroglu FA, Yaryura-Tobias JA. Exposure, response prevention, and cognitive therapy in the treatment of Body dysmorphic disorder. Behav Ther 1993; 24: 431–8.
9. Pope HG Jr, Phillips A, Olivardia R. The Adonis Complex: The Secret Crisis of Male Body Obsession, 2000; Free Press.
10. Phillips KA. The broken mirror: Understanding and treating body dysmorphic disorder. New York: Oxford University Press; 2005.
11. Body Dysmorphic Disorder (BDD) and Body Image Program at Butler Hospital (Providence. RI). [cited; Available from: http://www.bodyimageprogram.com.

Index

Page references in *italics* refer to tables or boxed material; those in **bold** to figures

Printed and bound by CPI Group (UK) Ltd, Croydon, CR0 4YY

18/10/2024

01776253-0020